The Nerve Growth Cone

The Nerve Growth Cone

Editors

Paul C. Letourneau, Ph.D.
Department of Cell Biology and Neuroanatomy
University of Minnesota
Minneapolis, Minnesota

Stanley B. Kater, Ph.D.
Department of Anatomy and Neurobiology
Colorado State University
Fort Collins, Colorado

Eduardo R. Macagno, Ph.D.
Department of Biological Sciences
Columbia University
New York, New York

Raven Press New York

Raven Press, Ltd., 1185 Avenue of the Americas, New York, New York 10036

Made in the United States of America

Library of Congress Cataloging-in-Publication Data

The Nerve growth cone / editors, Paul C. Letourneau, Stanley B. Kater, Eduardo R. Macagno.
    p.   cm.
    Based on the International Growth Cone Symposium held at the Cajal Neurobiology Institute in Madrid, Spain, Oct. 13–17, 1990.
    Includes bibliographical references and index.
    ISBN 0-88167-816-3
    1. Nerves—Growth—Congresses.   2. Nerves—Differentiation—Congresses.   I. Letourneau, Paul, MD.   II. Kater, Stanley B.
III. Macagno, Eduardo R.   IV. International Growth Cone Symposium
(1990 : Cajal Neurobiology Institute)
    [DNLM: 1. Nerve Fibers—physiology—congresses. 2. Nerve Fibers—ultrastructure—congresses.   WL 102.5 N455   1990]
    QP363.5.N45   1991
    612.8'1—dc20
    DNLM/DLC
    for Library of Congress   91-19165
                                                                                              CIP

9 8 7 6 5 4 3 2 1

Cover photo: *Whole-mount electron microscopy of a growth cone prepared by direct rapid-freezing and freeze-substitution. Two distinct cytoplasmic domains are present. The approximate boundary between the two domains is shown by the* dotted line. *The central (C) domain contains microtubules (mt), mitochondria (m), and numerous dense core vesicles. The peripheral (P) domain contains distinct microfilament bundles* (arrowheads) *that form the core of the majority of filopodia. A meshwork of microfilaments fills the cytoplasm between the filament bundles in the peripheral domain. Some of the microfilament bundles appear to terminate in discrete areas* (arrow) *that stain darkly compared with the surrounding cytoplasm. (From J Cell Biol 1989; 108: 95–109, with permission.)*

Contents

Section 1. Intrinsic Mechanisms of Growth Cone Motility

Section 4. The Growth Cone in Regeneration

Contributing Authors

Marvin E. Adams *Department of Biochemistry and Program in Neuronal Growth and Development, Colorado State University, Fort Collins, Colorado 80523*

Albert J. Aguayo *Centre for Research in Neuroscience, The Montreal General Hospital and McGill University, 1650 Cedar Avenue, Montreal, Quebec, Canada H3G 1A4*

John M. Aletta *Department of Pathology and Center for Neurobiology and Behavior, College of Physicians and Surgeons, Columbia University, 630 West 168th Street, New York, New York 10032*

Rosa-Magda Alvarado-Mallart *INSERM U. 106, Hôpital de la Salpétrière, 47, bld de l' Hôpital, 75651 Paris Cedex 13, France*

R. Armas-Portela *Centro de Biología Molecular, Universidad Autónoma de Madrid, E-28049 Madrid, Spain*

J. Avila *Centro de Biología Molecular, Universidad Autónoma de Madrid, E-28049 Madrid, Spain*

Herwig Baier *Max-Planck-Institut für Entwicklungsbiologie, Spemannstrasse 35, D-7400 Tübingen, West Germany*

James R. Bamburg *Department of Biochemistry and Program in Neuronal Growth and Development, Colorado State University, Fort Collins, Colorado 80523*

David Bentley *Department of Molecular and Cell Biology, University of California Berkeley, 519 Life Sciences Addition, Berkeley, California 94720*

Barbara W. Bernstein *Department of Biochemistry and Program in Neuronal Growth and Development, Colorado State University, Fort Collins, Colorado 80523*

Allan J. Bieber *Howard Hughes Medical Institute, Department of Molecular and Cell Biology, University of California Berkeley, 519 Life Sciences Addition, Berkeley, California 94720, and Department of Biological Sciences, Purdue University, West Lafayette, Indiana 47907*

Friedrich Bonhoeffer *Max-Planck-Institut für Entwicklungsbiologie, Spemannstrasse 35, D-7400 Tübingen, West Germany*

Paola Bovolenta *Neural Plasticity Laboratory, Instituto Cajal, C.S.I.C., Dr. Arce 37, 28002 Madrid, Spain*

Dennis Bray   *MRC Muscle and Cell Motility Unit, King's College London, 26–29 Drury Lane, London WC2B 5RL, England*

Garth M. Bray   *Centre for Research in Neuroscience, The Montreal General Hospital and McGill University, 1650 Cedar Avenue, Montreal, Quebec, Canada H3G 1A4*

Paul C. Bridgman   *Department of Anatomy and Neurobiology, Washington University School of Medicine, 660 South Euclid Avenue, St. Louis, Missouri 63110*

Donald W. Burmeister   *Department of Pharmacology and Center for Neurobiology and Behavior, Columbia University College of Physicians and Surgeons, 630 West 168th Street, New York, New York 10032*

J. D. Burrill   *Department of Biology and Neuroscience Program, University of Michigan, 3113 Natural Science/Kraus Building, Ann Arbor, Michigan 48109*

David A. Carter   *Centre for Research in Neuroscience, The Montreal General Hospital and McGill University, 1650 Cedar Avenue, Montreal, Quebec, Canada H3G 1A4*

Susannah Chang   *Department of Anatomy/Chemistry, University of Pennsylvania School of Medicine, Philadelphia, Pennsylvania 19104*

Lauren Davis   *Program in Neuronal Growth and Development, Department of Anatomy and Neurobiology, Colorado State University, Fort Collins, Colorado 80523*

Pierre N. E. De Graan   *Division of Molecular Neurobiology, Rudolf Magnus Institute and Institute of Molecular Biology and Medical Biotechnology, University of Utrecht, Padualaan 8, 3584 CH Utrecht, The Netherlands*

J. Díaz-Nido   *Centro de Biología Molecular, Universidad Autónoma de Madrid, E-28049 Madrid, Spain*

S. S. Easter, Jr.   *Department of Biology and Neuroscience Program, University of Michigan, 3113 Natural Science/Kraus Building, Ann Arbor, Michigan 48109*

Judith S. Eisen   *Institute of Neuroscience, University of Oregon, Eugene, Oregon 97403*

L. Frame   *Department of Cellular and Structural Biology, University of Colorado School of Medicine, 4200 East Ninth Avenue, Denver, Colorado 80262*

Willem Hendrik Gispen   *Division of Molecular Neurobiology, Rudolf Magnus Institute and Institute of Molecular Biology and Medical Biotechnology, University of Utrecht, Padualaan 8, 3584 CH Utrecht, The Netherlands*

Pierre Godement   *Universite Pierre et Marie Curie, Laboratoire de Neurophysiologie Ontogenetique, Bat B, 4e Etage, 9, quai St. Bernard, 75005 Paris, France*

Daniel J. Goldberg *Department of Pharmacology and Center for Neurobiology and Behavior, Columbia University College of Physicians and Surgeons, 630 West 168th Street, New York, New York 10032*

Corey S. Goodman *Howard Hughes Medical Institute, Department of Molecular and Cell Biology, University of California Berkeley, 519 Life Sciences Addition, Berkeley, California 94720*

Phillip R. Gordon-Weeks *Anatomy and Human Biology Group, King's College London, Strand, London WC2R 2LS, England*

Lloyd A. Greene *Department of Pathology and Center for Neurobiology and Behavior, Columbia University College of Physicians and Surgeons, 630 West 168th Street, New York, New York 10032*

Gabriele Grenningloh *Howard Hughes Medical Institute, Department of Molecular and Cell Biology, University of California Berkeley, 519 Life Sciences Addition, Berkeley, California 94720*

Xiaonan Gu *Department of Physiology and Biophysics, University of Miami School of Medicine, 1600 NW 10th Avenue, Miami, Florida 33136, and Department of Biology, University of California at San Diego, LaJolla, California 92093*

Susan P. Haffke *Neuroscience Program and the Department of Biochemistry/ Biophysics and Genetics, University of Colorado Medical School, 4200 East Ninth Avenue, Denver, Colorado 80262*

Richard L. Hawkins *Neuroscience Program and the Department of Biochemistry/Biophysics ad Genetics, University of Colorado Medical School, 4200 East Ninth Avenue, Denver, Colorado 80262*

S. Helmke *Department of Cellular and Structural Biology, University of Colorado School of Medicine, 4200 East Ninth Avenue, Denver, Colorado 80262*

B. A. de la Houssaye *Department of Cellular and Structural Biology, University of Colorado School of Medicine, 4200 East Ninth Avenue, Denver, Colorado 80262*

Craig E. Jahr *Section of Molecular Neurobiology, Howard Hughes Medical Institute, Yale School of Medicine, 333 Cedar Street, New Haven, Connecticut 06510, and Vollum Institute for Advanced Biomedical Research, Oregon Health Sciences University, Portland, Oregon 97201*

Katherine Kalil *Department of Anatomy and Neuroscience Training Program, University of Wisconsin, Bardeen Medical Laboratories, Madison, Wisconsin 53706*

Stanley B. Kater *Program in Neuronal Growth and Development, Department of Anatomy and Neurobiology, Colorado State University, Fort Collins, Colorado 80523*

Marcus Keep   *INSERM U. 106, Hôpital de la Salpétrière, 47, bld de l' Hôpital,
75651 Paris Cedex 13, France*

Alphonse Krystosek   *Neuroscience Program and the Department of
Biochemistry/Biophysics and Genetics, University of Colorado Medical School,
4200 East Ninth Avenue, Denver, Colorado 80262*

Lynn T. Landmesser   *Department of Physiology and Neurobiology, University
of Connecticut, Storrs, Connecticut 06269*

Paul C. Letourneau   *Department of Cell Biology and Neuroanatomy, University
of Minnesota, 4-135 Jackson Hall, 321 Church Street SE, Minneapolis,
Minnesota 55455*

R. Owen Lockerbie   *Department of Biochemistry and Program in Neuronal
Growth and Development, Colorado State University, Fort Collins, Colorado
80523, and Department of Cellular and Structural Biology, University of
Colorado School of Medicine, 4200 East Ninth Avenue, Denver, Colorado 80262*

K. Lohse   *Department of Cellular and Structural Biology, University of
Colorado School of Medicine, 4200 East Ninth Avenue, Denver, Colorado 80262*

Andrew Lumsden   *Division of Anatomy and Cell Biology, United Medical and
Dental Schools, Guy's Hospital, London SE1 9RT, England*

Eduardo R. Macagno   *Department of Biological Sciences, Columbia
University, New York, New York 10027*

S. Gary Mansfield   *Anatomy and Human Biology Group, King's College
London, Strand, London WC2R 2LS, England*

A. Martínez   *Centro de Biologia Molecular, Universidad Autonoma de Madrid,
E-28049 Madrid, Spain*

Adrian Mason   *Department of Physiology and Biophysics, University of Miami
School of Medicine, 1600 NW 10th Avenue, Miami, Florida 33136, and
University Department of Pharmacology, Oxford, England*

Carol Ann Mason   *Department of Pathology and Anatomy and Cell Biology,
Center for Neurobiology and Behavior, Columbia University, College of
Physicians and Surgeons, 630 West 168th Street, New York, New York 10032*

Ellen McGlade-McCulloh   *Department of Physiology and Biophysics,
University of Miami School of Medicine, 1600 NW 10th Avenue, Miami,
Florida 33136*

Paul G. McGuire   *Neuroscience Program and the Department of Biochemistry/
Biophysics and Genetics, University of Colorado Medical School, 4200 East Ninth
Avenue, Denver, Colorado 80262*

V. Miller   *Department of Cellular and Structural Biology, University of
Colorado School of Medicine, 4200 East Ninth Avenue, Denver, Colorado 80262*

Todd E. Morgan   *Department of Biochemistry and Program in Neuronal Growth and Development, Colorado State University, Fort Collins, Colorado 80523*

Kenneth J. Muller   *Department of Physiology and Biophysics, University of Miami School of Medicine, 1600 NW 10th Avenue, Miami, Florida 33136*

P. Negre-Aminou   *Department of Cellular and Structural Biology, University of Colorado School of Medicine, 4200 East Ninth Avenue, Denver, Colorado 80262*

Manuel Nieto-Sampedro   *Neural Plasticity Laboratory, Instituto Cajal, C.S.I.C., Dr. Arce 37, 28002 Madrid, Spain*

Ruth H. Nordlander   *Department of Oral Biology, The Ohio State University, 305 West 12th Avenue, Columbus, Ohio 43210*

Carolyn R. Norris   *Neuroscience Training Program, University of Wisconsin, 1300 University Avenue, Madison, Wisconsin 53706*

Timothy P. O'Connor   *Department of Molecular and Cell Biology, University of California Berkeley, 519 Life Sciences Addition, Berkeley, California 94720*

A. Beate Oestreicher   *Division of Molecular Neurobiology, Rudolf Magnus Institute and Institute of Molecular Biology and Medical Biotechnology, University of Utrecht, Padualaan 8, 3584 CH Utrecht, The Netherlands*

Karl H. Pfenninger   *Department of Cellular and Structural Biology, University of Colorado School of Medicine, 4200 East Ninth Avenue, Denver, Colorado 80262*

Kevin A. Phelan   *Department of Pathology and Center for Neurobiology and Behavior, College of Physicians and Surgeons, Columbia University, 630 West 168th Street, New York, New York 10032*

Susan H. Pike   *Institute of Neuroscience, University of Oregon, Eugene, Oregon 97403*

Mu-ming Poo   *Department of Biological Sciences, Columbia University, New York, New York 10027*

Mark Quillan   *Department of Biological Sciences, Columbia University, New York, New York 10027*

David W. Raible   *Department of Anatomy/Chemistry, University of Pennsylvania School of Medicine, 36th and Hamilton Walk, Philadelphia, Pennsylvania 19104*

Jonathan A. Raper   *Department of Anatomy/Chemistry, University of Pennsylvania School of Medicine, 36th and Hamilton Walk, Philadelphia, Pennsylvania 19104*

Vincent Rehder *Program in Neuronal Growth and Development, Department of Anatomy and Neurobiology, Colorado State University, Fort Collins, Colorado 80523*

Rodolfo J. Rivas *Department of Pharmacology and Center for Neurobiology and Behavior, Columbia University College of Physicians and Surgeons, 630 West 168th Street, New York, New York 10032*

M. Rocha *Centro de Biología Molecular, Universidad Autónoma de Madrid, E-28049 Madrid, Spain*

L. S. Ross *Department of Biology and Neuroscience Program, University of Michigan, 3113 Natural Science/Kraus Building, Ann Arbor, Michigan 48109*

Melitta Schachner *Department of Neurobiology, Swiss Federal Institute of Technology, 8093 Zurich, Switzerland, and University of Heidelberg, Heidelberg, West Germany*

Nicholas W. Seeds *Neuroscience Program and the Department of Biochemistry/ Biophysics and Genetics, University of Colorado Medical School, 4200 East Ninth Avenue, Denver, Colorado 80262*

Elliott H. Sherr *Department of Pathology and Center for Neurobiology and Behavior, College of Physicians and Surgeons, Columbia University, 630 West 168th Street, New York, New York 10032*

J. H. Pate Skene *Department of Neurobiology, Duke University, Durham, North Carolina 27710*

Stephen J Smith *Section of Molecular Neurobiology, Howard Hughes Medical Institute, Yale School of Medicine, 333 Cedar Street, New Haven, Connecticut 06510, and Department of Molecular and Cellular Physiology, Beckman Center, Stanford University Medical School, Stanford, California 94305*

Constantino Sotelo *INSERM U. 106, Hôpital de la Salpétrière, 47, bld de l' Hôpital, 75651 Paris Cedex 13, France*

Kathryn W. Tosney *Department of Biology, University of Michigan, Natural Science Building, Ann Arbor, Michigan 48109*

Menno van Lookeren Campagne *Division of Molecular Neurobiology, Rudolf Magnus Institute and Institute of Molecular Biology and Medical Biotechnology, University of Utrecht, Padualaan 8, 3584 CH Utrecht, The Netherlands*

Shala Verrall *Neuroscience Program and the Department of Biochemistry/ Biophysics and Genetics, University of Colorado Medical School, 4200 East Ninth Avenue, Denver, Colorado 80262*

Manuel Vidal-Sanz *Centre for Research in Neuroscience, The Montreal General Hospital and McGill University, 1650 Cedar Avenue, Montreal, Quebec, Canada H3G 1A4*

Acknowledgments

This book would not have been possible without the financial support of several organizations that sponsored the International Growth Cone Symposium. These include: the National Science Foundation, the National Institutes of Health, and Raven Press; NATO in Brussels, Belgium; and the Instituto Cajal, the Consejo Superior de Investigaciones Cientificas, and the Fundacion Banco Bilbao Vizcaya in Spain. Many individuals provided important assistance in conducting the meeting and preparing this book, including Jose Borrell, Alberto Ferrus and Manuel Nieto-Sampedro at the Instituto Cajal, and Patricia Haugen, University of Minnesota, Vincent Rehder, Colorado State University, and Laura Wolszon, Columbia University. The excellent introductory chapters of each section were written by James Bamburg, Colorado State University, Lloyd Greene and Carol Mason, Columbia University, and Ken Muller, University of Miami. Planning, preparation, and conduct of the meeting and this book were also supported by NIH grants HD19950 and NS24403 to P. Letourneau; NIH grant NS–20336 and NSF grant BNS–88–18970 to E. Macagno.

The Nerve Growth Cone

SECTION 1

Intrinsic Mechanisms of Growth Cone Motility

The Nerve Growth Cone, edited by P. C. Letourneau,
S. B. Kater, and E. R. Macagno, Raven Press, Ltd.,
New York © 1992.

1

Introduction

James R. Bamburg

*Department of Biochemistry and Program in Neuronal Growth and Development,
Colorado State University, Fort Collins, Colorado 80523*

The discovery of the neuronal growth cone in 1890 by Ramón y Cajal (1) provided the critical piece of evidence that led to the acceptance of the theory that neurons developed as single cells. This put to rest the opposing theory that neurons were composed of tubes of fused cells that developed in a completely unique manner from other tissues. Subsequent efforts during the past 100 years have dealt with deciphering the mechanisms by which the growth cone interacts with its environment in laying down the circuitry necessary for proper functioning of the nervous system.

The growth cone has fascinated scientists for a century. Even when severed from the cell body, the growth cone continues to extend filopodia and lamellipodia and migrate in a directed fashion (2). Although the ability of the severed growth cone to migrate and lay down new neurites will eventually terminate because of the lack of raw materials normally provided by the cell body, its ability to perform these functions transiently implies that the essential components for extension and guidance are locally regulated. For growth cones to move in a directed fashion implies that the environmental signals, arriving as soluble factors (3) or as part of a matrix that contacts the growth cone directly (4), interact with specific receptors on the growth cone and that these interactions result in transmembrane signals that lead to a reorganization of the adjacent cytoskeleton. The cytoskeletal alterations result in changes in expansive and contractile forces (5) that can alter the pathway of growth. Although our current knowledge of events linking membrane receptors to the cytoskeletal reorganization and generation of the forces for growth is far from complete, substantial progress has been made on several fronts, which are described in this volume.

The first section of this book deals with some of the intrinsic mechanisms involved in the motile process. This section begins with a chapter by Dennis Bray, one of the modern pioneers of growth cone research, whose observations during the past 20 years have provided much of the foundation for current research in this field. This chapter provides some of these historic observations and gives an overview of some of the questions addressed in subsequent chapters in this volume.

The application of computer-enhanced differential interference contrast video-microscopy to growth cones has given us a picture of the real-time dynamics of some of the processes that take place during the advance of the neuronal growth cone. Several of the chapters in this section of the book (chapters by Smith and Jahr, Bridgman, and Goldberg et al.) use this technique to examine neuronal growth cones. Although there are several general observations that provide some unifying concepts of growth cone motility from all these studies, the nature of the neurons used and the substratum on which they grow can strongly influence growth cone behavior and may account for some of the different interpretations in "push" versus "pull" models. Confocal microscopy of living neurons that have been fluorescently labeled with membrane-associated dyes has been valuable in examining neuronal growth patterns in brain slices (Smith and Jahr chapter), an environment that comes closer to providing a natural substratum for growth than those commonly used for *in vitro* culture. This technique opens the door to *in vivo* studies of labeled growing neurons in organisms not adaptable to direct microscopic study, such as those discussed in Section 3 of this book.

Other chapters in this first section discuss how the cytoskeletal proteins, actin and tubulin, are transported to the growth cone and how the assembly of these components into microfilaments and microtubules might be regulated (chapters by Bamburg et al., Gordon-Weeks and Mansfield, and Diaz-Nido et al.). How membrane addition takes place in the growth cone is also addressed in one chapter (Pfenninger et al. chapter). The dynamics of the neuronal growth associated protein (GAP-43) in the process of neurite outgrowth is discussed in this section as well (Campagne et al. chapter); a chapter in a later section returns to the topic of GAP-43 in regenerating nerves and the signals that regulate its reexpression (Skene chapter).

Although an understanding of these intrinsic mechanisms of growth is essential to prediction of growth behavior, it appears that multiple inputs through a number of receptors must be integrated to give the final response. Thus, changes in any of the environmental cues, some of them that may be brought about by the ability of the growth cone to modify its own environment (Seeds et al. chapter), and the nature of the signaling pathways available in a particular neuron, make even a simplistic understanding of growth cone behavior in response to a signal a nontrivial process. Given the substantial amount of cross-talk that occurs between signal transduction pathways (6), molecules that integrate the stimulatory and inhibitory growth responses from the environment (see chapters in Section 2) must exist, among these being free calcium (Davis et al. chapter).

The localization and function of conventional myosin in the growth cone is addressed in the chapter by Bridgman. In Section 2 of this volume, the chapter by Phelan et al. reports on the identification of a protein that cross-reacts with antibodies to minimyosin (myosin I) and that has been postulated to provide the force for filopodial extensions and contraction (7,8). Certainly, additional work in this area is necessary to clarify the nature and regulation of the contractile motors involved with actin filaments in growth cone motility.

Whether developing neurites have the ability to branch at points other than the

30. Forscher P, Smith SJ. Actions of cytochalasins on the organization of actin filaments and micro-tubules in a neuronal growth cone. *J Cell Biol* 1988;107:1505–1516.
31. Bridgman PC, Dailey ME. The organization of myosin and actin in rapid frozen nerve growth cones. *J Cell Biol* 1989;108:95–109.
32. Letourneau PC, Shattuck TA. Distribution and possible interactions of actin-associated proteins and cell adhesion molecules of growth cones. *Development* 1989;105:505–519.
33. Fukui Y, Lynch TJ, Brzeska H, Korn ED. Myosin I is located at the leading edge of locomoting *Dictyostelium* amoebae. *Nature* 1989;341:328–331.
34. Oster G, Perelesen AS. The physics of cell motility. *J Cell Sci Suppl* 1987;8:35–54.
35. Bray D. Mechanical tension produced by nerve cells in tissue culture. *J Cell Sci* 1979;37:391–410.
36. Lamoureux P, Buxbaum RE, Heidemann SR. Direct evidence that growth cones pull. *Nature* 1989;340:159–162.
37. Denerll TJ, Lamoureux P, Buxbaum RE, Heidemann SR. The cytomechanics of axonal elongation and retraction. *J Cell Biol* 1989;109:3073–3083.
38. Bray D. Axonal growth in response to experimentally applied tension. *Dev Biol* 1984;102:379–389.
39. Marsh L, Letourneau PC. Growth of neurites without filopodial or lamellipodial activity in the presence of cytochalasin B. *J Cell Biol* 1984;99:2041–2047.
40. Lamoureux P, Steel VL, Regal C, Adgate L, Buxbaum RE, Heidemann SR. Extracellular matrix allows PC12 neurite elongation in the absence on microtubules. *J Cell Biol* 1990;110:71–79.
41. Nakai J. Studies on the mechanism determining the course of nerve fibres in tissue culture. *Z Zellforschung* 1960;51:427–449.
42. Letourneau PC. Cell-to-substratum adhesion and guidance of axonal elongation. *Dev Biol* 1975;44:92–101.
43. Letourneau PC. Cell–substratum adhesion of neurite growth cone and its role in neurite elongation. *Exp Cell Res* 1978;124:127–138.
44. Wessells NK, Nuttall RP. Normal branching, induced branching, and steering of cultured parasym-pathetic motor neurons. *Exp Cell Res* 1978;115:111–122.
45. Goldberg DJ, Burmeister DW. Looking into growth cones. *Trends Neurosci* 1989;12:503–506.

The Nerve Growth Cone, edited by P. C. Letourneau,
S. B. Kater, and E. R. Macagno, Raven Press, Ltd.,
New York © 1992.

3

Rapid Induction of Filopodial Sprouting by Application of Glutamate to Hippocampal Neurons

Stephen J Smith and Craig E. Jahr

*Section of Molecular Neurobiology, Howard Hughes Medical Institute,
Yale School of Medicine, New Haven, Connecticut 06510*

Neuronal activity can alter synaptic structure and connectivity in both developing (23,27) and mature nervous systems (5,10,11). So far, however, this conclusion has been based mainly on comparisons of multiple specimens after differing sensory or electrical stimulation treatments. Recently, it has also been shown that glutamate and its analogues can affect the structure of isolated neurons in cell culture (1,4,17, 20) and can alter the course of development *in vivo* (6). These effects of glutamate, however, are either slowly developing or require comparison of multiple specimens. We now describe observations of structural remodeling of individual living neurons occurring within a few seconds of glutamate application. These effects may reflect a cellular mechanism by which synaptic activity could very promptly alter neuronal structure.

RESULTS

Figure 1A is a photomicrograph of a neuron in culture meeting the criteria we used to select cells for experimentation. Its form resembles that of a CA1 hippocampal cell as observed *in situ* (2,21). The cell body is roughly triangular, with an elongated apex terminating in an apical dendrite, a bifurcated dendrite in this example. In addition, there are processes resembling basal dendrites and a single axon identifiable by its small, constant diameter and relatively great length. Such cells were usually observed only in close association with protoplasmic astrocytes: In Fig. 1A the neuron is growing on the surface of an extensively spread-out astrocyte, of which only a portion is visible.

Figures 1B–K shows a sequence of digital video micrographs at higher magnification of the same neuron as in Fig. 1A. Now only a portion of the cell body and apical dendrite is visible. Arrows in Fig. 1B indicate small filopodial protrusions

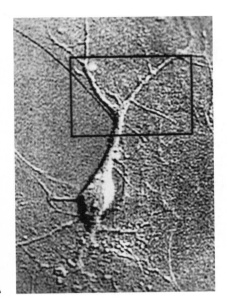

A

FIG. 1. Response of a rat hippocampal neuron in cell culture to a pulse of glutamate applied from a micropipette. **A:** Low-magnification view showing cell body, dendrites, and initial segment of axon (*arrow*). *Open rectangle* indicates dendritic segment measured for graph in Fig. 2 **B–K:** Sequence of higher magnification images from apical dendrite area indicated by rectangular outline in **A.** Timing of the sequence is expressed relative to the onset of a 30-sec pressure (0.5 atm) application of glutamate (1 mM). Tip of the micropipette (3-μm outer diameter) is visible in **C** through **J.** *Arrowheads* in **D, E, F, and G** indicate the tip of one filopodium that sprouted from this dendrite in response to glutamate application. It is readily evident in this sequence that numerous other filopodia exhibit similar behavior in response to this treatment.

often observed on these neurons. Electron microscopy indicates that dendritic filopodia in these cultures are approximately 100 nm in diameter and consist of a bundle of actin filaments surrounded by plasma membrane (3,8,18). The small diameter of these processes precludes straightforward resolution of their true diameter by visible-light microscopy, but as evident from Fig. 1B, they are readily detected using digital video contrast enhancement.

The sequence of images in Fig. 1B–K illustrates an experiment in which glutamate (100 μM) was applied by pressure from a micropipette. As in 42 of 161 similar experiments, the result of glutamate application was a prompt and reversible elongation of one or more of the dendritic filopodia. The relative stability of dendritic structure before glutamate application is indicated by the similarity of Fig. 1B and C. Figure 1D shows that elongation of filopodia can be detected readily only 4 sec after the onset of glutamate application. Figures 1E, F, and G represent the maximum extension, which occurred within 10 to 15 sec of glutamate application. The rapid reversibility of glutamate-induced protrusion is evident in the sequence of Fig. 1G–J. Figure 1G was obtained just before termination of a 30-sec pulse of glutamate application; Figs. 1H and I were obtained 2 sec and 8 sec, respectively, after termination. Figure 1J shows that glutamate-induced extension was essentially reversed within 30 sec of glutamate termination. Comparison of J and K in Fig. 1 again illustrates the stability of dendritic form under baseline conditions. Careful examination of Fig. 1 indicates that a small reduction in the apparent width of the dendrite also occurred as a result of glutamate application.

Measurements taken from the same image sequence represented in Fig. 1 are

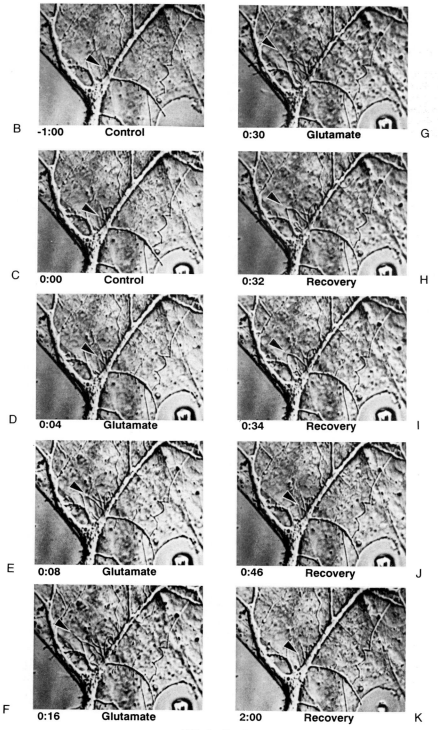

FIG. 1. *Continued.*

summarized in Fig. 2. Lengths of a filopodium and widths of the parent dendrite are plotted as functions of time before, during, and after glutamate application. Figure 2 shows that there are baseline variations in filopodial length but that these are negligible compared with the extension induced by glutamate application. This graph confirms that both the protrusion in response to glutamate application and retraction in response to glutamate removal can begin with delays of as little as 2 sec. Maximum rates of protrusion and retraction are on the order of 2 μm/sec. The data in

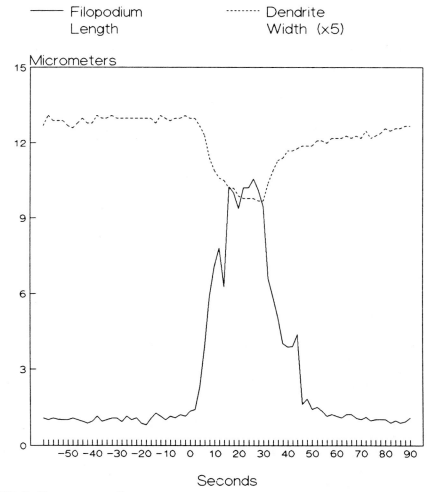

FIG. 2. Measurements of structural response to 0.1 glutamate neuron from neonatal rat hippocampus. Length of the filopodium indicated by the arrow in Fig. 1 was measured by hand-tracing, using a mouse and graphic overlay on the video image processor screen. Dendrite width was measured automatically by a scanning program from the digitized image of the dendrite within the rectangular box in Fig. 1. Pressure-pipette application of glutamate begins at the time indicated zero seconds and ends at thirty seconds.

The Nerve Growth Cone, edited by P. C. Letourneau,
S. B. Kater, and E. R. Macagno, Raven Press, Ltd.,
New York © 1992.

4

Actin Dynamics in Neuronal Growth Cones

James R. Bamburg, R. Owen Lockerbie, Barbara W. Bernstein,
Todd E. Morgan, Marcia Whitney, and Marvin E. Adams

*Department of Biochemistry and The Program in Neuronal Growth and Development,
Colorado State University, Fort Collins, Colorado 80523*

It has been almost 20 years since actin was first identified in growing neurons by
Fine and Bray (1). Since then we have learned much about the organization of actin
in neurons at different stages of development and about some of the proteins that
regulate the assembly and membrane attachment of filamentous actin (F-actin). Recent reviews (2–5) discussing the postulated roles for actin and actin binding proteins in neurons and other nonmuscle cells should be consulted for detailed information. In this chapter, we will confine our remarks to a discussion of actin transport
and assembly dynamics in developing neurons of the chick and the role of one
protein, actin depolymerizing factor, which we believe plays a major role in both of
these processes.

Actin microfilaments comprise one of the three major classes of cytoskeletal
filaments, the other two being the microtubules and the neuronal class of intermediate filaments, the neurofilaments. Both neurofilaments and microtubules are major
longitudinal structural components of the developing axon. Neurofilaments seldom
extend into the growth cone, whereas microtubules often extend through the central
regions of the growth cone and can be seen terminating near the leading edge of the
advancing growth cone, the region where actin filaments comprise the majority of
the cytoskeleton (6,7). Actin filaments are often found as bundles of parallel filaments that form the core of filopodia (microspikes), and they also occur in a meshwork within the lamellipodia and distal portion of the growth cone. Actin, presumably in the filamentous form, also is found in high concentration underneath the
axolemma, where it forms a cortical skeleton, which, along with the longitudinal
arrangement of the microtubules and neurofilaments, gives the axons and dendritic
fibers their characteristic cylindrical shapes.

In most nonmuscle cells, a substantial pool of unassembled actin exists, which is
believed to be in a dynamic equilibrium with the actin in the filament pool. Because
intracellular ionic conditions are such that more than 98% of the actin should be in
the assembled form and because often less than 50% is actually assembled, other

actin assembly regulatory factors must exist. The role of the actin assembly process in neurite growth has been investigated by using drugs that inhibit the process of actin assembly. Some of the fungal metabolites, called *cytochalasins*, have been shown to inhibit subunit addition to the preferred growth end (+ end) of the polar actin filaments and cause a net actin depolymerization. Growth cones treated with cytochalasin B undergo a rapid cessation of filopodial activity, followed by filopodial withdrawal (8). Although neurite growth can continue in the absence of filopodia both *in vitro* (9) and *in vivo* (10), the growth is undirected. Thus, filopodial activity must be important in pathfinding but not in the general addition of material into the neurite cytoskeleton. Presumably membrane signal transduction pathways, activated by surface adhesion molecules or other receptor cues, serve to regulate both actin binding to the neuronal membrane and localized assembly of the actin filaments, leading to selective outgrowth along a tension-generated pathway dependent on the actin filaments (11).

Because axons lack the machinery for *de novo* protein synthesis, all proteins of the axoplasm are derived from protein synthesis occurring within the cell body and the transport of the material down the axon. Several rates of active transport have been identified (12,13), each containing its own unique mixture of axoplasmic proteins. The majority of the actin in most axons moves down the axon with the slow component b (SCb) of transport (about 2–5 mm/day). This is a somewhat faster rate than the slowest component (SCa), which usually carries the bulk of the neurofilament proteins and tubulin (the major microtubule protein). The finding that the components of the cytoskeleton were carried by these slowest components of transport and that the labeled proteins move in a relatively discrete band prompted Lasek (14) to postulate that the components of the cytoskeleton were transported as assembled cytoskeletal structures with some slippage possible between the different elements. However, recent studies on the transport and assembly of tubulin, neurofilament proteins, and actin (reviewed in refs. 15,16; see also refs. 17,18) support a model in which the axonal cytoskeleton is immobile and the cytoskeletal protein subunits are transported in an unassembled (or very dynamic) form. The cytoskeletal protein subunits in this model have the capability to exchange with their assembled counterparts along the axon at sites where filament dynamics are allowed (e.g., the (+) or distal end of the microtubules). Although results from pulse-chase experiments indicate that actin rapidly equilibrates between a soluble and sedimentable pool in the cell body (19), how the newly synthesized actin is transported into and down the axon remains largely unknown.

In 1980, we reported on the isolation and characterization of a 19-kDa actin depolymerizing factor (ADF) from chick embryo brain (20), the encoding cDNA of which has since been cloned, sequenced, and expressed (21). This protein has been found in high amounts in most embryonic tissue, but brain and spinal cord contain the most, approximately 0.3 to 0.4% of the total protein (22). ADF has a weak actin severing activity and sequesters actin monomers in a 1:1 complex with a K_d of about 0.1 μM (23,24). The complex can be specifically cross-linked by the homobifunctional sulfhydryl cross-linking reagent, *p*-phenylenedimaleimide (25). Localization of ADF in cells and tissues by indirect immunofluorescence has shown that ADF is rather diffuse in most cells (as expected for a soluble actin monomer binding protein), but it shows high concentration in ruffling membranes and neuronal growth cones. Developmental studies on the distribution of ADF in rat cerebellum by both light and electron microscopic immunocytochemical methods showed that ADF is widely distributed in the cerebellum of newborn rats (26). By 6 days of development, ADF immunoreactivity was found to be especially concentrated in Purkinje cell bodies; by 10 days, Purkinje cell dendrites were intensely labeled. In 14- and 35-day-old rats, the entire molecular layer is immunoreactive, as are fibers in the white matter, but the granule cells in both the external and internal layers do not contain significant amounts of ADF immunoreactivity. At the ultrastructural level, Purkinje cell bodies of 14-day rats were labeled, both in the nucleus and cytoplasm. The dendrites were stained throughout their entire arborization, with intense staining surrounding the microtubules, but Purkinje cell axons were not immunoreactive for ADF at this stage of development. The climbing and mossy fibers of the cerebellum did contain ADF, as did the cell bodies of the Bergmann astrocytes, but the Bergmann fibers and the oligodendrocytes in 14-day rat cerebellum did not contain ADF immunoreactivity.

We have investigated the developmental expression of ADF and its mRNA in chick muscle and in cultured myocytes (27). ADF levels in muscle decline from 0.2% of the total tissue protein at 10 days embryonic development to undetectable levels by 14 days posthatching, remaining at this low level throughout subsequent development. The ADF mRNA follows the same pattern, suggesting that the regulation is transcriptionally controlled. In myocyte cultures, ADF mRNA levels do not decline as *in vivo*, and levels of immunoreactive ADF increase over a period of 2 weeks, a time of intense myocyte fusion and sarcomere formation. The increase in immunoreactive ADF is due to the formation of a new isoform that we isolated and characterized as inactive in depolymerizing filamentous actin *in vitro*. This isoform contains an incorporated phosphate, and it represents a posttranslationally modified form of ADF, produced, we believe, by calcium/calmodulin-dependent protein kinase II, which can phosphorylate ADF *in vitro* (T. Morgan, M. Browning, and J. Bamburg, *unpublished observations*). The levels of active ADF found in both muscle tissue and cultured myocytes correlate well with the levels of total actin remaining in the unassembled state. Thus ADF is an important actin assembly regulatory protein in developing muscle and brain, and its activity is controlled by both pretranslational and posttranslational mechanisms.

RECENT RESULTS

To understand better the role of ADF in neuronal development, John Bray, Paul Fernyhough, Dennis Bray, and I undertook a study on the axonal transport of ADF (28). In particular we wished to see in which component of transport ADF is carried and to quantify its amount relative to actin. The chicken sciatic nerve was selected as the system in which to study this transport. [^{35}S]-Methionine was injected into the ventral horn of the lumbar spinal cord to label the pool of motor neurons supplying the sciatic nerve. At various times, animals were sacrificed and the sciatic nerve was removed and cut into segments for analysis. In some experiments the nerve was crushed 2 cm from the cord to collect the rapidly transported components in the segment proximal to the lesion. No ADF or actin was detected in the rapid transport component. After 4 days, it was possible to identify the peaks of radioactivity associated with both SCa and SCb. We elected to use segments taken from animals 4 days after labeling because this allowed both components of slow transport to be recovered separately. The sciatic nerve segments were pulverized in liquid nitrogen and the nerve powder extracted with a Tris buffer for 30 min before centrifugation at 100,000 g. The supernatant was freeze dried, and both supernatant and pellet fractions were dissolved in a solution of urea and nonionic detergent before separating the proteins by 2D gel electrophoresis. Immunoblots of 2D gels, used to locate ADF, profilin, and cofilin, were run with nonequilibrium pH gradient gel electrophoresis for the first dimension. Other 2D gels, where isoelectric focusing was used for the first dimension, were run to examine the actin. Of these labeled and identified proteins carried by slow axonal transport, only ADF and actin were highly labeled and present in significant amounts, mostly in SCb, but with some in SCa also. The ratio of these two proteins was determined by quantifying the radioactivity in each species and correcting for their different methionine content. The ADF:actin molar ratio in slow axonal transport is about 1:1, suggesting that the actin might be transported in a complex with ADF. Extraction of sciatic nerve in the presence of p-phenylenedimaleimide, the ADF–actin cross-linking reagent, resulted in the formation of a 1:1 complex between ADF and actin. When the cross-linking reagent was added after extraction in a large volume of buffer, much less of the covalent complex was formed, suggesting that the ADF–actin complex existed before extraction. Thus, we believe that actin is transported in slow axonal transport as an ADF–actin complex, and not as assembled filaments.

Previous studies on the dynamics of the ADF–actin complex have shown that labeled actin in the complex rapidly exchanges with unlabeled actin (25). This has been demonstrated *in vivo* by fixing fibroblasts 15 min after microinjecting them with fluorescein-actin complexed to ADF. Fluorescent actin filaments were observed throughout the cell. Given the rapidity of this exchange with the F-actin pool in cells, one would expect a change in the ratio of specific activity of ADF to actin as the ADF–actin complex travels down the axon during axonal transport. Our analyses to date have only examined this ratio in the peak of slow transport at 4 days postinjection. Analysis of more distal segments at later time points might provide useful information on the dynamics of this exchange process in axons.

Additional evidence from ongoing experiments that supports the finding that actin is transported in an unassembled form has come from studies on cultured neurons from dissociated chick dorsal root ganglia. Neurons are loaded with fluorescently labeled actin or phalloidin before neurite outgrowth by triturating trypsin-treated ganglia in a solution containing either rhodamine-labeled actin (Rh-actin) or rhodamine-phalloidin (Rh-P). Phalloidin is a small cyclic peptide with a high binding affinity for F-actin. We have then followed the distribution of fluorescence in the ruffling lamellipodium, growth cones, and neurites, as these cells differentiate after their plating on glass coverslips in the presence of nerve growth factor (Fig. 1). Neurons loaded with Rh-P had little if any fluorescence associated with the ruffling lamellipodium or with growth cones. A small amount of fluorescence was sometimes observed in the proximal segment of the neurite fiber, but seldom were neurites labeled throughout their length. We assume that the small amounts of Rh-P loaded into cells bind to F-actin within the soma and stay associated with F-actin segments of various lengths throughout the observation times used. Similar assumptions have been made by others who have used Rh-P as a tag to study the redistribution of F-actin during cell division (29).

In neurons loaded with Rh-actin to the same fluorescence intensity as those containing Rh-P, fluorescence is associated first with the leading edge of the ruffling lamellipodium, then with the growth cones that form later, and finally with the entire neurite fiber that follows. These observations were made in living cells, but photobleaching was so rapid the cells had to be photographed with very high-speed film (Kodak Tmax 3200). Cells that were fixed with glutaraldehyde, extracted with Triton X-100, reduced with sodium borohydride, and preserved in glycerol containing a photobleaching protectant had a greater fluorescence intensity and were more stable under observation but yielded the same results. Our interpretation of these results is that phalloidin stabilization of F-actin retards the translocation of the actin into the neurite, suggesting that only the monomeric form of actin is able to translocate rapidly to appropriate locations in cells to reassemble into the dynamic filaments of the growth cones and lamellipodia. The intensity of the ADF immunocytochemical staining that surrounds microtubules in some processes of cerebellar neurons (26) suggests that this transport might be microtubule-based.

The levels of total and unassembled actin in chick growth cone particles have been compared with those in synaptosomes from adult chicken brain. Growth cone particles were isolated from 18-day embryonic chick brain using a procedure developed for embryonic rat brain (30), and preparations have been characterized for their content of GAP-43 and c-src, as well as ultrastructurally. Actin comprises about 3.5% of the total protein in growth cones as compared with only about 1% in synaptosomes. In synaptosomes, about 50 to 60% of the actin is F-actin, whereas growth cones in suspension have only about 20–25% of the actin as F-actin when lysed into identical buffers without a calcium chelating agent. When lysed into buffer containing 1-mM EGTA, the F-actin level in growth cone particles was found to be 54%, whereas the F-actin level in synaptosomes was not significantly changed. Thus, F-actin in growth cones is more susceptible to calcium-induced depolymerization than is actin in synaptosomes. Even so, actin in synaptosomes is dynamic and can respond to depolarization by undergoing cycles of assembly and disassembly (31). Growth cones plated on a polylysine substrate have 15 to 20% more F-actin than their counterparts in suspension when lysed into buffer without calcium chelator, indicating that actin assembly can be locally regulated here as

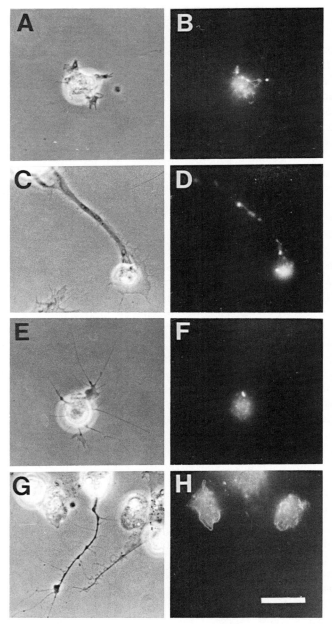

FIG. 1. Phase contrast (**A,C,E,G**) and fluorescence (**B,D,F,H**) photomicrographs of dissoci-ated chick embryonic dorsal root ganglia neurons loaded with rhodamine-actin (**A–D**) or rhoda-mine-phalloidin (**E–H**) before placing in cell culture on glass coverslips. Cells were loaded by trituration of ganglia and cultured as described previously (22). Not all cells incorporate fluores-cent label (see **G** and **H**). Notice labeled actin extends into many processes from the time they are formed. Rhodamine-phalloidin, however, does not typically appear in the processes when they first extend and is seen only occasionally in neurites at early stages of growth. Photo-graphs were taken on Nikon Diaphot microscope with DM 100 objective and Kodak Tmax 3200 film, processed at the ASA of 1600. Calibration bar equals 20 μm.

well, presumably through transmembrane signaling induced by membrane adhesion.

Both ADF and profilin have been examined in growth cone particles by immunoblotting methods. Very little free profilin was found, although we detected a 58-kDa species that was immunoreactive with both antiprofilin and antiactin antibody. This species probably represents a covalent complex between profilin and actin, possibly formed by transglutaminase, which is present in neurons (32). None of this higher-molecular-weight actin immunoreactivity was found in synaptosomes. Levels of ADF were much higher in growth cones (0.4–0.5% of total protein) than in synaptosomes (0.2% of total protein) but are not high enough to totally account for all the unassembled actin. However, levels of ADF are sufficient to account for the dynamic pool of actin that assembles in response to growth cone adhesion to polylysine.

The finding that ADF activity in cultured myocytes was regulated by posttranslational modification of ADF, probably through calcium/calmodulin kinase II, prompted us to search for the phosphorylated form of ADF in embryonic chick brain and in growth cone particles. We have partially purified a modified form of ADF from embryonic chick brain, which has identical electrophoretic mobility on 2D gels (nonequilibrium pH gradient gel electrophoresis and SDS-PAGE) and yields identical peptides after cyanogen bromide digestion to the phosphorylated myocyte ADF. Growth cone particles also contain an ADF immunoreactive species with identical 2D gel mobility. Therefore, the local regulation of actin assembly that occurs in nerve terminals is controlled, at least in part, by ADF, and the activity of ADF is locally controlled, presumably through the activity of the calcium/calmodulin-dependent protein kinase II.

FUTURE DIRECTIONS

If, as we suspect, actin is transported in the slow component of axonal transport in the unassembled form, as a complex with ADF, how is this complex maintained and transported as a discrete component? The same question arises concerning the transport of the other cytoskeletal components, microtubule and neurofilament proteins. One possible answer to this question might be that all the components of the axonal cytoskeleton are packaged in a large transport complex that moves along preexisting cytoskeletal elements either with its own motor or via a unidirectional facilitated diffusion mechanism. One possibility for such a complex has been identified by Weisenberg and co-workers (33). Although this complex did not contain substantial amounts of actin, it did contain tubulin and neurofilament proteins and demonstrated movement along microtubules *in vitro* at a rate similar to SCa of axonal transport. These particles were given the name SCAPs (for *slow component a particles*). It is possible that the particles isolated by Weisenberg and colleagues (33) represent the core components of a transport particle and that the ADF–actin complex is more loosely associated and lost on isolation. Possible future experiments might involve reconstituting these particles with fluorescently labeled tubulin and examining associations that occur between this complex and a biotinylated ADF–actin complex *in vitro*. If binding of the ADF–actin to the SCAPs can be demonstrated, cotransport studies could be done *in vivo* and *in vitro*. Alternatively, a separate transport complex might exist for actin that can move at a faster velocity than tubulin and neurofilament proteins in many axons.

A major area for future study is the role of the extracellular matrix and cell adhesion molecules on the organization of the growth cone actin filament network. Many proteins that are known to link actin filaments, either directly or indirectly, to integral membrane proteins have been identified in growth cones; among these are α-actinin, vinculin, talin, fodrin, and ankyrin. However, little is known at the molecular or ultrastructural level concerning how each of these proteins serves this function. In addition, as the nature of the interactions with the substratum are vitally important in neuronal guidance and synaptogenesis, much additional work is necessary to determine which components of the transmembrane actin filament anchoring network are important at each of the different stages of neurite outgrowth during the developmental process. We also need to delineate the differences that occur in these assemblies between dendritic and axonal growth cones. We are beginning to explore the roles of these different proteins by using growth cone particles adhered to different substrata. Platinum rotary replicas of the deep-etched dorsal and ventral surfaces of growth cones have been obtained for growth cone particles adhered to polylysine coverslips (Fig. 2). These surfaces were obtained by placing a second polylysine-coated coverslip over the sample for 5 min before shearing open the growth cones by prying the coverslips apart. Growth cones of neurons plated directly on gold electron microscope grids coated with formvar, carbon, and polylysine have also been examined by whole-mount transmission electron microscopy after glutaraldehyde fixation, tannic acid treatment, osmification, and uranyl acetate staining (Fig. 3). By combining these methods with immunogold localization of particular membrane-associated actin-binding proteins, we hope to be able to determine which membrane anchoring complexes are important in actin organization during different stages of outgrowth. For these studies, growth cone particles that represent a more homogeneous and defined subpopulation will be required.

Of particular interest in nerve growth is the role of actin and actin binding proteins in the consolidation process that occurs at the junction between the growth cone and the neurite fiber. Within the neurite, actin filaments are most concentrated in the cortex where they are thought to play a role in maintenance of the cylindrical shape of the cell. As the growth cone advances, it seems likely that the actin involved in the filopodial bundles and lammelipodial meshwork becomes reorganized into the cortical actin web underlying the membrane of the neurite process. Little is currently known concerning the origin of the actin in the cortical network and how dynamically this actin behaves with respect to the pool of newly transported actin. Axonal transport studies have demonstrated a preferential labeling of this cortical actin pool by the components of SCb (34). Whether this represents an actual exchange of labeled protein with the actin filaments themselves or an association of

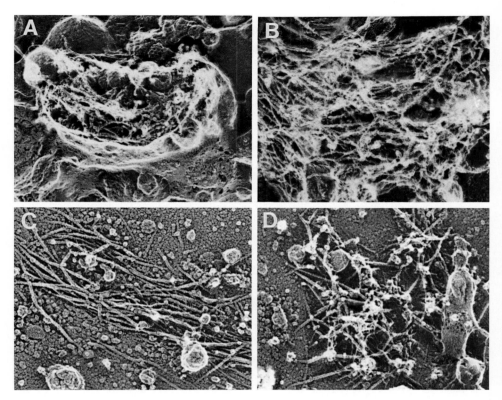

FIG. 2. Platinum replicas of deep-etched, physically ruptured growth cone particles. Chick brain growth cone particles were prepared by the method of Lockerbie and Pfenninger (30) and sedimented onto polylysine-coated glass coverslips. After a 30-min incubation at 37°C, the growth cone particles were physically ruptured and the exposed internal surfaces prepared for ultrastructural analysis by the method of Isobe and Shimada (35). **A** and **B:** View of lower coverslip showing growth cones that have patches of membrane removed. **C** and **D:** View of membrane patches that adhered to the upper coverslip. Magnifications: **A,C,D** = 54,200; **B** = 65,000.

these cortical filaments with a mobile actin pool and other proteins in the SCb is not known.

To understand the local regulation of actin assembly in neuronal growth cones, we need to achieve a better picture of the membrane signal transduction events that provide the cues to which actin assembly is but one response. We also need to understand better the dynamic interrelationships between the different actin binding proteins present in the growth cone. Most of the progress in this area will come by combining *in vitro* analysis of the actin binding properties of the proteins with *in vivo* studies of their regulation by local signal transduction pathways. The use of molecular biological approaches to overexpress or underexpress the protein of interest within neurons will provide some of the key evidence for the role of these

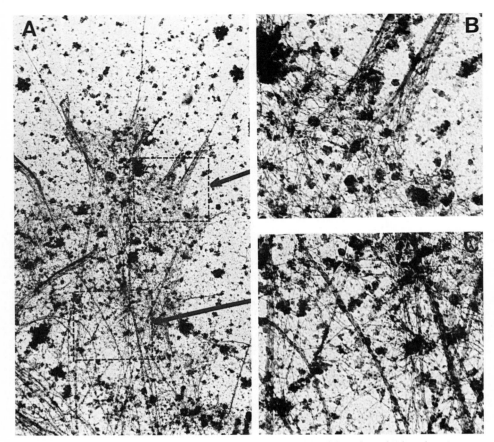

FIG. 3. Whole-mount transmission electron micrographs of chick embryonic dorsal root ganglion neuronal growth cone. Neuron was cultured on formvar, carbon, and polylysine-coated gold EM grid, fixed and extracted simultaneously, and stained as described by Letourneau (7). **A:** Leading edge and central region of growth cone at 16,400 magnification showing prominent microtubules and actin filament bundles in the filopodia. **B** and **C:** Higher magnification (50,600) of the marked regions showing the actin filament meshwork that is not readily visible in the boxed areas (*arrows*) of **A**.

proteins, but because of a high degree of redundancy in the actin-regulating machinery of the cell, multiple protein deletions may be necessary before the role of even one of these proteins becomes clear. We are currently using this approach with ADF, the cDNA of which has been cloned behind an inducible promoter for transfection of neurons and other cell types.

ACKNOWLEDGMENTS

This work was supported in part by grants GM35126, NS28338 from the National Institute of Health, and INT-8814146 from the National Science Foundation.

REFERENCES

1. Fine RE, Bray D. Actin in growing nerve cells. *Nature* 1971;234:115–118.
2. Bamburg JR, Bernstein BW. Actin and actin-binding proteins in neurons. In: Burgoyne RD, ed. *The neuronal cytoskeleton.* New York: Wiley-Liss, 1990:121–159.
3. Mitchison T, Kirschner M. Cytoskeletal dynamics and nerve growth. *Neuron* 1989;1:761–772.
4. Smith SJ. Cytoskeletal dynamics and nerve growth. *Science* 1988;242:708–715.
5. Pollard TD, Cooper JA. Actin and actin-binding proteins. A critical evaluation of mechanisms and functions. *Annu Rev Biochem* 1986;55:987–1035.
6. Yamada KM, Spooner BS, Wessells NK. Ultrastructure and function of growth cones and axons of cultured nerve cells. *J Cell Biol* 1971;49:614–635.
7. Letourneau PC. Differences in the organization of actin in the growth cones compared with the neurites of cultured neurons from chick embryos. *J Cell Biol* 1983;97:963–973.
8. Forscher P, Smith SJ. Actions of cytochalasins on the organization of actin filaments and microtubules in a neuronal growth cone. *J Cell Biol* 1988;107:1505–1516.
9. Marsh L, Letourneau PC. Growth of neurites without filopodial or lamellipodial activity in the presence of cytochalasin B. *J Cell Biol* 1984;99:2041–2047.
10. Bentley D, Toroion-Raymond A. Disoriented pathfinding by pioneer neuron growth cones deprived of filopodia by cytochalasin treatment. *Nature* 1986;323:712–715.
11. Lamoureux P, Buxbaum RE, Heidemann SR. Direct evidence that growth cones pull. *Nature* 1989;340:159–162.
12. Black MM, Lasek RJ. Slow components of axonal transport: two cytoskeletal networks. *J Cell Biol* 1980;86:616–623.
13. Willard M, Cowan WM, Vagelos PR. The polypeptide composition of intraaxonally transported proteins: evidence for four transport velocities. *Proc Natl Acad Sci USA* 1974;71:2183–2187.
14. Lasek RJ. Polymer sliding in axons. *J Cell Sci Suppl* 1986;5:161–179.
15. Bamburg JR. The axonal cytoskeleton: stationary or moving matrix? *Trends Neurosci* 1988;11:248–249.
16. Hollenbeck PJ. The transport and assembly of the axonal cytoskeleton. *J Cell Biol* 1989;108:223–227.
17. Okabe S, Hirokawa N. Turnover of fluorescently labelled tubulin and actin in the axon. *Nature* 1990;343:479–482.
18. Lim SS, Edson KJ, Letourneau PC, Borisy GG. A test of microtubule translocation during neurite elongation. *J Cell Biol* 1990;11:123–130.
19. Clark SE, Moss DJ, Bray D. Actin polymerization and synthesis in cultured neurons. *Exp Cell Res* 1983;147:303–314.
20. Bamburg JR, Harris HE, Weeds AG. Partial purification and characterization of an actin depolymerizing factor from brain. *FEBS Lett* 1980;121:178–182.
21. Adams ME, Minamide LS, Duester G, Bamburg JR. Nucleotide sequence and expression of a cDNA encoding chick brain actin depolymerizing factor. *Biochemistry* 1990;29:7414–7420.
22. Bamburg JR, Bray D. Distribution and cellular localization of actin depolymerizing factor. *J Cell Biol* 1987;105:2817–2825.
23. Hayden SM. Interaction of actin depolymerizing factor with monomeric and filamentous actin. Ph.D. Thesis, Colorado State University, Fort Collins, CO, 1988.
24. Bamburg JR, Minamide LS, Morgan TE, Hayden SM, Giuliano KA, Koffer A. Purification and characterization of low molecular weight actin depolymerizing proteins from brain and cultured cells. *Methods Enzymol* 1991;196: (*in press*).
25. Giuliano KA, Khatib FA, Hayden SM, et al. Properties of purified actin depolymerizing factor from chick brain. *Biochemistry* 1988;27:8931–8938.
26. Léna JY, Bamburg JR, Rabié A, Faivre-Sarrailh C. Actin depolymerizing factor (ADF) in the cerebellum of the developing rat: a quantitative and immunocytochemical study. *Neuroscience* 1991; (*in press*).
27. Morgan TE. Regulation of the amount and activity of actin depolymerizing factor in developing brain and muscle. Ph.D. Thesis, Colorado State University, Fort Collins, CO, 1990.
28. Bray JJ, Fernyhough P, Bamburg JR, Bray D. Actin depolymerizing factor in axons is a component of slow axonal transport. *J Neurochem* 1991; (*in press*).
29. Cao L, Wang Y.-L. Mechanism of the formation of contractile ring in dividing cultured animal cells. I. Recruitment of preexisting actin filaments into the cleavage furrow. *J Cell Biol* 1990;110:1089–1095.

30. Lockerbie RO, Miller VE, Pfenninger KH. Regulated plasmalemmal expansion in the nerve growth cone. *J Cell Biol* 1990.
31. Bernstein BW, Bamburg JR. Cycling of actin assembly in synaptosomes and neurotransmitter release. *Neuron* 1989;3:257–265.
32. Byrd JC, Lichti U. Two types of transglutaminase in the PC12 pheochromocytoma cell line. Stimulation by sodium butyrate. *J Biol Chem* 1987;262:11699–11705.
33. Weisenberg RC, Flynn J, Gao B, et al. Microtubule gelation–contraction: essential components and relation to slow axonal transport. *Science* 1987;238:1119–1122.
34. Heriot K, Gambetti P, Lasek RJ. Proteins transported in slow components a and b of axonal transport are distributed differently in the transverse plane of the axon. *J Cell Biol* 1985;100:1167–1172.
35. Isobe Y, Shimada Y. Organization of filaments underneath the plasma membrane of developing chicken skeletal muscle cells *in vitro* revealed by the freeze-dry and rotary replica method. *Cell Tissue Res* 1986;244:47–56.

The Nerve Growth Cone, edited by P. C. Letourneau,
S. B. Kater, and E. R. Macagno, Raven Press, Ltd.,
New York © 1992.

5

Functional Anatomy of the Growth Cone in Relation to its Role in Locomotion and Neurite Assembly

Paul C. Bridgman

Department of Anatomy and Neurobiology, Washington University School of Medicine, St. Louis, Missouri 63110

Research in the past several years has defined two functional roles for growth cones in nerve growth: First, they act as a locomotory organelle with both protrusive and tension-producing activity that regulates the rate and direction of growth, and second, they function as the site of neurite assembly that results in elongation. This separation of growth cone function into two related but distinct activities represents a refinement of the views of growth cone function that previously existed.

The work of Bray and colleagues (3,5) had previously defined the role of the growth cone as an organelle responsible for regulating growth through the production of tension. From this work, it was postulated that filopodial contraction resulted in a pulling force on the neurite and that this was the driving force behind neurite elongation (4). One of the first indications that neurites can elongate without the motile and tension-producing activity of the growth cone came from experiments using cytochalasin B to disrupt actin filaments (23). Under these conditions, growth cone shape was severely disrupted, and the motile activities ceased. However, if the substrate was sufficiently adhesive, neurite elongation continued but at a slower rate and in a disoriented fashion. This result suggested that the tension-producing activity of the growth cone was primarily responsible for regulating growth rate and direction but was not essential for elongation. However, total inhibition of neurite elongation does result when the microtubule-disrupting agents colchicine or nocodazole are focally applied to the growth cone, suggesting that microtubule polymerization is necessary for elongation and that the growth cone is the site of microtubule assembly (2). Support for the possibility that the growth cone represents the site of neurite assembly also came from observations made using video-enhanced differential interference contrast (DIC) microscopy (1,14). A sequence of events was observed that suggested that the growth cone progressively transforms into the neurite. This suggested that the growth cone represented the nascent form of

the neurite. The authors of these studies were unable to observe filopodial contraction and therefore suggested that the production of tension either does not occur or is
not important for growth or guidance. However, pertinent to this point are the observations from another study (12). A retrograde flow of peripherally located F-
actin was observed. Subsequent experiments have shown that this flow is apparently
coupled to the movement of cell surface proteins (13). It has been suggested that
this activity is somehow linked to the generation of tension and forward movement
of the growth cone (28). A direct demonstration that growth cones do produce
tension and that the presence of tension correlates with the growth phase has also
come recently (17). The pull the growth cone exerts on the neurite and cell body
was measured using the displacement of glass micro-needles. Taken together, these
studies suggest that the growth cone is both a locomotory organelle that produces
tension on the neurite and is also the site of neurite assembly.

Integration of the locomotion/assembly functions to bring about normal directed
nerve axon growth presents an intriguing and perhaps unique cell biological problem that clearly needs further investigation to understand fully the underlying mechanisms. With this in mind, we and others have approached these problems using
various microscopy and labeling techniques. This has resulted in the identification
of different anatomically distinct regions or domains within growth cones. The delineation of these domains appears to correlate with the regions of the growth cones
responsible for the two different functions indicated above. Determination of the
cytoskeletal organization in these two different regions should give insight into the
mechanisms that underlie their associated function.

CYTOPLASMIC DOMAINS: HOW ARE THEY DEFINED IN THE LIVING GROWTH CONE?

When observing cultured rat sympathetic neuron growth cones grown on laminin
substrates using video-enhanced DIC microscopy, two distinct regions or domains
are readily apparent that differ in their organelle content, thickness, and motile
activity (Fig. 1). At the base of the growth cone contiguous with the neurite cylinder
is a relatively thick, organelle-rich region. Mitochondria are usually present and
undergo a variety of movements and changes in shape. Other smaller membranous
organelles are also present and are often seen to undergo rapid random motions, as
well as directed movements along distinct tracks or pathways that are presumably
microtubules. Because of the location and similarity to the perinuclear region seen
in other types of cultured cells, we have referred to this region as the central or
C-domain. This region of the growth cone remains after cytochalasin treatment and
therefore may represent the distal-most site of neurite assembly. Surrounding the
C-domain is a thin, highly dynamic region of cytoplasm that usually appears devoid
of organelles when viewed with DIC microscopy. This region includes broad
lamellae and varying numbers of filopodia and is referred to as the peripheral or
P-domain. Activity in this region includes protrusions and retractions by both

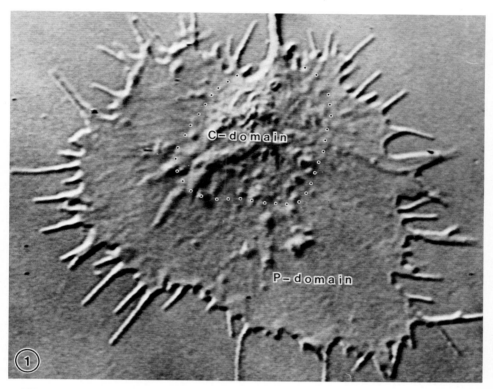

FIG. 1. Video-enhanced DIC image of a growth cone from rat superior cervical ganglion neurons grown on laminin substrates. Two distinct cytoplasmic domains are apparent: a thin peripheral (P) region surrounds a thicker organelle-rich central (C) region. The circle of dots demarcates the approximate border between domains.

lamellae and filopodia and a slow continuous, radially oriented retrograde flow, which becomes obvious in time-lapse observations (Fig. 2). Similar observations on growth cones of cultured *Aplysia* neurons have resulted in the independent identification of the same two domains, suggesting that this organization can be generalized to most well-spread growth cones (11).

WHAT IS THE COMPOSITION AND GENERAL ORGANIZATION OF THE DIFFERENT DOMAINS?

Staining of growth cones with fluorescent derivatives of phalloidin to determine the distribution of F-actin reveal that the P-domain is especially rich in actin filaments (Fig. 3). (7,12). This includes bundles of filaments within filopodia and an extensive network of radially oriented filaments within lamellae. Whole-mount

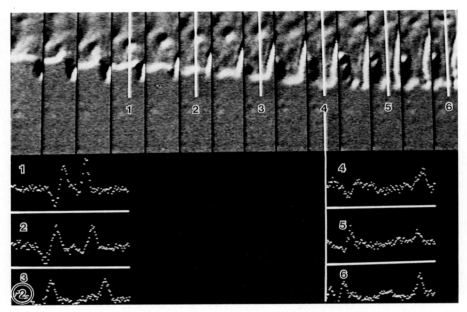

FIG. 2. Video-enhanced DIC time-lapse sequence from a growth cone showing protrusion of the leading edge and the retrograde flow that occurs within the P-domain. Contrast profiles of indicated images are shown. Time between images is 7 seconds.

electron microscopy of rapid frozen, freeze-substituted growth cones reveals additional details about the cytoplasmic organization that complements the light microscopy observations (Fig. 4) (7).

In whole mounts, the P-domain is mainly characterized by the abundance of microfilaments that have been identified as actin filaments. Bundled actin filaments form the core of most filopodia and sometimes radiate from the base of the filopodia into the lamellae for 0.5 to 1.0 μm. Lamellipodia contain a dense interwoven meshwork of actin filaments that has varying degrees of orientation. Sometimes filaments appear to radiate from the leading edge roughly parallel to each other, but more frequently they appear to form an intricate network. The details of filament organization are often hard to discern in whole mounts of intact cells because the granular "ground substance" and plasma membrane tend to obscure the filaments.

The C-domain also contains actin filaments but in lower concentrations and in more distinct bundles than in the P-domain. Immunofluorescence observations reveal varying numbers of microtubules that usually enter the C-domain from the neurite and then splay out in a variety of different patterns (8). Often microtubules will show one or more tight turns as if they were meeting resistance to their elongation. Some microtubules penetrate into the P-domain, often aligning with filopodia.

Staining with the fluorescent lipophilic dye, $DiOC_6$ reveals the distribution of membranous organelles (8). Organelles are concentrated within the C-domain. However, occasionally brightly stained "fingers" radiate from the C-domain and

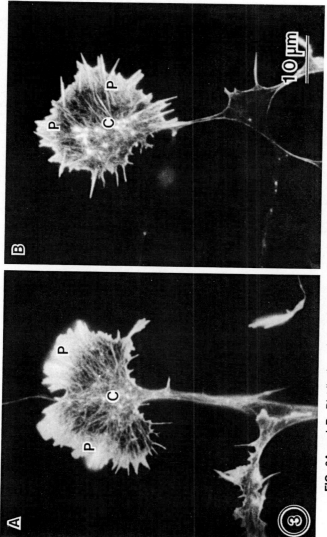

FIG. 3A and B. Distribution of growth cone actin filaments as determined by staining with rhodamine-phalloidin. The relatively thin P-domain shows a high concentration of actin filaments compared with the C-domain. (From ref. 7, with permission.)

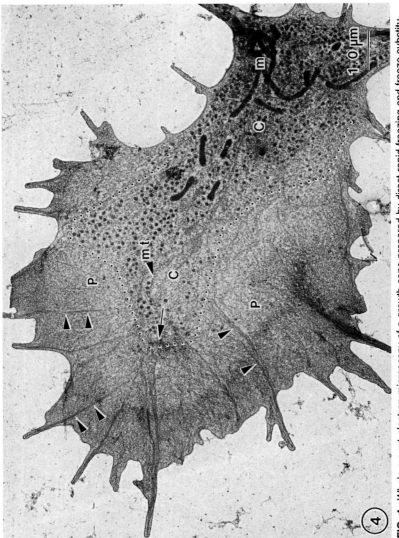

FIG. 4. Whole-mount electron microscopy of a growth cone prepared by direct rapid-freezing and freeze-substitution. Two distinct cytoplasmic domains are present. The approximate boundary between the two domains is shown by the *dotted line*. The central (C) domain contains microtubules (mt), mitochondria (m), and numerous dense core vesicles. The peripheral (P) domain contains distinct microfilament bundles (*arrowheads*) that form the core of the majority of filopodia. A meshwork of microfilaments fills the cytoplasm between the filament bundles in the peripheral domain. Some of the microfilament bundles appear to terminate in discrete areas (*arrow*) that stain darkly compared with the surrounding cytoplasm. (From ref. 7, with permission.)

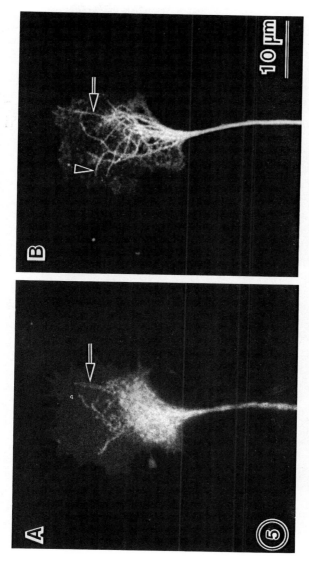

FIG. 5. Fluorescent images of a growth cone consecutively stained with DiOC$_6$ (**A**) and anti-tubulin antibodies (**B**). DiOC$_6$ fluorescent processes often colocalize with distal segments of microtubules (*arrows*), although some microtubule segments are not associated with DiOC$_6$ fluorescence (*arrowhead*). (From ref. 8, with permission.)

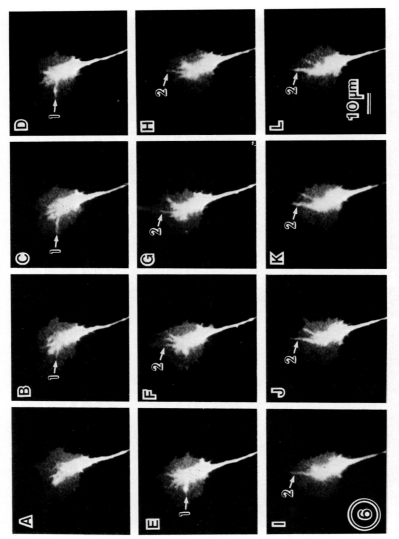

FIG. 6. Time-lapse sequence of a DiOC$_6$-stained living growth cone showing extension, retraction, and thickening of fluorescent processes. Process 1 extended toward the margin and immediately retracted. Process 2 extended as a thin process into the base of a filopodium and became thicker; it was initially distinct from the fluorescent mass (**G–H**) until the latter began to advance into the processes (**I–L**). Total sequence time was 11 min at 1-min intervals. (From ref. 8, with permission.)

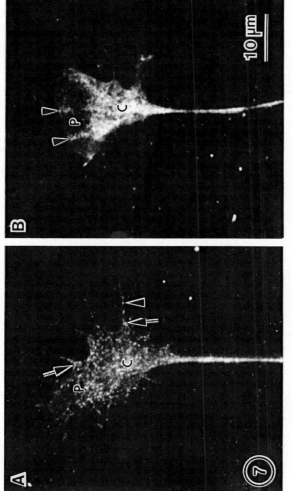

FIG. 7. Fluorescent images of growth cones stained with antibodies to myosin. Staining is brightest in the C-domain and is often punctate when precisely focused. Small spots of stain can also be seen distributed throughout the P-domain and are especially bright at the base of some filopodia (*arrows*). Small spots of stain can sometimes be seen along the length of filopodia (*arrowhead* in **A**). In growth cones with broad lamellipodia, staining was more intense in areas of the P-domain that appeared to be ruffling (*arrowheads* in **B**). (From ref. 7, with permission.)

project into the P-domain, sometimes extending all the way to the leading edge of the lamellae. Double fluorescence staining of microtubules and membranes reveals that the fingers of $DiOC_6$ fluorescence correspond with microtubule projections into the P-domain (Fig. 5). Observations on living growth cones have revealed that the fingers are highly dynamic; they extend, retract, move laterally, and are often swept back at the same rate as the retrograde flow of actin (Fig. 6) (8). Much of the dynamic behavior of the fingers is similar to that observed for microtubules undergoing growth with dynamic instability characteristics (24), although it is apparent that their behavior is also influenced by interaction with actin filaments. The fingers have been identified by whole-mount electron microscopy to consist mainly of long, thin membrane tubes that are aligned with peripheral microtubule segments (9). The thin strands of membrane are continuous with a branching network of membranes in the C-domain with the morphological characteristics normally associated with smooth endoplasmic reticulum (9). Less frequently, other membranous organelles are also seen along microtubules such as the blind-ended tubes and dense core vesicles.

Immunofluorescence staining of myosin reveals a punctate distribution; the staining is most intense in the C-domain probably because of its thickness; bright spots of stain can also be seen within the P-domain, often at the base and along the length of filopodia (Fig. 7) (7; see also refs. 18 and 25). Actin binding proteins including filamin, α-actinin, vinculin, and talin also appear to be concentrated in the P-domain, whereas fodrin is most concentrated in the C-domain (19,29).

Immunoelectron microscopy of myosin using colloidal gold markers confirms the punctate distribution seen by immunofluorescence and gives additional information about the relative concentration of myosin in different regions of the growth cone (7). Myosin is present in both domains in roughly equal amounts, but its distribution is nonuniform; it is more concentrated at the border between the P- and C-domains and is also consistently concentrated at the base of filopodia.

IS THE PERIPHERAL DOMAIN RESPONSIBLE FOR GROWTH CONE LOCOMOTORY ACTIVITY?

Locomotion involves both protrusion of the leading edge of the growth cone and the production of tension to pull the main cytoplasmic mass and trailing neurite forward. The protrusive activity of the peripheral domain is obvious in observations of living growth cones (see Fig. 2); however, the evidence for P-domain involvement in the generation of the pulling force is at present mostly circumstantial. Because the P-domain is very rich in actin filaments and disruption of actin filaments with cytochalasin abolishes the retrograde flow and the generation of tension, it has been suggested that the P-domain is the main site of tension production. The force necessary for the production of tension could conceivably come from the interaction of myosin with actin, because myosin is present in this region (7). The pulling force would result if actin was coupled to receptors for cell substrate molecules, which were in turn interacting with the appropriate molecules fixed on the substrate. Consistent with this possibility is the relatively high concentration of integrin receptors present in the P-domain (19,31). However, much work needs to be done to determine whether this model for production of tension is correct. For instance, it is not clear whether the conventional form of myosin that has been detected in growth cones is in sufficient quantities or in the right place to generate the retrograde flow. Other forms of myosin could be involved, but to date, nonconventional forms of myosin have not been positively identified in growth cones. The mechanism of tension production will be important to define in future research.

DOES ACTIN FILAMENT ORGANIZATION REFLECT THE FUNCTION OF THE PERIPHERAL DOMAIN?

Despite the uncertainty regarding the mechanism of tension production, it has been assumed that actin filaments are involved because depolymerization of actin results in cessation or disruption of normal growth (23) and a decrease in tension (10). Similarly, the exact mechanism by which protrusion occurs remains unknown, but it is clear that actin filaments are necessary for this activity (23,30). Because of the involvement of actin filaments in both processes, it is important to determine the precise structural arrangement and polarity of actin filaments within growth cones and in particular within the P-domain. Previous work has shown that actin filaments are organized in a manner that appears similar to that seen in the periphery of motile nonneuronal cells (20). However, the precise 3-dimensional organization of actin filaments has not been fully worked out, mainly because different ultrastructural methods have given different results (26) and growth cone F-actin seems particularly labile. Nevertheless, it was clear from these previous studies that most filopodia have a core of bundled actin, whereas lamellae are filled with a distinct meshwork of filaments that has varying degrees of radial orientation. In nonneuronal cells, decoration of actin filaments with myosin S1 or heavy meromyosin (HMM) has been used to show that the "barbed" or fast-growing end of the filament is distally located (toward the leading edge) and the "pointed" end is roughly oriented toward the C- or perinuclear domain (27). However, the amount of data on polarity is somewhat limited and has usually been restricted to a few filaments splaying out from the leading edge. The polarity of actin filaments in growth cones has not been described [although some data have been presented on neuroblastoma cells (27)]. Actin filament polarity will be important for determining the direction of filament growth during polymerization and for assessing the expected types of interaction that would result from myosin-mediated activity. For these reasons we have spent a considerable amount of time studying the organization and polarity of actin filaments in growth cones with several different electron microscopy techniques, including negative stain (21) and, more recently, freeze-etch. Preliminary results suggest that actin filaments within filopodia are primarily oriented with their barbed end at the distal most tip, but a few filaments enter the base of a filopodia with the opposite orientation. Similarly, the filaments radiating from the leading edge of a lamellae are almost exclusively oriented with their barbed ends located distally, but this uniformity in orientation is lost several tenths of a micrometer from the leading edge. This suggests that the plasma membrane at the leading edge may be the key element in determining actin filament orientation. The relatively uniform orientation of filaments at the periphery of lamellae and within filopodia is consistent with a mechanism in which actin polymerization drives protrusion. However, the mixed polarity farther from the leading edge and at the base of filopodia is consistent with actin–myosin interactions that lead to complex movements and the production of tension. More difficult to explain is the retrograde flow of actin that is apparent throughout the P-domain.

IS THE CENTRAL DOMAIN RESPONSIBLE FOR NEURITE ASSEMBLY?

The once-held belief that neurite elongation results from the sequential addition or assembly of new materials at the cell body [reviewed by Grafstein and Forman (15)] has recently been challenged by several different types of experiments; this includes the observation that microtubules do not move in mass down the neurite but are stationary (22). This result, combined with those on the sensitivity of the growth cone to microtubule depolymerizing agents (2), suggests that the construction of the neurite occurs at its distal end and that the growth cone is the specific site of assembly. Neurites are cylindrical structures that contain bundles of microtubules, closely associated neurofilaments, and an outer sheath of actin filaments. Membranous organelles are distributed along the neurite closely associated with microtubules. At the growth cone, expansion of the neurite should result in the splaying of microtubules and an accumulation of organelles in the C-domain. Simply on morphological grounds, it is apparent that the C-domain resembles a nascent form of the neurite. Its components are the same, with a different organization; microtubules transition from bundled to splayed and the association with organelles is not as tightly organized. The C-domain is also relatively stable compared with the P-domain; low concentrations (0.1 μg/ml) of nocodazole that cause depolymerization of P-domain microtubules do not cause loss of microtubules from the C-domain (M. Dailey and P. Bridgman, *unpublished results*). In addition, the C-domain and elongation is not abolished by cytochalasin treatment, which has dramatic effects on the P-domain (12,23). Therefore, it seems reasonable to conclude that the initial site of neurite assembly is the C-domain. One test of this possibility would be to amputate the growth cone from its neurite and then observe whether the isolated growth cone can continue to locomote and form a neurite. Preliminary experiments of this nature suggest that under appropriate conditions, growth cones can continue to show locomotion and formation of new neurites. The final length of the new neurite is roughly proportional to the original size of the growth cone, suggesting that the growth cone is transformed into the neurite (6).

The Nerve Growth Cone, edited by P. C. Letourneau,
S. B. Kater, and E. R. Macagno, Raven Press, Ltd.,
New York © 1992.

6

Assembly of Microtubules in Growth Cones: The Role of Microtubule-Associated Proteins

P. R. Gordon-Weeks and S. Gary Mansfield

*Anatomy and Human Biology Group, King's College London,
London WC2R 2LS, England*

The growth cone's remarkable ability to find its way through the complex terrain of the developing nervous system and successfully locate its synaptic partner has been surmised since the time of its discovery by Ramón y Cajal (1). This navigational feat is based on the possession, by growth cones, of a system of surface receptors for extrinsic guidance cues that are coupled to a cytoskeleton capable of motility by mechanisms that have yet to be elucidated (2). As well as pathfinding activities and synaptogenesis, growth cones are also involved in growth of the neurite, and in this respect they differ from other motile entities such as fibroblasts in culture or chemotaxing leucocytes (3). Growth is used here in the sense of the addition of new material, because as the growth cone advances, it builds behind it the extending neurite. This involves the assembly of the cytoskeleton of the neurite and the addition of new surface and internal membrane systems and other elements of the cytoplasm. In the axon, the cytoskeleton is assembled from components brought down from the cell body, their site of synthesis, by axonal transport (4). In mature axons and dendrites, the cytoskeleton may consist of microtubules, neurofilaments, and microfilaments. Of these three filamentous systems, we are now beginning to make some headway in understanding how microtubules are assembled in the growing neurite, and this area is the topic of the research in our laboratory.

Microtubules in Growing Neurites

In the growing neurite, as in most mature axons and dendrites, microtubules are a dominant feature and are often observed in bundles running parallel to the longitudinal axis of the neurite. Although individual microtubules in growing neurites can be as long as 100 μm, many do not extend the full length of the neurite (which may be many millimeters in length) and may be contained entirely within the neurite. Two functions of microtubules within neurites have been identified: a specific one, the

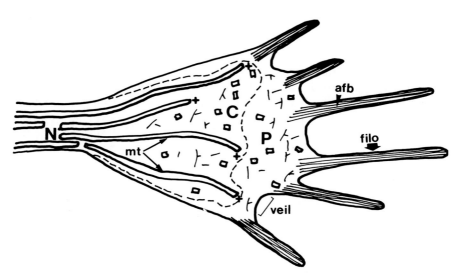

FIG. 1. Schematic diagram of a growth cone showing the microtubule and microfilament cyto-skeleton. The small squares represent the soluble tubulin pool, while the short line segments are non-bundled F-actin. The plus signs show the location of the "plus" ends of the micro-tubules. C, central domain; N, neurite; P, peripheral domain; afb, actin filament bundle; filo, filopodium; mt, microtubule.

substrate for fast axonal (and dendritic) transport; and a more general one, the main-tenance of the shape and structural integrity of the neurite. At the distal end of the neurite, where it enlarges into the growth cone, the individual microtubules of the bundle diverge like the ribs of a fan to extend into the central (C) domain of the growth cone (Fig. 1). Microtubules only rarely extend beyond the C-domain and into the peripheral (P) region of the growth cone, or P-domain, where the cyto-skeleton is mainly composed of microfilaments, and have never been found in the filopodia (5) (Fig. 1). As they diverge from each other on entering the C-domain, microtubules may have a winding course at their distal ends, whereas in the neurite they are straight (6). Furthermore, there is a marked preference for smooth endo-plasmic reticulum and vesicles to be associated with the straight regions but not the winding regions (6).

Microtubule Assembly in Growth Cones

The microtubules that enter the growth cone from the neurite shaft are all oriented with their so-called plus ends, the end at which tubulin subunit addition takes place preferentially, distally (7) (Fig. 1). We now know from recent work that micro-tubule elongation takes place in the growth cone by the addition of tubulin onto the distal ends of the neurite microtubules that enter the C-domain of the growth cone.

It has been known for some time that neurite advance is critically dependent on microtubule assembly because neurite extension in cultured neurons can be inhibited or reversed by the addition of agents that interfere with microtubule assembly/disassembly (8,9). More recent experiments have shown that it is the assembly of microtubules in the growth cone, rather than the cell body or neurite, that is important for neurite extension. The evidence for this derives from a number of observations that, although indirect, are collectively compelling. First, as discussed above, only the "plus" ends of the neurite microtubules extend into the growth cone. This is true of both axonal and dendritic growth cones despite the fact that in the shafts of dendrites a significant proportion of the microtubules are oriented with their "plus" ends proximal (10). Second, the direct application onto the growth cone by micropipette of agents that depolymerize or stabilize microtubules prevents neurite growth (11). Furthermore, the growth cone is the most sensitive region of the neuron to these agents by orders of magnitude (11). Third, a large assembly-competent pool of tubulin in the growth cone is the immediate source of tubulin for microtubule elongation (12,13). This was first shown by observing the effects of the agent taxol on growth cones in culture (12). Taxol lowers the critical concentration point for tubulin assembly within cells and thus forces the soluble pool of tubulin to form microtubules. The effect of taxol treatment on growth cones is to assemble the soluble pool of tubulin onto the "plus" ends of the microtubules that enter the C-domain from the neurite shaft (12,13). At high concentrations of taxol (low µM), when this effect goes to completion, microtubule loops appear in the C-domain of the growth cone because of the large volume of the soluble tubulin pool. This effect has also been seen in growth cones isolated from developing brain as a subcellular fraction (13; see review in ref. 14). Normally, microtubules are absent from these growth cones for reasons that are not clear, but they appear on incubation in taxol because of the presence of the large pool of soluble tubulin (13).

The soluble pool of tubulin in the growth cone can be visualized in cultured neurons using certain antibodies to tubulin (15). These label both the microtubules and the soluble tubulin, which, unlike the microtubules, is distributed throughout the P- and C-domains, including the filopodia. As described above, taxol treatment accelerates the assembly of the soluble pool of tubulin onto the ends of the microtubules in the growth cone forming loops in the C-domain. This process exhausts the pool of soluble tubulin and consequently results in a loss of the staining of the P-domain and filopodia with tubulin antibodies (15). If neuronal cultures are incubated in microtubule assembly buffer and detergent before fixation, the soluble pool of tubulin is removed, leaving behind the cytoskeleton including the microtubules. Under these circumstances, only the microtubules are seen in growth cones after immunofluorescence with tubulin antibodies (P. Gordon-Weeks, *unpublished observation*).

In the neurite itself we now know that microtubules are stationary. This was recently demonstrated by Okabe and Hirokawa (16), who microinjected fluorescently labeled tubulin into neurons in culture and followed the recovery of fluorescence after photobleaching short segments of the neurite. Bleached zones in the neurite remained stationary, despite the fact that the neurite was extending, and slowly recovered their fluorescence, indicating that although neurite microtubules are dynamically exchanging tubulin subunits, they are not moving. This result has recently been independently confirmed (17). By measuring the recovery times after photobleaching in PC12 pheochromocytoma cells (a cell line resembling sympathetic neurons), Lim and colleagues (18) have shown that microtubules are more dynamic in the growth cone than in the neurite or cell body, an observation in keeping with a predominant assembly in the growth cone.

These studies provide a view of microtubule assembly in extending neurites in which microtubules are formed and elongated in the growth cone and deposited in the neurite as the growth cone advances, like the laying of a cable by a cable-laying ship. The immediate source of the tubulin to support microtubule formation is the large pool of soluble tubulin in the growth cone. Microtubules are clearly necessary in the neurite both to provide structural support and for the substrate of fast axonal (and dendritic) transport. Unlike the neurite shaft, however, the growth cone is a highly motile structure, and it seems that the presence of excessive numbers of microtubules compromises motility (12). This observation and the fact that the large pool of tubulin in the growth cone is assembly competent and yet remains unassembled (12,13,15), despite the presence of the "plus" ends of microtubules (7), implies that microtubule assembly in the growth cone is precisely controlled (3).

Control of Microtubule Assembly in Growth Cones

On the basis of our knowledge of microtubule assembly *in vitro*, several factors may be involved in the control of microtubule assembly in growth cones. These are Ca^{2+}, GTP, posttranslational modification of tubulin, and microtubule-associated proteins (MAPs).

Calcium has been known for some time to depolymerize microtubules *in vitro*; however, it is unlikely that the concentration of Ca^{2+} in growth cones is sufficiently high, under normal circumstances, to affect microtubule polymerization (19). In some circumstances, however, such as growth cone collapse, Ca^{2+} levels may rise dramatically in the growth cone (20), and microtubule numbers may then be expected to decline (21). Guanosine triphosphate is known to be essential for tubulin polymerization, but nothing is known about the distribution of this molecule within growth cones.

Several posttranslational modifications of tubulin have been identified including phosphorylation, acetylation, and a reversible removal of the C-terminal tyrosine of α-tubulin by specific enzymes (22). Although the function of these modifications has not been established, it is possible that they may affect microtubule assembly either directly or through modifying the binding of MAPs, which may themselves alter microtubule assembly.

Microtubule-associated proteins have been shown to affect microtubule dynamics profoundly both *in vitro* and *in vivo*, and they are candidates, therefore, for controlling microtubule assembly in growth cones.

RECENT STUDIES

Posttranslational Modifications of Tubulin

With a few minor exceptions, most of the genes for α-tubulin code for a protein with a carboxy-terminal tyrosine (22). This tyrosine can be selectively removed by a specific tubulin tyrosine carboxypeptidase (23) or added by a specific tubulin tyrosine ligase (24,25). These posttranslational modifications are unique to tubulin. Most of the α-tubulin in growth cones is carboxy-terminal tyrosinated, as indicated by biochemical experiments with isolated growth cones (15,26). Furthermore, immunofluorescence studies of cultured neurons using antibodies specific for either tyrosinated or detyrosinated α-tubulin support this finding (18,27–29). For instance, in dorsal root ganglion cells in culture, the majority of the axonal growth cones (these cells do not have dendrites) stain for antibodies specific for tyrosinated α-tubulin but not for detyrosinated α-tubulin (27). This is also the case with PC12 growth cones (18), and the axonal and dendritic growth cones of cerebral cortical neurons in culture (28,29).

The function of these posttranslational modifications of tubulin are not known, but it has been found that α-tubulin becomes detyrosinated and acetylated sometime after assembly in nonneuronal cells (31). A similar event occurs in neurons and neuroblastoma cells extending neurites in culture (18,27–29). When the growth cone has moved on and the microtubules have become incorporated into the neurite cytoskeleton the α-tubulin is detyrosinated at its carboxy terminal and acetylated (18,27–29). These posttranslational modifications of tubulin correlate with an increase in the stability of the microtubules to depolymerization by cold shock and microtubule depolymerizing agents such as nocodazole, but they are not causal to microtubule stability (31). The events that stabilize microtubules to depolymerization are not known. Once they have become incorporated into the neurite cytoskeleton, although immobile, microtubules can still exchange tubulin subunits at their "plus" ends (32) and here also the added α-tubulin is initially tyrosinated at its carboxy terminal and unacetylated (33).

It is likely that microtubules in growth cones are dynamically unstable, that is to say, they are alternately growing slowly and shrinking back rapidly (34). Although dynamic instability has been directly observed in some cell types (35), it has not been looked for systematically in growth cones. However, in a recent study (36) of *Aplysia* neurons observed in culture with video-enhanced microscopy, microtubules showing dynamic instability were observed in growth cones, although the authors were not able to rule out forward sliding of the microtubules. The proposal that growth cone microtubules are undergoing dynamic instability is also consistent with the observation that these microtubules are turning over more rapidly than in other regions of the growing neuron (18) and that these microtubules are largely composed of tyrosinated α-tubulin (see above), which correlates with microtubule instability. Recently we have found that the distal regions of microtubules in the growth cones of neurons growing in culture, but not the microtubules in the neurite shaft, depolymerize in microtubule assembly buffers containing detergents, a finding that also suggests that these microtubules are relatively labile (P. Gordon-Weeks, *unpublished observations*).

Tyrosinated α-tubulin is no less able to polymerize than detyrosinated α-tubulin. However, if the carboxy-terminal tyrosine is phosphorylated, assembly is markedly impaired (37). Even if assembly occurs, the binding of MAPs may be altered by phosphorylation, and this in turn may lead to less stable microtubules (see below). Experiments with isolated growth cones have shown that tubulin can be phosphorylated on tyrosine residues in the growth cone, but the location of the tyrosine within the molecule is not known (38,39). Nor has the tyrosine kinase been identified, although pp60^{c-src}, a tyrosine kinase, is present in an active form in growth cones (40). However, pp60^{c-src} is mainly associated with the plasma membrane, and it is not clear what access the kinase would have to soluble tubulin. Preliminary experiments by us in collaboration with J. Diaz-Nido and J. Avila (Madrid) have shown that α-tubulin can be phosphorylated at the carboxy-terminal tyrosine in isolated growth cones in which the ATP pools have been radiolabeled with ^{32}P-orthophosphate (*unpublished observations*). Phosphorylation of the carboxy-terminal tyrosine of α-tubulin by a specific membrane kinase is an attractive means of influencing microtubule assembly and has the advantage that it provides a route for extrinsic guidance factors to affect neurite elongation via membrane signal transduction. Future experiments will need to identify the kinase responsible.

Microtubule-Associated Proteins

Although direct evidence is lacking, several independent observations point to a role for certain MAPs in neurite extension (41). For instance, some of the high-molecular-weight MAPs, including MAP 2 and MAP 1B [a.k.a. MAP 5 (42), MAP 1.2 (43), MAP 1x (44)] and also tau, have been found in growth cones by immunocytochemistry (15,45,46). Most MAPs are under strong developmental regulation in neurons (41), for instance, MAP 1B, or have juvenile forms that are truncated versions of the adult proteins produced by differential splicing of RNA transcripts, such as tau and MAP 2 (47,48). Furthermore, when PC12 cells are induced to form neurites in culture by the action of nerve growth factor, MAP 1B and tau are rapidly up-regulated, suggesting that they are required for neurite outgrowth (49–51). MAP 1B is posttranslationally phosphorylated by a casein kinase II–like activity (52), and there is strong developmental down-regulation of the phosphorylated form (53,54). Interestingly, it is the phosphorylated form of MAP 1B that is most strongly induced during neurite outgrowth (43,52), and recently we have found that MAP 1B is phosphorylated in both isolated growth cones and the growth cones of rat cerebral cortical neurons in culture (55). In some axons in culture, the phosphorylated form of MAP 1B is distributed in a striking gradient, which is highest distally and lowest near the cell body, whereas the nonphosphorylated form is distributed throughout the neuron (55). The phosphorylated form of MAP 1B has also been found in high levels in growing axons *in vivo* (53,57). Tau

(15) and MAP 1B (55) but not MAP 2 (15) are present in growth cones in excess over their tubulin binding sites and may have roles in growth cones unrelated to microtubules. For instance, they may interact with the actin cytoskeleton, a suggestion supported by the observation that tau can bind to actin (56). Collectively these results suggest an important role for tau and MAP 1B, particularly the phosphorylated form of MAP 1B (see also the chapter by Diaz-Nido et al.), in neurite outgrowth, which may be unrelated to the ability of these proteins to act as microtubule cross-linkers (57).

In Alzheimer's disease, in which it is thought there is a massive attempt at axonal and dendritic regeneration, it is interesting to note that there is an accumulation of hyperphosphorylated tau and MAP 1B (58,59).

These observations have led to the idea that during neurite outgrowth, a set of MAPs is required that is different, either by differential splicing or posttranslational modification, from those present in the mature neurite (41). Although the function of most MAPs is not understood, it is assumed that these two sets of MAPs have functions that relate to the differing requirements of an extending neurite in the developing nervous system and a more stable one in the adult.

In addition to microtubule elongation at the growth cone, the presence of microtubules entirely within extending neurites may indicate that microtubules are also formed *de novo* in growth cones. This presumably requires a form of microtubule organizing center (MTOC), such as that found associated with centrosomes (60). However, there have been very few signs of these in neurites or growth cones. By definition, MTOCs contain MAPs, and it is interesting to note in this context that some MAP 1B antibodies cross-react with centrosomes (61).

FUTURE PROSPECTS

Naturally, the experiments described here, while providing answers to some questions, engender more. For instance, how is the soluble tubulin in the growth cone maintained and delivered to the growth cone from the cell body where, at least in axons, it is synthesized? Perhaps it comes down in the so-called "slow component a particles" described by Weisenberg and co-workers (62), which may correspond to the motile varicosities seen in some cultured neurites (63). Another basic question is how is microtubule assembly coupled to growth cone motility (3,34)? One indication that these events are linked is the observation that the formation of microtubule loops after taxol treatment is associated with the collapse of the growth cone (12,15,28,29).

In the near future we can expect a deeper understanding of the molecular aspects of neurite extension to derive from further study of the assembly of microtubules in growth cones and in particular in the role of MAPs in controlling assembly. MAPs almost certainly have other roles in growth cone behavior, such as linking microtubules to actin filaments and as microtubule motors (64), and these areas also are certain to yield exciting discoveries. Ultimately we will have a molecular description of how extrinsic guidance cues influence these important events that occur within growth cones.

ACKNOWLEDGMENTS

The work in my laboratory is supported by the MRC, Wellcome Trust, British Council, and the Royal Society.

REFERENCES

1. Ramón y Cajal S. A quelle époque apparaissent les expensions des cellules nerveuses de la molle épinière du poulet? *Anat Anz* 1890;21:609–613, 631–639.
2. Dodd J, Jessell TM. Axon guidance and the patterning of neuronal projections in vertebrates. *Science* 1988;242:692–699.
3. Gordon-Weeks PR. Growth at the growth cone. *Trends Neurosc* 1989;12:238–240.
4. Lasek RJ. Translocation of the axonal cytoskeleton and axonal locomotion. *Proc Trans R Soc Lond (SerB)* 1982;299:313–327.
5. Gordon-Weeks PR. The ultrastructure of the neuronal growth cone: new insights from subcellular fractionation and rapid freezing studies. *Electron Microsc Rev* 1988;1:201–219.
6. Cheng TPO, Reese TS. Polarized compartmentalization of organelles in growth cones from developing optic tectum. *J Cell Biol* 1985;101:1473–1480.
7. Baas PW, White LA, Heidemann SR. Microtubule polarity reversal accompanies regrowth of amputated neurites. *Proc Natl Acad Sci USA* 1987;84:5272–5276.
8. Yamada KM, Spooner BS, Wessells NK. Axon growth: roles of microfilaments and microtubules. *Proc Natl Acad Sci USA* 1970;66:1206–1212.
9. Daniels M. Colchicine inhibition of nerve fiber formation *in vitro*. *J Cell Biol* 1972;53:164–176.
10. Baas PW, Deitch JS, Black MM, Banker GA. Polarity orientation of microtubules in hippocampal neurons: uniformity in the axon and nonuniformity in the dendrite. *Proc Natl Acad Sci USA* 1988;85:8335–8339.
11. Bamburg JR, Bray D, Chapman K. Assembly of microtubules at the tip of growing axons. *Nature* 1986;321:788–790.
12. Letourneau PC, Ressler AH. Inhibition of neurite initiation and growth by taxol. *J Cell Biol* 1984; 98:1355–1362.
13. Gordon-Weeks PR. The cytoskeletons of isolated, neuronal growth cones. *Neuroscience* 1987; 21:977–989.
14. Lockerbie RO. Biochemical pharmacology of isolated neuronal growth cones: implications for synaptogenesis. *Brain Res Rev* 1990;15:145–165.
15. Gordon-Weeks PR, Mansfield SG, Curran I. Direct visualisation of the soluble pool of tubulin in the neuronal growth cone: immunofluorescence studies following taxol polymerisation. *Dev Brain Res* 1989;49:305–310.
16. Okabe S, Hirokawa N. Turnover of fluorescently labelled tubulin and actin in the axon. *Nature* 1990;343:479–482.
17. Lim S-S, Edson JE, Letourneau PC, Borisy GG. A test of microtubule translocation during neurite elongation. *J Cell Biol* 1990;111:123–130.
18. Lim S-S, Sammak PJ, Borisy GG. Progressive and spatially differentiated stability of microtubules in developing neuronal cells. *J Cell Biol* 1989;109:253–263.
19. Silver RA, Lamb AG, Bolsover SR. Calcium hotspots caused by L-channel clustering promote morphological changes in neuronal growth cones. *Nature* 1990;343:751–754.
20. Bandtlow CE, Schmidt MF, Kater SB, Schwab ME. Inhibition of neurite growth by a CNS myelin-specific protein (NI-35) is correlated to changes of $[Ca^{2+}]$. *Cell Biol Int Rep* 1990;14: Abstr. Suppl. S138.
21. Lankford KL, Letourneau PC. Evidence that calcium may control neurite outgrowth by regulating the stability of actin filaments. *J Cell Biol* 1989;109:1229–1243.

tion of these cells with cloned cDNAs coding for certain MAPs (22,23), which induces stabilization of microtubules.

Interestingly, the tubulin binding ability of MAPs, and therefore their effects on microtubule assembly and stabilization, can be modulated by both the binding of other regulatory molecules to MAPs and posttranslational modifications of MAPs. Of particular interest in this regard is the binding of calcium/calmodulin to MAPs, as it competitively inhibits the association of MAPs with tubulin, possibly because both calcium/calmodulin and tubulin compete for a common binding site on MAPs (24–26). This may constitute an important regulatory mechanism, because MAPs may interact with calmodulin and tubulin alternatively, depending on the free-calcium concentration, thus favoring or suppressing microtubule instability in response to signal transduction pathways from those extracellular signals (growth factors, hormones, neurotransmitters, neuromodulators, adhesion molecules) that control calcium level fluctuations.

Reversible posttranslational modifications of MAPs, mainly phosphorylation–dephosphorylation, may also affect tubulin binding (17,18,27,28) and consequently regulate microtubule dynamics in response to those extracellular signals that control the activity of the different MAP kinases and phosphatases. As a case in point, calcium/calmodulin-dependent phosphorylation of several MAPs leads to microtubule disassembly (29).

Additionally, posttranslational modifications of the tubulin molecule may also modify the dynamic properties of microtubules. For example, it has been suggested that acetylation and detyrosination of α-tubulin may be involved in the stabilization of axonal microtubules (9,11,30).

Here we have chosen a rather simple model (neuroblastoma cells) to study neurite growth and to analyze the contribution of some of the regulatory mechanisms mentioned above, mainly those involving MAPs and posttranslational modifications, to the control of microtubule assembly, dynamics, and stabilization within developing neurites.

Phosphorylation of β3-Tubulin and MAP1B Accompanies Neurite Outgrowth

We have used two clonal cell lines, N2A and NIE-115, derived from the same murine neuroblastoma tumor C-1300 (5,6,31), throughout this study. These cells are considered as transformed neural crest precursors of sympathetic neurons and can be maintained in *in vitro* culture as proliferating undifferentiated cells. After serum withdrawal from the culture medium, these cells differentiate into amitotic cells expressing certain neuronal characteristics, including the growth of axon-like processes (5,6,31).

Neurite outgrowth in these neuroblastoma cells is accompanied by a net increase in assembled microtubules. Whereas $15\% \pm 9\%$ of total tubulin is polymerized in undifferentiated NIE-115 cells, $65\% \pm 10\%$ of total tubulin is in the assembled form

in differentiated NIE-115 cells. This increase in the proportion of polymerized tubulin is not due to any increase in the total amount of tubulin (about 4 pg ± 1 pg/
cell) but might result from posttranslational modifications of microtubule proteins.

The phosphorylation of a β-tubulin isoform and a high-molecular-weight MAP
tentatively identified as MAP1 in differentiating neuroblastoma cells had been previously described (32). We have determined that the Class III β-tubulin (the product
of the Mβ6 gene) is that phosphorylated in neurons, probably by a casein kinase II–
related enzyme (28,33,34). As for the high-molecular-weight MAP that becomes
phosphorylated in neuroblastoma cells, we have found that it corresponds to
MAP1B, as determined from immunoprecipitation and coassembly with tubulin and
phosphopeptide mapping, and that it is also phosphorylated by a casein kinase II–
related enzyme (35).

The increase in phosphorylated MAP1B parallels neurite growth and is not due to
any increase in the synthesis of this protein but to augmented phosphorylation (Fig.
1). Interestingly, MAP1B phosphorylation has also been observed when pheochromocytoma PC12 cells are induced to extend axon-like processes on NGF (nerve
growth factor) treatment, although, in this case, variations in the steady-state levels
of the protein are observed (36).

Notwithstanding the fact that both β3-tubulin and MAP1B are phosphorylated by
a casein kinase II–related enzyme, there are some important differences between
β3-tubulin and MAP1B phosphorylation. First, β3-tubulin phosphorylation is significantly inhibited when differentiating neuroblastoma cells are treated with micro-
tubule-depolymerizing drugs (32–34), whereas MAP1B phosphorylation is essentially unaffected under the same conditions (32,35). Second, assembled tubulin is a

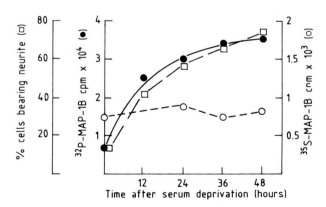

FIG. 1. Increase in the level of phosphorylated MAP1B during neuroblastoma cell differentiation. Phosphorylation and synthesis of MAP1B were determined by immunoprecipitation of
aliquots of N2A neuroblastoma cell extracts labeled with ³²PO₄ and [³⁵S]-methionine after 0 to
48 hr of serum withdrawal, as indicated in ref. 35. Whereas no change in the rate of MAP1B
synthesis (○) is observed, an increase in MAP1B phosphorylation (●) that parallels the increase in the percentage of neurite-bearing cells (□) is found.

better substrate for casein kinase II *in vitro* than unassembled tubulin, and phosphorylated β3-tubulin is largely restricted to assembled microtubules *in situ* in neuroblastoma cells (34). Third, the kinetics of β3-tubulin phosphorylation is delayed with respect to that of the net microtubule assembly that takes place in differentiating neuroblastoma cells (34), whereas MAP1B phosphorylation precedes the increase in microtubule assembly that accompanies neurite outgrowth both in neuroblastoma and pheochromocytoma cells (35,36). Taken together, these results suggest that β3-tubulin phosphorylation probably takes place after the association of β3-tubulin with assembled microtubules. However, MAP1B phosphorylation could be a prior step to the polymerization of microtubules within the growing neurite.

The association of phosphorylated MAP1B with major sites of microtubule assembly is supported by immunocytochemical studies. Thus, phosphorylated MAP1B is largely concentrated to a perinuclear spot that corresponds to the centrosome, the major microtubule-organizing center in undifferentiated neuroblastoma cells, whereas it is quite prominent within developing neurites, mainly in growth cones, in differentiating neuroblastoma cells (Fig. 2). Interestingly, the association of phosphorylated MAP1B with centrosomes in nonneural cells has also been described, based not only on immunocytochemical studies (16,18,20) but also on

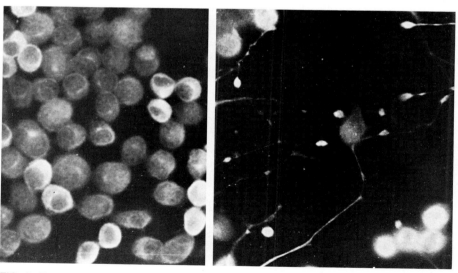

FIG. 2. Distribution of phosphorylated MAP1B in undifferentiated and differential N2A neuroblastoma cells. Immunofluorescent staining pattern of undifferentiated (*left*) and differentiated (*right*) N2A neuroblastoma cells incubated with a mouse monoclonal antibody to phosphorylated MAP1B and a fluorescein-conjugated goat antimouse immunoglobulin. Preferential localization of phosphorylated MAP1B in a perinuclear spot (which corresponds to the centrosome) in undifferentiated cells and in neurites and growth cones of differentiated cells is shown.

biochemical analyses of purified centrosome preparations (36a). In fact, nonneural cells contain phosphorylated MAP1B, as determined from phospholabeling and immunoprecipitation studies, at a notably lower level than that found in differentiated neuroblastoma cells (28). Thus, there seems to be a correlation between the amount of phosphorylated MAP1B and the requirements for microtubule assembly, which are larger in neural cells extending many processes with numerous bundles of microtubules than in nonneural cells, in which a substantially lower number of microtubules are nucleated by the centrosome. Of particular interest, in this regard, is the fact that exhaustive phosphatase treatment of centrosomes *in situ* blocks microtubule growth, a finding suggesting that phosphorylated sites on centrosome-associated phosphoproteins (perhaps including MAP1B) may be required for microtubule nucleation (37). Accordingly, the large increase in MAP1B phosphorylation that occurs in differentiating neuroblastoma cells might be a mechanism to augment the assembly of microtubules within growing neurites.

In addition to the results obtained with neuroblastoma cells, we have found that MAP1B is a major phosphoprotein associated with microtubule preparations obtained from either cultured neurons or developing rat brain (28). These biochemical studies have also indicated that phosphorylated MAP1B is enriched in white matter regions of the brain (28), which agrees well with the immunohistochemical studies showing the presence of phosphorylated MAP1B within growing axons in the developing nervous system (38,39). These data are consistent with the view that phosphorylated MAP1B might promote microtubule assembly during axonal outgrowth in developing neurons.

The mechanisms responsible for the activation of the casein kinase II–related enzyme(s) involved in MAP1B and β3-tubulin phosphorylation remain to be established. However, we have observed a translocation of casein kinase II from the nucleus to the cytoplasm, which could partially account for the activation occurring in differentiating neuroblastoma cells (40).

Calcium Effects on Neurite Outgrowth and Microtubule Protein Phosphorylation

Developing neurons receive numerous signals from extracellular molecules that modulate neurite outgrowth. It has been suggested that changes in intracellular calcium levels may mediate the growth modulatory effects of at least some of these molecules (41–43). There seems to be an optimal level of calcium for neurite outgrowth; no growth is observed below it, and both growth inhibition and neurite regression take place above it (43).

We have analyzed the mean free-calcium concentration in undifferentiated and differentiating neuroblastoma cells by fura-2 fluorimetry. Figure 3 shows that differentiating neuroblastoma cells contain higher calcium levels than undifferentiated cells. This could be due to the increased cellular adhesion to the substrate (the extracellular matrix-coated plastic dish in *in vitro* culture), which occurs after serum

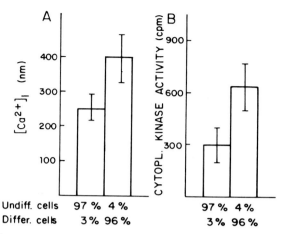

FIG. 3. Increase in cytosolic free-calcium level and casein kinase II activity on neuroblastoma cell differentiation. The cytosolic free calcium level ([Ca^{2+}]i, nM) of N2A neuroblastoma cells grown either in presence (*left*) or in absence (*right*) of serum was determined by fura-2 fluorimetry. Cytosolic casein kinase II activity of N2A neuroblastoma cells grown either in presence (*left*) or in absence (*right*) of serum was determined using brain MAP1B as a substrate after partial purification of the kinase by heparin-sepharose chromatography. The proportion of undifferentiated and differentiated (neurite-bearing) cells in each culture condition is also shown.

deprivation, possibly resulting from the withdrawal of proteases present in serum, and which act on substrate adhesion molecules. The interactions of substrate adhesion molecules with the substrate may affect intracellular second-messenger systems in a similar way to that found *in vitro* for several neural cell adhesion molecules (i.e., increasing calcium influx) (44). The relatively high calcium level found in differentiating neuroblastoma cells seems to be important for neurite outgrowth, as the lowering of intracellular calcium concentration on treatment with the potent calcium chelator, quin-2, causes neurite outgrowth inhibition (data not shown).

As for the effects of raising intracellular calcium above standard levels on neurite outgrowth *in situ*, we have studied differentiating neuroblastoma cells in culture medium containing a high level of potassium and depleted of sodium, which activates voltage-dependent calcium influx as described before (45). The rise in intracellular calcium causes a block in neurite outgrowth, finally resulting in neurite regression. These results are similar to those observed when colcemid is included in the normal culture medium of neuroblastoma cells (Table 1), thus suggesting that a primary effect of increased intracellular calcium may be the depolymerization of microtubules.

To test whether the calcium-induced microtubule disassembly in neuroblastoma cells depends on calmodulin, as it had been indicated by other authors for nonneural cells (46), we have used the potent calmodulin inhibitor calmidazolium. The addition of calmidazolium to normal culture medium does not affect neurite outgrowth

TABLE 1. *Effects of different culture conditions on neurite outgrowth and appearance of growth cones in mouse neuroblastoma cells[a]*

| | Neurite | | Presence of growth cones |
	Outgrowth	Regression	
Normal medium	+	−	+
Normal medium + cytochalasin B	+	−	−
Normal medium + colcemid	−	+	+
Normal medium + calmidazolium	+	−	±
High-K⁺ medium	−	+	+
High-K⁺ medium + calmidazolium	±	±	±

[a]Mouse neuroblastoma cells were incubated in serum-free medium (normal medium) and either treated with the different drugs indicated or transferred to sodium-depleted high-potassium medium. Addition of calmidazolium to high-potassium medium partially reverses the effects of this medium on neurite growth and growth cone appearance.

but makes growth cones considerably smaller (Table 1). This effect is similar to that found when neuroblastoma cells are treated with cytochalasin B, a drug that depolymerizes actin microfilaments (4,6). These results suggest that under normal conditions, calmodulin may be required to activate actin-dependent motility as it has been previously proposed by other authors (47,48). The addition of calmidazolium to the high-potassium medium also results in growth cone retraction, although at a lower extent than in normal medium. Furthermore, calmidazolium partially reverses the neurite regression, which is otherwise observed in high-potassium medium (Table 1). Consequently, the calcium-induced microtubule depolymerization underlying neurite regression may depend on calmodulin.

FUTURE DEVELOPMENTS

We propose, as a tentative hypothesis (Fig. 4), that microtubule dynamics and stabilization within growing neurites are mainly governed by the influences of certain regulatory molecules and posttranslational modifications on the binding of MAPs to tubulin.

At the leading edges of growth cones, and as a consequence of calcium channel clustering (49,50), the free-calcium level would be high enough (or calcium transients would be frequent enough) to favor actin assembly and actin–myosin interactions, thus stimulating growth cone motility, as well as favoring dynamic microtubule organization. A putative role for calmodulin in promoting growth cone motility through stimulation of filopodia formation has been proposed (47,48). It has been hypothesized that phosphoinositide turnover and cytoplasmic $[C^{2+}]$ are increased at growth cone edges as a consequence of the binding of certain signaling molecules to specific receptors on the growth cone surface. This would lead to the activation of protein kinase C, which could phosphorylate GAP-43 (neuromodulin), a calmodulin binding protein highly enriched in axonal growth cones, thus releasing high concentrations of calcium/calmodulin locally at growth cone edges (47,48).

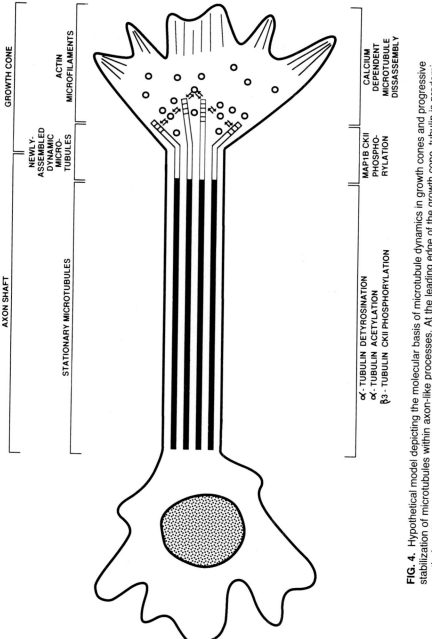

FIG. 4. Hypothetical model depicting the molecular basis of microtubule dynamics in growth cones and progressive stabilization of microtubules within axon-like processes. At the leading edge of the growth cone, tubulin is predominantly found in the soluble form (O), possibly because calcium/calmodulin prevents its association with MAPs. At the growth cone base, tubulin may bind to phosphorylated MAP1B (and other MAPs), so that its assembly into microtubules is promoted. Futher posttranslational modifications of tubulin may result in the stabilization of microtubules within the axon.

The dynamic instability of growth cone microtubules might also depend on modulation of MAP activities by the binding of calcium/calmodulin to MAPs. MAP1B, the major MAP present in neuroblastoma cells, binds to calcium/calmodulin, as previously described for MAP2 and tau (26). Calcium/calmodulin might interfere with the binding of MAP1B (and other MAPs) to tubulin. Furthermore, MAP1B phosphorylation by casein kinase II may also be impaired under these conditions, because elevated calcium levels inhibit casein kinase II. Similarly, calcium/calmodulin-dependent phosphorylation of other MAPs [tau proteins are also present in neuroblastoma cells (51)] may play an additional role in the microtubule instability at growth cones.

In the growth cone base, free-calcium level might be low enough (or calcium transients rare enough) to allow the binding of MAP1B and other MAPs to tubulin, enhancing microtubule stability. MAP1B phosphorylation by a casein kinase II–related enzyme could also lead to the stimulation of microtubule assembly.

Growth cone microtubules seem to assemble through the addition of tubulin molecules to their uniformly polarized distal "plus" ends (52). Microtubules with uniform polarity are also observed in immature growing dendrites, although some microtubules with opposite polarity appear in mature dendrites (52). The molecular basis for the uniform microtubule polarity during neurite outgrowth remains unknown. It has been proposed that stable "seeds" may nucleate axonal microtubules (11). Perhaps phosphorylated MAP1B might participate in the building of these microtubule-nucleating elements. Additionally, there might be MAPs that specifically promote tubulin polymerization at the microtubule "plus" ends. A 215-kDa MAP with this ability has been isolated from *Xenopus* eggs, and immunologically related proteins have been detected in nerve cells (53), although it is not yet known whether such proteins are actually present at growth cones.

Of relevance for microtubule stabilization and consolidation of neurite form would be the presence of capping structures that prevent the depolymerization of particular growth cone microtubules, in a similar manner to the relative stabilization of mitotic spindle microtubules by kinetochores. This would stabilize neurite outgrowth in a particular direction (12).

As the growth cone advances, microtubule stabilization could be consolidated. Assembled tubulin within the axon shaft could serve as a substrate for posttranslational modifications including β3-tubulin phosphorylation and α-tubulin acetylation and detyrosination, which might result in further stabilization of axonal microtubules. This stabilization and the lower calcium level might cause a reorganization of actin microfilaments in such a way that the neurite loses contact with the substratum and its protusive activity.

Thus, the presence of high concentrations of MAPs (mainly MAP1B), their posttranslational modifications (mainly phosphorylation), the influence of regulatory molecules (such as calmodulin), and the posttranslational modifications of tubulin might account for the high dynamics of microtubules in growth cones and their progressive stabilization within the axon. The control of microtubule protein processing enzymes (e.g., protein kinases and phosphatases) and other regulatory molecules by second messengers (including calcium level fluctuations) generated on the binding of signaling molecules to growth cone surface receptors may provide a link between the extracellular factors and intracellular events that determine growth cone activity and neuritic stabilization.

As numerous signaling molecules alter intracellular calcium level, this is a particularly important parameter, as has been previously stressed (41–43). According to the model depicted in Fig. 4, free calcium may participate in the control of microtubule disassembly and assembly, thus regulating the balance between neurite plasticity and stability. This could serve as a mechanism for neurotransmitters and other signaling molecules to mold neuronal shape. It would be important not only during neuronal morphogenesis, but also in adult neurons, as transient events of microtubule disassembly could promote neuronal shape modifications underlying neuronal plasticity. Finally, abnormal calcium/calmodulin-induced disassembly of microtubules, resulting in neurite regression, could also be involved in excitatory amino acid neurotoxicity and other neurodegenerative disorders.

REFERENCES

1. Ramón y Cajal S. A quelle epoque apparaissent les expansions des cellules nerveuses de la moelle epinere du poulet. *Anat Anzerger* 1890;5:609–613.
2. Mitchison T, Kirschner M. Cytoskeletal dynamics and nerve growth. *Neuron* 1988;1:761–772.
3. Smith S. Neuronal cytomechanics: the actin-based motility of growth cones. *Science* 1988;242:708–715.
4. Marsh L, Letourneau PC. Growth of neurites without filopodial or lamellipodial activity in the presence of cytochalasin B. *J Cell Biol* 1984;99:2041–2047.
5. Seeds NW, Gilman AG, Amanos T, Nirenberg M. Regulation of axon formation by clonal lines of a neural tumor. *Proc Natl Acad Sci USA* 1970;66:160–167.
6. Yamada KM, Spooner BS, Wessels MK. Axon growth: role of microfilaments and microtubules. *Proc Natl Acad Sci USA* 1970;66:1206–1212.
7. Daniels MP. The role of microtubules in the growth and stabilization of nerve fibers. *Annu NY Acad Sci* 1975;253:535–544.
8. Bamburg JR, Bray D, Chapman, K. Assembly of microtubules at the tip of growing axons. *Nature* 1986;321:788–790.
9. Lim SS, Sammak PJ, Borisy GG. Progressive and spatially differentiated stability of microtubules in developing neuronal cells. *J Cell Biol* 1989;109:253–263.
10. Okabe S, Hirokawa N. Turnover of fluorescently labelled tubulin and actin in the axon. *Nature* 1990;343:479–482.
11. Baas PW, Black MH. Individual microtubules in the axon consist of domains that differ in both composition and stability. *J Cell Biol* 1990;111:495–509.
12. Kirschner M, Mitchison T. Beyond self-assembly: from microtubules to morphogenesis. *Cell* 1986;45:329–342.
13. Schulze E, Kirschner M. Microtubule dynamics in interphase cells. *J Cell Biol* 1986;102:1020–1031.
14. Schulze E, Kirschner M. Direct observation of microtubule dynamics in living cells. *Nature* 1988;344:356–359.
15. Bré MH, Kreis TE, Karsenti E. Control of microtubule nucleation and stability in MDCK cells: the occurrence of non centrosomal, stable detyrosinated microtubules. *J Cell Biol* 1987;105:1283–1296.
16. Olmsted JB. Microtubule-associated proteins. *Annu Rev Cell Biol* 1986;2:421–457.
17. Matus A. Microtubule-associated proteins: their potential role in determining neuronal morphology. *Annu Rev Neurosci* 1988;11:29–44.
18. Díaz-Nido J, Hernández MA, Avila J. Microtubule proteins in neuronal cells. In: Avila J, ed. *Microtubule proteins*. Florida, CRC Press, 1990.

19. Bré MH, Karsenti E. Effects of brain microtubule-associated proteins on microtubule dynamics and the nucleating activity of centrosomes. *Cell Motil Cytoskel* 1990;15:88–98.
20. Díaz-Nido J, Avila J. Characterization of proteins immunologically related to brain microtubule-associated protein MAP1B in non-neural cells. *J Cell Sci* 1989;92:607–620.
21. Drubin DG, Kirschner, MW. Tau protein function in living cells. *J Cell Biol* 1986;103: 2739–2746.
22. Kanai Y, Takemura R, Oshima T, *et al*. Expression of multiple tau isoforms and microtubule bundle formation in fibroblasts transfected with a single tau cDNA. *J Cell Biol* 1989;109:1173–1184.
23. Lewis SA, Ivanov LE, Lee GH, Cowan NJ. Organization of microtubules in dendrites and axons is determined by a short hydrophobic zipper in microtubule-associated proteins MAP2 and tau. *Nature* 1989;342:498–505.
24. Lee YC, Wolff J. Calmodulin binds to both microtubule associated protein 2 and tau proteins. *J Biol Chem* 1984;259:1226–1230.
25. Kumagai H, Nishida E, Kotani S, Sakai H. On the mechanism of calmodulin-induced inhibition of microtubule assembly *in vitro*. *J Biochem* 1986;99:521–525.
26. Vera JC, Rivas CI, Maccioni RB. Heat-stable microtubule protein MAP-1 binds to microtubules and induces microtubule assembly. *FEBS Lett* 1988;232:159–162.37.
27. Jameson L, Frey T, Zeebag B, *et al*. Inhibition of microtubule assembly by phosphorylation of microtubule-associated proteins. *Biochemistry* 1980;19:2472–2479.
28. Díaz-Nido J, Serrano L, Hernández MA, Avila J. Phosphorylation of microtubule proteins in rat brain at different developmental stages: comparison with that found in neuronal cultures. *J Neurochem* 1990;54:211–222.
29. Yamamoto Y, Fukunaga K, Goto S, *et al*. Calcium/calmodulin-dependent regulation of microtubule formation via phosphorylation of MAP2, tau factor and tubulin, and comparison with the cyclic AMP–dependent phosphorylation. *J Neurochem* 1985;44:759–764.
30. Cambray-Deakin MA, Burgoyne RD. Posttranslational modifications of α-tubulin: acetylated and detyrosinated forms in axons of rat cerebellum. *J Cell Biol* 1987;104:1569–1574.
31. Eddé B, De Neuchaud B, Denoulet P, Gros F. Control of isotubulin expression during neuronal differentiation of mouse neuroblastoma and teratocarcinoma cell lines. *Dev Biol* 1987;123:549–558.
32. Gard DL, Kirschner M. A polymer-dependent increase in phosphorylation of β-tubulin accompanies differentiation of a mouse neuroblastoma cell line. *J Cell Biol* 1985;100:764–774.
33. Serrano L, Díaz-Nido J, Wandosell F, Avila J. Tubulin phosphorylation by casein kinase II is similar to that found *in vivo*. *J Cell Biol* 1987;105:1731–1739.
34. Díaz-Nido J, Serrano L, López-Otín C, Vandekerckhove J, Avila J. Phosphorylation of a neuronal-specific β-tubulin isotype. *J Biol Chem* 1990;265:13949–13954.
35. Díaz-Nido J, Serrano L, Méndez E, Avila J. A casein kinase II–related activity is involved in phosphorylation of microtubule-associated protein MAP1B during neuroblastoma cell differentiation. *J Cell Biol* 1988;106:2057–2065.
36. Aletta JM, Lewis SA, Cowan NJ, Greene LA. Nerve growth factor regulates both the phosphorylation and steady-state levels of MAP-1.2. *J Cell Biol* 1988;106:1573–1581.
36a. Domínguez, JE, Avila J, Karsenti E. A protein related to brain MAP1B is localized to the centrosome in mammalian cells. *J Cell Biol* 1989;109:77a.
37. Centonze VE, Borisy, GG. Nucleation of microtubules from mitotic centrosomes is modulated by a
38. Sato-Yoshitake R, Shiomura Y, Miyasaka H, Hirokawa N. Microtubule-associated protein 1B: molecular structure, localization, and phosphorylation-dependent expression in developing neurons. *Neuron* 1989;3:229–238.
39. Schoenfeld T, McKerracher L, Obar R, Vallee RB. MAP1A and MAP1B are structurally related microtubule associated proteins with distinct developmental patterns in the CNS. *J Neurosci* 1989; 9:1712–1730.
40. Serrano L, Hernández MA, Díaz-Nido J, Avila J. Association of casein kinase II with microtubules. *Exp Cell Res* 1989;181:263–272.
41. Mattson MP, Kater SB. Calcium regulation of neurite elongation and growth cone motility. *J Neurosci* 1987;7:4034–4043.
42. Mattson MP. Neurotransmitters in the regulation of neuronal cytoarchitecture. *Brain Res Rev* 1988; 13:179–212.
43. Lipton SA, Kater SB. Neurotransmitter regulation of neuronal outgrowth, plasticity and survival. *Trends Neurosci* 1989;12:265–270.
44. Schuch U, Lohse MJ, Schachner M. Neural cell adhesion molecules influence second messenger systems. *Neuron* 1989;3:13–20.

45. Mattson MP, Guthrie PB, Kater SB. A role for sodium-dependent calcium extrusion in protection against neuronal excitotoxicity. *FASEB J* 1989;3:2519–2526.
46. Keith CH, DiPaola M, Maxfield F, Shelanski M. Microinjection of calcium/calmodulin causes a local depolymerization of microtubules. *J Cell Biol* 1983;97:1918–1924.
47. Liu Y, Stosm DR. Regulation of free-calmodulin levels by neuromodulin: neuron growth and regeneration. *Trends Pharmacol Sci* 1990;11:107–111.
48. Van Hooff, Oestreicher AB, De Graan PN, Gispen WH. Role of the growth cone in neuronal differentiation. *Mol Neurobiol* 1989;3:101–133.
49. Connor JA. Digital imaging of free calcium changes and of spatial gradients in growing processes in single, mammalian central nervous system cells. *Proc Natl Acad Sci USA* 1986;83:6179–6183.
50. Silver RA, Lamb AG, Bolsover SR. Calcium hotspots caused by L-channel clustering promote morphological changes in neuronal growth cones. *Nature* 1990;343:751–754.
51. Drubin D, Kobayashi S, Kirschner M. Association of tau protein with microtubules in living cells. *Ann NY Acad Sci* 1986;466:257–268.
52. Baas PW, Black MM, Banker GA. Changes in microtubule polarity orientation during the development of hippocampal neurons in culture. *J Cell Biol* 1989;109:3085–3094.
53. Gard DL, Kirschner M. A microtubule-associated protein from *Xenopus* eggs that specifically promotes assembly at the plus end. *J Cell Biol* 1987;105:2203–2211.

The Nerve Growth Cone, edited by P. C. Letourneau,
S. B. Kater, and E. R. Macagno, Raven Press, Ltd.,
New York © 1992.

8

Video Microscopic Analysis of Events in the Growth Cone Underlying Axon Growth and the Regulation of these Events by Substrate-Bound Proteins

Daniel J. Goldberg, Donald W. Burmeister, and Rodolfo J. Rivas

*Department of Pharmacology and Center for Neurobiology and Behavior,
Columbia University College of Physicians and Surgeons,
New York, New York 10032*

The growth cone has been likened to a "leukocyte on a leash" (1), crawling ahead and pulling the axon out behind it. This simile is instructive, for it calls attention to the morphological and behavioral resemblance between the growth cone and migratory cells. If new membrane and cytoskeleton were assembled in the axon and cell body, the simile would be entirely apt. However, it is now known that most insertion of new membrane (2) and net assembly of microtubules (3) occurs within the growth cone. Observations of growth cones at high power and in real-time (rather than in time-lapse) show the growth cone sending out plasma membrane, which then gradually matures morphologically into new neurite (4). What was growth cone becomes neurite as new growth cone forms in front. We thus prefer to liken neurite growth to the construction of a tall building.

The significance to us of the difference in similes is how it has shaped our thinking, in two important ways, about events in the growth cone. First, just as a building rises in stages—the steel skeleton and external walls preceding the floors and internal walls—the axon grows in stages, with plasma membrane advancing first and then being filled by membranous organelles, cytoplasm, and lengthening microtubules (4). Thus, we have been trying to study each of the stages independently with the hope of then fitting them back together into a satisfying explanation of growth cone functioning. Second, we have tended not to view the growth cone as a crawling structure and, thus, have deemphasized its pulling of trailing materials forward and have been more sensitive to the possible importance of trailing materials moving forward under their own steam. Discussion [the so-called push–pull debate (5)] and useful experimentation (6,7) have been engendered; through the dust kicked up we think we can sometimes see the outlines of a resolution. It is our

79

feeling that this resolution will be framed in terms of the stages of growth cone transformation into axon and will clarify and make more detailed our understanding of how growth cones work.

Our figurative as well as literal view of the growth cone has been a function of the way we have studied it, using high-resolution, high-magnification, real-time video microscopy. By allowing us to detect far more of the membranous organelles and their movements in the living growth cone than possible with conventional light microscopy, video microscopy has impressed on us the stepwise nature of axon elongation. The technique we have used was invented in 1980 by Robert Allen and is called *video-enhanced contrast-differential interference contrast* (VEC-DIC) microscopy (8). DIC (Nomarski) microscopy is useful for viewing organelles in living cells; they stand out as if in relief. But the limit of resolution for the light microscope is 0.22 μm, about the diameter of a mitochondrion. VEC-DIC microscopy allows much more light to pass through the system, thus increasing the potential detectability of objects smaller than the limit of resolution by increasing the amount of light they scatter. The special video camera subtracts the increased background light that would otherwise obscure the light from the in-focus objects (i.e., it greatly enhances the contrast of those objects). Structures well below the limit of resolution, such as the 30 to 100-nm vesicles with which many growth cones are filled, become visible. Even elements of the cytoskeleton can sometimes be detected (8). Viewing the scene at a magnification of 7,000 to 10,000 on a television monitor rather than at 600 to $1,000 \times$ in the microscope accentuates the difference between VEC-DIC and DIC microscopy. An Edward Hopper street scene becomes a Bruegel.

We have studied neurons from the central nervous system of the marine slug *Aplysia*. Though the neurons are very large, their growth cones are not exceptionally sized. They are, however, richly endowed with vesicles that, in the peptidergic neurons, are large, so internal events are easy to monitor. In addition, they tolerate well the intense light used in VEC-DIC microscopy, and events are slower and thus perhaps more easily deciphered at the 20 to 23°C at which they are viewed than at the 35 to 37°C at which avian and mammalian growth cones must be viewed. But the latter can be informative subjects of VEC-DIC microscopy (9,10), even in our hands (see below).

GROWTH SEQUENCE

All axonal growth from these cells that we have observed is achieved by a sequence of three morphologically defined steps in the growth cone (Fig. 1). Plasma membrane projects forward by the protrusion of digitate filopodia and sheet-like veils from the organelle-rich central region (C region) of the growth cone. Protruding veils fill in the space between neighboring filopodia. They act independently of one another, so that a veil on one side of a filopodium may be advancing while one on the other side is stationary or retracting. The protruded membrane (P region) is flat and nearly devoid of membranous organelles. The second step involves the

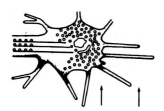

Protrusion

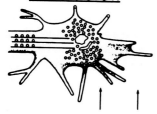

Engorgement

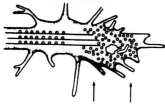

Consolidation

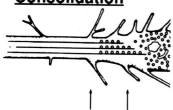

FIG. 1. Sequence of morphological transformations of the growth cone underlying axon elongation. See text for details. (From ref. 31, with permission.)

engorgement of the veils with cytoplasm, membranous organelles, and microtubules entering from the central region. Small vesicles enter first, followed by larger mitochondria. Organelles appear to move forward both by directed transport (presumably along microtubules) and by Brownian motion. Eventually the engorged veils become a new C region, still laterally spread on the substrate but more voluminous. Lastly, in the step we call *consolidation*, this new C region narrows laterally to become cylindrical, and the movement of membranous organelles changes from being predominantly Brownian to almost exclusively bidirectional fast transport. Further maturation—for example, increases in the stability and cross-linking of microtubules (11)—probably takes place after consolidation, but this is beyond our purview, because it is with consolidation that the nascent region of neurite ends its transient existence as growth cone.

The same sequence of events has been described in neurites of differentiated PC12 cells and rat sympathetic neurons in culture (10), and most other neurites studied in culture have growth cones of similar morphology (e.g., ref. 9) and thus, very likely, grow in the same way. Filopodia with veils or broader lamellipodia have also been observed in numerous *in vivo* situations (12–14), so we suspect that this sequence of events is rather general.

But it is likely not universal. In some circumstances, the growth cone of a rat sympathetic neurite growing extremely rapidly in culture has a broad lamellipodium without filopodia and truly looks like an autonomous structure that maintains its identity as the neurite lengthens behind it (15). Consolidation is clearly occurring, but visible protrusion and engorgement steps seem to be missing. Yet, obviously, advance of plasma membrane and organelles is occurring; we suspect the mechanisms underlying their advance (see below) are the same as in the more common situation when protrusion and engorgement are visually definable. At the other end of the spectrum from this type of growth cone with its expanse of specialized growth cone cytoplasm (dense actin network poor in microtubules and membranous organelles) are apparently blunt-ended growth cones of axons growing in straight paths along defined fiber tracts *in vivo* (12). This form is also suggestive of an absence of protrusion and engorgement. Most of these observations have been of fixed stained material at rather low resolution, so it is uncertain that growth cones were captured when the neurites were actually growing or that small protrusions were visualized. Current work being done in several laboratories involving the use of confocal microscopy to observe living stained axons growing *in vivo* could settle this question. But should one call these neuritic endings growth cones? They may be more relevant to the question of whether neuritic growth requires a growth cone than to the question of how growth cones mediate neuritic growth. Lastly, there is a new report of "saltatory" growth of grasshopper axons *in vivo* (16). Here, a small swollen growth cone suddenly appears at the distal end of a filopodium, with the filopodium subsequently thickening into a neuritic process. It is as if the growth cone has jumped from one end of the filopodium to the other. Undoubtedly, a neurite forming from a single filopodium rather than a veil or veils and neighboring filopodia is different from what we typically see in our studies. But, the underlying events must be similar in that the filopodium, which is the protrusive element, undergoes engorgement (i.e., it is invaded by microtubules and membranous organelles from the old central region). That filopodia may be subject to ingress of microtubules will be discussed below.

PROTRUSION

We have tried to study the growth cone by using procedures by which we can trigger a particular step. So far, this approach has been applied to protrusion, the advance of the plasma membrane, and engorgement, the advance of membranous organelles and microtubules. Protrusion of filopodia seems likely to be caused by polymerization of actin. Filopodia have a core bundle of actin filaments (17), resembling structures such as vertebrate intestinal microvilli (18) and the acrosomal process of invertebrate sperm (19). Extension of the latter has been shown to be driven by explosive actin polymerization (19). The rich network of actin filaments within the veil is much less ordered than in the filopodium (17) and, thus, less strongly implies a primary role for polymerization in triggering veil protrusion. But one observation that suggests the importance of actin polymerization in veil protrusion is that conditions inside the forming veil seem to be conducive to actin polymerization. In one of our studies, two-thirds of the forming veils that were observed had bordering filopodia that were growing along with them, sometimes at the same rate (4) (Fig. 2a). Also, growing veils often develop nubs, some of which grow into filopodia (Fig. 2b). In this they resemble the axonal excrescences that we have observed to serve as filopodia factories shortly after axon transection (Fig. 2c).

To what internal signals does the growth cone respond by issuing protrusions? For example, what triggers a growth cone to project many filopodia (as, presumably, exploratory structures) on reaching a "decision point" *in vivo* where possible pathways must be selected among (12)? A rise in intracellular $[Ca^{2+}]$ may be one such signal. Ca^{2+} would seem to be suitable for triggering directional responses to focal environmental stimuli, for it acts locally (i.e., when a rise in $[Ca^{2+}]_i$ is confined to one area of the growth cone, the protrusion emerges from that area). We have shown this by reducing $[Ca^{2+}]_o$ sufficiently to block protrusion from *Aplysia* growth cones *in vitro* and then applying Ca^{2+} to one area of the growth cone with a micropipette (20). A protrusion usually forms only from that area (Fig. 3). Silver and co-workers have shown that patches of L-type Ca channels are in the growth cones of neuroblastoma cells and that protrusions form preferentially near these patches when electrical activity causes localized intracellular hotspots of Ca^{2+} (21). Lankford and Letourneau (9) have shown the network of actin filaments of the P region to be the most sensitive target of action of Ca^{2+}, although they were studying the destructive effects of high $[Ca^{2+}]$ on the network. It is perhaps of relevance here that GAP-43, which is one of the most abundant membrane proteins in vertebrate growth cones, is preferentially associated with the network of actin filaments in the protrusive structures of the growth cone (22) and causes massive protrusion of filopodia when transfected into fibroblasts (23). GAP-43 binds calmodulin and releases it when phosphorylated by protein kinase C, or when $[Ca^{2+}]$ rises, and it has been suggested that it serves to sharpen the spatial and temporal resolution of Ca^{2+} signals in the growth cone (24). It should be emphasized that, although focal increases in Ca^{2+} probably serve as one type of signal for protrusion, they are unlikely to be essential. Fura measurements did not detect changes in $[Ca^{2+}]_i$ underlying spontaneous protrusions from neuroblastoma growth cones (25).

Although filopodia are typically seen with various microscopic techniques to be filled with actin filaments and devoid of microtubules and membranous organelles, there may be situations in which they admit or are formed with microtubules, and

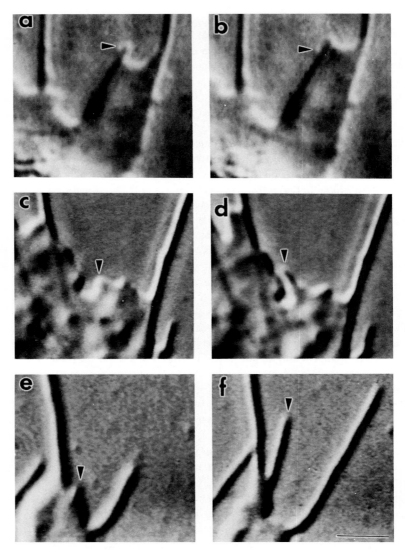

FIG. 2. Filopodia and veils often protrude together. A veil and one of its neighboring filopodia both extend past a particle (*arrowheads*) on the substrate in the 7 sec between *a* and *b*. Filopodia also grow from nubs on forming veils (*c* and *d*). In this, the veil resembles the axonal excrescence from which filopodia extend soon after transection of the axon (*e* and *f*). Bar, 2 μm.

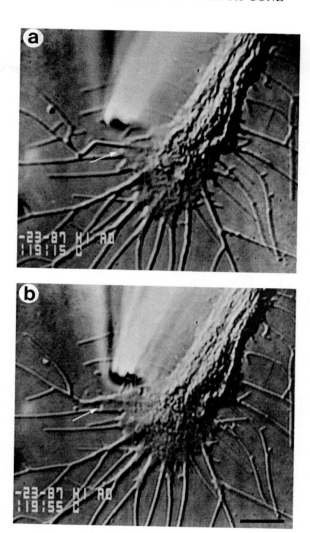

FIG. 3. Ca^{2+} can act locally to cause veil formation. *a:* A micropipette containing 1-M CaCl has just been moved next to a growth cone that lost its veils by being exposed to bathing medium containing $22\times$ reduced $[Ca^{2+}]$, and a new veil is beginning to grow (*arrow*). *b:* 40 sec later the veil (*arrow*) has reached its full extent, and no other veils have formed. Bar, 5 μm. (From ref. 20, with permission.)

this may be important for growth. Many of the filopodia that form soonest after axon transection of *Aplysia* neurons in culture exhibit abundant bidirectional transport of swellings at rates of a few microns per second (Fig. 4). What appear by VEC-DIC microscopy to be single membranous organelles can sometimes be seen to travel smoothly from the axon into and along the filopodium. Transport of membranous organelles in animal cells is known to occur along microtubular tracks, and we have found preliminarily that the filopodial transport of swellings and individual

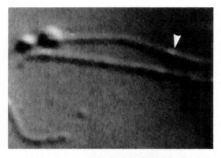

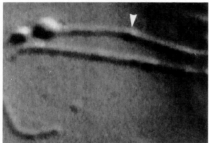

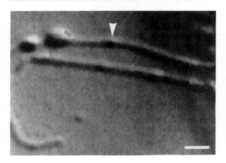

FIG. 4. Newly formed filopodia display rapid particle transport. A particle (*arrowheads*) rapidly translocates along a filopodium, which had protruded several minutes before from an *Aplysia* axon (out of view to the right), which had been transected in culture. Two very large particles are to the *left* in that filopodium, and several particles can be seen in the other filopodium in view. There is less than a 2-sec interval between the top and bottom panels. Bar, 1 μm.

organelles is prevented by pre-treating the axon with nocodazole, a drug that prevents microtubule polymerization. Thus, microtubules may be commonly found in these newly formed filopodia, although this remains to be proven. Sheetz and colleagues (26) attributed the movement that they observed of swellings in filopodia of mouse cerebral neurons in culture to actin filaments rather than microtubules. Two recent studies, including the aforementioned observations of grasshopper growth cones *in vivo*, suggested that contact of a filopodium with another cell can result in the proximo-distal thickening of that filopodium into a neurite (16,27). This would be an important mode of orienting growing neurites to appropriate landmarks. Entry of microtubules into the filopodium could initiate the thickening. Alternatively, the thickening may simply be the unrecognized movement of a thin veil up the filopodium, followed by its conventional engorgement, a process that we can see with VEC-DIC microscopy in culture. Analysis at higher resolution of the contact-mediated filopodial thickening will be required to decide between these alternatives.

ENGORGEMENT

Aplysia growth cones can be studied *in vitro* in conditions in which they have large protruded areas of veil and lamellipodium (P regions) that engorge only very slowly but can be triggered to undergo rapid and complete engorgement. This has facilitated the use of drugs and fluorescent stains to study the roles of the cytoskeleton in this step. Why the cytoskeleton? All the steps of the growth sequence involve shape changes, and engorgement and consolidation also involve changes in the organization of membranous organelles; these are cellular events controlled by the cytoskeleton. Neurofilaments do not enter the leading edge of the growth cone (17), so we confine our interest to actin filaments and microtubules.

If one is inclined to view the dense network of actin filaments of the P region as functioning to pull the rest of the growth cone forward, perhaps the most surprising result of these studies is that elimination of this network facilitates, rather than blocks, engorgement (28). We have found that dihydrocytochalasin B, which diminishes the lamellipodial actin network, triggers an engorgement that matches normal engorgement in speed and extent (Fig. 5). This suggests that the membranous organelles of the C region are steadily impelled forward by forces other than the pull of the peripheral network of actin filaments; the network actually resists this advance. The density of the weave of the network and the proximity of the dorsal and ventral plasma membranes (0.1–0.2 μm separation) (28,29) probably restrict the entry of membranous organelles. This implies that a critical event in triggering engorgement is weakening of the actin network at the interface between C and P regions.

What other forces might be directly responsible for the forward movement of the membranous organelles? Brownian motion and fast axonal transport, which moves membranous organelles along microtubules, are the likely candidates. The C region of the growth cone is seemingly much richer in microtubules than the P region (although some microtubules can be seen penetrating well beyond the C region), and microtubules seem to advance along with the membranous organelles during engorgement (28). One might suspect that the organelles would advance even without the microtubules, as they should tend to fill any newly accessible cytoplasmic space in the P region simply by Brownian motion. But we find that if polymerization of microtubules is prevented with colcemid or nocodazole, engorgement occurring naturally or in response to dihydrocytochalasin is blocked (30). Whether this means that membranous organelles only move forward by fast axonal transport is unclear. Microtubules may facilitate their entry in other ways, for example, by forming a space-filling structural network that widens the separation between dorsal and ventral plasma membranes.

Engorgement, then, involves and requires net microtubule elongation into the P region and probably also requires weakening of the network of actin filaments at the distal margin of the C region. It is perhaps most straightforward to think that entry of microtubules into the P region is restricted by the actin network and that weakening of the network is the primary event in triggering engorgement (28,31). How-

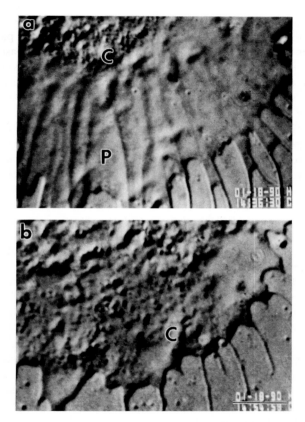

FIG. 5. Dihydrocytochalasin B causes engorgement. *a*: Shortly before application of 1 μM dihydrocytochalasin B, there is a large P region poor in membranous organelles. *b*: 17 min after application, the membranous organelles (C marks the distal border) have moved forward to almost fill the former P region. Bar, 5 μm.

ever, it also seems possible that microtubules are free to enter the unengorged P region but do not persist. Frequent transient excursions of microtubules deep into lamellipodia of living motile fibroblasts have been detected by video-intensified fluorescence microscopy (32). The increase in microtubules in the P region during engorgement might then result from stabilization and retention of these penetrating microtubules. Weakening of the actin network might either cause or be caused by this stabilization; in either case, it would be necessary for advance of the membranous organelles.

SUBSTRATE-BOUND GROWTH-PROMOTERS ACCELERATE ENGORGEMENT

One of the most attractive aspects to us of the analysis of growth cone function described in the previous sections is that it provides a framework for understanding how macromolecules in the environment influence the growth cone to affect neuritic growth. Such molecules are critically important in determining the path of growth of an axon and the synaptic connections it will form. At the most basic level, such molecules promote or inhibit neurite growth. Laminin, a large, multichain glycoprotein, is the most widely used and studied of growth promoters that act when bound to the surface over which the neurite is growing. It greatly enhances the neuritic growth of many types of neurons when used to coat culture plates (33,34) and probably does so also for axons that encounter it *in vivo* in the extracellular matrix or on the surface of support cells such as Schwann cells (35). Although several substrate-bound neurite growth promoters have been identified and molecular details of their structures and of their binding to neurons have been elucidated (36), it is unclear how this binding leads to the promotion of neurite growth.

A common assumption (as noted in ref. 33) has been that these proteins mediate the adhesion of the growth cone to the immobile substrate, allowing it to pull itself and the neurite forward. It should come as no surprise that we do not find this an entirely satisfying explanation. Nor are we alone, for others have found that the strength of adhesion does not necessarily correlate with the extent of growth (37, 38). For example, many neurons adhere well to polylysine but grow poorly on it.

We have been able to gain some insight into this issue by directing our experimental approach toward determining which of the steps in the growth sequence is a primary target of action for substrate-bound growth promoters. The growth of *Aplysia* axons in culture is greatly accelerated by the presence on the substrate of an as yet unpurified high-molecular-weight (>100 kDa) protein (or proteins) from *Aplysia* blood or defined medium conditioned by exposure to *Aplysia* ganglia. Axons that have grown little on polylysine can be stimulated to rapid growth on acute addition of growth-promoting medium. VEC-DIC microscopy reveals effects on the growth cone within 2 to 5 min.

The first effect on the growth cone is typically a massive stimulation of engorgement (Fig. 6). It is clear that this is a primary effect. The growth cones on polylysine do not seem deficient in either the production or retention of protrusions. It is easy to find growth cones, as the one in Fig. 6, with large lamellipodia tipped by multiple filopodia. These are stable and seem attached to the substrate, for they do not shake or curl back toward the C region, as is typical for unattached protrusions. But they engorge slowly, if at all. The acceleration of engorgement caused by acute addition of growth-promoting medium almost always precedes visible effects on protrusion or consolidation. Considerable, occasionally total, engorgement of the lamellipodium happens before the margins of its veils advance farther. The acceleration of engorgement is thus not secondary to effects on the other steps of the growth sequence (e.g., of consolidation squeezing materials forward).

Various experiments make it clear that the *Aplysia* growth-promoting protein has this acute effect on the growth cone by binding to the substrate. We have recently sought to determine whether a similar protocol, in which the material is added acutely rather than as a precoating for the culture dish, could be used to analyze the mechanism of action of a substrate binding promoter of neurite growth, laminin, about which there is much molecular information. It can; acute addition of laminin

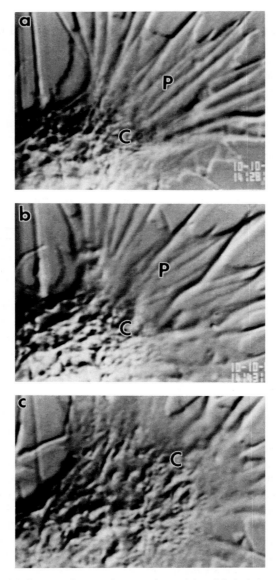

FIG. 6. Substrate-binding, neurite growth-promoting activity of *Aplysia* hemolymph causes engorgement. An *Aplysia* growth cone in defined medium on polylysine maintains a large P region, which undergoes no engorgement during the 15 min between *a* and *b*. C denotes the distal edge of the C (central, engorged) region. *c:* 15 min after the addition of dialyzed hemolymph, membranous organelles have moved forward almost to fill the former P region. The distal margin of the P region has extended only a little and so there is little P region remaining. Bar, 5 μm.

to cultures of neonatal rat sympathetic neurons on polylysine rapidly accelerates their growth. Laminin can thus be studied like a drug, and rapid effects readily assessed.

Our results so far indicate that engorgement is a primary target for laminin in the rat growth cones, just as it is for the *Aplysia* protein in the *Aplysia* growth cones. Large lamellipodia remain basically unchanging until the addition of laminin provokes engorgement within minutes.

Based on our knowledge of the cytoskeletal events underlying engorgement, discussed in the previous section, it appears that a primary consequence of the binding of laminin or the *Aplysia* protein to receptive neurites is the promotion of the elongation and/or stabilization of microtubules in the growth cone and the (at least localized) weakening of the peripheral network of actin filaments. This is markedly different from the rapid response elicited by nerve growth factor, which is the only other growth-promoting protein whose rapid effects on the growth cone have been studied. Growth cones of rat sympathetic neurons or differentiated PC12 cells are blunt and quiescent in the absence of nerve growth factor, and their earliest response to the addition of nerve growth factor is the protrusion of filopodia, veils, and lamellipodia (i.e., a restoration of the actin motility apparatus) (see chapter by Phelan et al.).

We offer here four models to explain the rapid effects on the growth cone that we have described (Fig. 7). The first three posit the actin network as the primary target for the substrate protein, presenting three alternative explanations for how the substrate protein could weaken that network. In one of these, pulling against the substrate is important. The fourth involves a direct effect of the substrate protein on microtubules.

The first two models rely on the substrate protein linking to the ventral cortical network of actin filaments in the P region of the growth cone. It has been suggested that a substrate such as polylysine is relatively ineffective in promoting neurite growth, because it does not link to the cortical network of actin filaments (39). Efficient growth promoters on the substrate, such as laminin and fibronectin, are thought to link to this network via their specific membrane receptors (40). What are the consequences of this linking?

There is evidence that the network of actin filaments in the P region is continually moving toward the C region (28), with subunits continually being added to the distal ends of filaments at the margin of the growth cone and coming off the proximal ends in the transitional area between P and C regions (Fig. 7I) (41). If this is true, an actin filament should shorten proximodistally when it links to the immobile substrate, because it is no longer moving in new subunits to the P-C transitional region to replace those continually lost. If numerous actin filaments bind to the substrate and shorten, the network will weaken in this region. A nice feature of this explanation is that it predicts a weakening localized to the region where it would be required rather than a global effect on the network, which might impair needed protrusive and motile activities. Another feature is that protrusion should accompany the engorgement, because the continual addition of subunits at the distal end will no

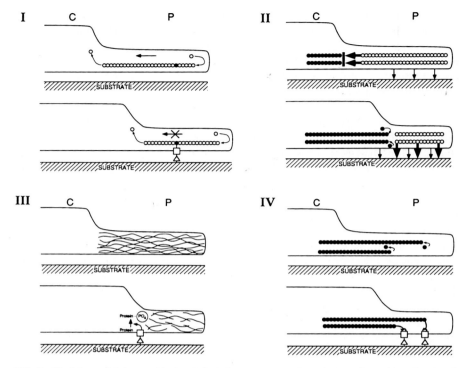

FIG. 7. Models explaining rapid stimulation of engorgement by substrate-bound neurite growth promoters. See text for details.

longer be compensated for by rearward movement. This coupling of the two steps would be an efficient means for the substrate protein to stimulate elongation. Unfortunately, we typically see engorgement start before advance of the distal margin. But because the array of filaments is more uniformly longitudinal in the filopodia than the veils (17), one might expect filopodia to extend first, and in fact, net filopodial lengthening often closely follows the start of engorgement. The linking of the motile cortical actin network to the immobile substrate would cause it to pull on the substrate, and a development of tension would correlate with elongation. However, this pull on the substrate would not, in a nontrivial way, be a cause of the engorgement or protrusion, but rather a fellow result of the linking. It is not the generation of tension but the actin cycling that is critical here.

The generation of tension *is* critical in the second model (Fig. 7II), which is an adaptation of the ideas of Heidemann and co-workers. They presented evidence suggesting that the actin network generates tension that is supported by the neuritic microtubules and by the substrate (42,43). If laminin mediates the binding of the actin network to the substrate, tension should be more effectively transmitted to the substrate, thus relieving some of the load on the microtubules. Heidemann's group hypothesizes that a relief of compression on the microtubules will cause them to polymerize (42–44). Here, localized "weakening" is achieved by transfer of force elsewhere in the growth cone; the pull on the substrate removes the resistance to microtubule elongation.

The third model is quite different from the preceding two, for here the substrate protein activates biochemical pathways to weaken the actin network of the P region (Fig. 7III). It has been known for many years that various types of cells in culture change from a flattened to a rounded morphology when exposed to treatments that will activate protein kinase A (45). This change is probably caused by diminishment of the actin network. Engorgement can be thought of as this type of shape change. Consonant with this idea is the finding of Forscher and colleagues (46) that stimulation of protein kinase A causes a rapid loss of actin activity in the P region and then engorgement; we have found that stimulation of protein kinase C also causes engorgement. Perhaps then, the substrate protein causes network weakening and engorgement by stimulating protein phosphorylation. This seems less appealing than the preceding models, because it does not imply a localized weakening of the actin network and, as yet, is not grounded in data demonstrating rapid effects on phosphorylation by laminin-type molecules.

Last is the possibility that the primary target of action of the substrate protein is the microtubule rather than the actin filament (Fig. 7IV). Here, microtubules are assumed to be penetrating continually into the P region but retracting rapidly. Binding of the substrate protein to its receptor would coalesce a macromolecular assemblage capable of capturing the ends of microtubules and stabilizing them. Apparent insertion of microtubules into newly formed contacts in the P region of locomoting fibroblasts has been reported (47). Weakening of the actin network and entry of organelles is secondary to the stabilization of microtubules in this scheme.

These models seem testable. The experimental assessment of model IV should be most straightforward: observation of the behavior of microtubules in the living growth cone and a determination of how that behavior is changed by acute administration of substrate factor. Inhibitors of protein kinases could be used to assess model III. Growth cone particles in culture (48) might be useful in determining whether molecules like laminin cause rapid changes in phosphorylation, especially in actin-associated proteins. Models I and II both require that the growth-promoting molecule be bound to an immobile substrate; models III and IV do not. Thus, experiments in which small beads coated with the growth-promoting molecule were applied to the upper surface of the P region, where they would move rearward by linking to the moving cortical actin network (49), should be instructive. Triggering of engorgement by such beads would weigh heavily against models I and II. The ability to literally look into living growth cones with video microscopy should continue to be an important asset in understanding how molecules in the environment promote and inhibit growth and thus shape the circuitry of the brain.

ACKNOWLEDGMENTS

The research from our laboratory discussed in this article was supported by grants from the NIH, the Stifel Paralysis Research Foundation, and the Paralyzed Veterans of America—Spinal Cord Research Foundation.

REFERENCES

1. Pfenninger KH. Molecular biology of the nerve growth cone: a perspective. *Adv Exp Med Biol* 1984;181:1–14.
2. Pfenninger KH, Maylié-Pfenninger M-F. Lectin labeling of sprouting neurons. II. Relative movement and appearance of glycoconjugates during plasmalemmal expansion. *J Cell Biol* 1981;89:547–559.
3. Bamburg JR, Bray D, Chapman K. Assembly of microtubules at the tip of growing axons. *Nature* 1986;321:788–790.
4. Goldberg DJ, Burmeister DW. Stages in axon formation: observations of growth of *Aplysia* axons in culture using video-enhanced contrast-differential interference contrast microscopy. *J Cell Biol* 1986;103:1921–1931.
5. Bray D. Growth cones: do they pull or are they pushed? *Trends Neurosci* 1987;10:431–434.
6. Letourneau PC, Shattuck TA, Ressler AH. "Pull" and "push" in neurite elongation: observations on the effects of different concentrations of cytochalasin B and taxol. *Cell Motil Cytoskel* 1987;8:193–209.
7. Lamoureux P, Buxbaum RE, Heidemann SR. Direct evidence that growth cones pull. *Nature* 1989;340:159–162.
8. Allen RD. New observations on cell architecture and dynamics by video-enhanced contrast optical microscopy. *Annu Rev Biophys Chem* 1985;14:265–290.
9. Lankford KL, Letourneau PC. Evidence that calcium may control neurite outgrowth by regulating the stability of actin filaments. *J Cell Biol* 1989;109:1229–1243.
10. Aletta JM, Greene LA. Growth cone configuration and advance: a time-lapse study using video-enhanced differential interference contrast microscopy. *J Neurosci* 1988;8:1425–1435.
11. Lim S-S, Sammak PJ, Borisy GG. Progressive and spatially differentiated stability of microtubules in developing neuronal cells. *J Cell Biol* 1989;109:253–263.
12. Tosney KW, Landmesser LT. Growth cone morphology and trajectory in the lumbosacral region of the chick embryo. *J Neurosci* 1985;5:2345–2358.
13. Roberts A, Taylor JSH. A study of the growth cones of developing embryonic sensory neurites. *J Embryol Exp Morphol* 1983;75:31–47.
14. Harris WA, Holt CE, Bonhoeffer F. Retinal axons with and without their somata growing to and arborizing in the tectum of *Xenopus* embryos: a time-lapse video study of single fibres *in vivo*. *Development* 1987;101:123–133.
15. Kleitman N, Johnson MI. Rapid growth cone translocation on laminin is supported by lamellipodial not filopodial structures. *Cell Motil Cytoskel* 1989;13:288–300.
16. O'Connor TP, Duerr JS, Bentley D. Pioneer growth cone steering decisions mediated by single filopodial contacts. *J Neurosci* 1990;10:3935–3946.
17. Letourneau PC, Ressler AH. Differences in the organization of actin in the growth cones compared with the neurites of cultured neurons from chick embryos. *J Cell Biol* 1983;97:963–973.
18. Tilney LG, Mooseker M. Actin in the brush border of epithelial cells of the chicken intestine. *Proc Natl Acad Sci USA* 1971;68:2611–2615.
19. Tilney LG, Hatano S, Ishikawa H, Mooseker M. The polymerization of actin: its role in the generation of the acrosomal process of certain echinoderm sperm. *J Cell Biol* 1973;59:109–126.
20. Goldberg DJ. Local role of Ca^{2+} in formation of veils in growth cones. *J Neurosci* 1988;8:2596–2605.
21. Silver RA, Lamb AG, Bolsover SR. Calcium hotspots caused by L-channel clustering promote morphological changes in neuronal growth cones. *Nature* 1990;343:751–754.
22. Allsopp TE, Moss DJ. A developmentally regulated chicken neuronal protein associated with the cortical cytoskeleton. *J Neurosci* 1989;9:13–24.

from fetal rat brain and demonstrated that second messengers, such as Ca^{2+} and cyclic adenosine $3',5'$-monophosphate (cyclic AMP), are affecting the phosphorylation of various proteins in growth cone membranes. Gordon-Weeks and Lockerbie (20) isolated in bulk and characterized neuronal growth cones from neonatal rat forebrain, showing that uptake and release mechanisms for GABA are present (21).

Studies on the protein and lipid phosphorylation in SPM isolated from the cerebral cortex of adult rat indicate a function of the PKC-mediated phosphorylation of B-50 in membrane signal transduction of the presynaptic terminal (9). An inverse relationship between changes in B-50 phosphorylation and the degree of phosphatidylinositol 4,5 biphosphate (PIP_2) labeling is demonstrated in a variety of paradigms. From these studies we developed a working hypothesis for B-50 in neuronal membrane function suggesting that increased B-50 phosphorylation inhibits the PIP kinase activity, thus giving a feedback inhibition to the Ca^{2+} or receptor-stimulated polyphosphoinositide hydrolysis at the membrane (9).

Outline of the Studies

We explored the role of B-50 in the neuronal growth cones from two viewpoints. Because growth cones develop ultimately to presynaptic terminals, we examined the function of B-50 in membrane signal transduction and report of experiments on effects of (extra)cellular signals on the B-50 phosphorylation in growth cone membranes and in isolated intact growth cones. The second approach is studying changes in localization of B-50 in neuronal cell cultures of various developmental stages and *in situ* in the developing brain.

RESULTS

Role of B-50 in Signal Transduction in the Growth Cone

We showed that the nerve growth cone membranes isolated from fetal and neonatal rat brain are enriched in B-50. The B-50 phosphorylation in these growth cone membranes *in vitro* is inhibited by $ACTH_{1-24}$ and stimulated by phorbol diesters, indicating that PKC is the active protein kinase. In addition $ACTH_{1-24}$ stimulated the PIP_2 formation in growth cone membranes, suggesting the possibility of an inverse relationship between the degree of B-50 phosphorylation and PIP_2 labeling as shown for adult presynaptic membranes (6).

The question arose whether B-50 phosphorylation in intact nerve growth cones would respond to extracellular agents. To explore this, intact growth cones were isolated from the brain of 5-day-old rats (20) and studied after prelabeling with $[^{32}P]$-orthophosphate, using an immunoprecipitation method to monitor selectively the degree of B-50 phosphorylation. Phorbol 12,13-dibutyrate and dioctanoyl glycerol, activators of PKC, stimulate B-50 phosphorylation in the intact growth cones, confirming that PKC is involved in B-50 phosphorylation (6).

Depolarization induced by 30 mM K^+ produces a transient rise in B-50 phosphorylation. This response to K^+ depolarization is also demonstrated in adult rat brain preparations, such as the hippocampal slice (22) and isolated synaptosomes. The effect of K^+ depolarization on B-50 phosphorylation in growth cones can be blocked partially by atropine (0.1–1 mM). The suggestion of involvement of muscarinic receptors is supported by the finding that carbachol, a cholinergic receptor agonist, enhances B-50 phosphorylation in a concentration-dependent manner (50% at 1 mM). The carbachol (1 mM) stimulation can be blocked by atropine (0.1 μM). The carbachol stimulation can be further increased by concurrent K^+ depolarization. These results show that B-50 phosphorylation by PKC may mediate signal transduction in growth cones (6,23).

CAM Binding of Endogenous B-50 in Isolated Growth Cone Membranes

B-50, which is identical to neuromodulin, has been described as an atypical CAM binding protein (11). In contrast to other CAM binding proteins, purified B-50 as well as B-50 solubilized from cortical membranes has a higher affinity for CAM in the absence of Ca^{2+} ions than in their presence. Liu and Storm (11) proposed that in growth cones, B-50, forming a local store, may regulate the availability of CAM for processes important for growth cone motility and outgrowth. Because binding of CAM to endogenous B-50 in native neuronal membranes has not been demonstrated, we examined this interaction in isolated growth cone membranes and, for reasons of comparison, in SPM. To assess the physiological relevance, CAM/B-50 binding was studied in the presence and absence of free Ca^{2+} ions and detected by the use of the homo-bifunctional cross-linker disuccinimidyl suberate (DSS). With this tool a covalent bound B-50/CAM complex can be formed, which is detectable by sodium dodecyl sulphate polyacrylamide gel electrophoresis (SDS-PAGE) and Western blots. Before the experiment, the membranes were washed four times in a buffer containing alternating EGTA or $CaCl_2$ to dissociate and remove endogenously bound CAM.

In the first set of experiments using purified B-50 and CAM, we found that B-50/CAM complex formation requires the presence of B-50, CAM, and DSS and the absence of Ca^{2+} during the incubation (24). The complex is detected in 11% SDS-PAGE as a protein band migrating with apparent molecular weight of 70 kDa. This is a value close to the sum of the apparent molecular weights of B-50 and CAM. The 70 kDA protein was shown by Western blotting to cross-react with antibodies specific for B-50 and a second set of antibodies specific for CAM. Both sets of antibodies detect also on the blot their homologous antigen in the presence and absence of Ca^{2+} ions. Formation of the 70 kDa complex is immunodetected only in the absence of Ca^{2+}

With growth cone membranes and SPM, the B-50/CAM complex cannot be detected by protein silver staining, because in these preparations there are already too many proteins present in the 70 kDA range. In the second set of experiments, we used growth cone membranes or SPM to form the complex under identical conditions as previously. We found on Western immunoblot that both sets of antibodies cross-reacted with a 70-kDa protein band only if the incubation was performed in the absence of Ca^{2+} (24). The formation is more easily detected when exogenous CAM was added. It is possible to show, by varying the Ca^{2+} concentration in the medium, that the amount of B-50/CAM complex in the membranes decreases as the Ca^{2+} concentration increases from 10^{-7} to 10^{-5} M, a range similar as reported for the dissociation of the complex formed from the purified CAM and B-50 (11) and close to physiological Ca^{2+} concentrations in the growth cones.

Role of B-50 in Nerve Growth Factor Induced Neuronal Differentiation of Rat Pheochromocytoma PC12 Cells

PC12 cells have been intensively studied as a model for the mechanism of neuronal differentiation. When rat PC12 cells are cultured in the presence of nerve growth factor (NGF), the cells stop proliferating and differentiate to a phenotype resembling cholinergic sympathetic neurons, elaborating neuritic extensions (25). B-50 has been identified in both undifferentiated and NGF-treated PC12 cells (6). Treatment of PC12 cells with NGF for 2 days results in a 2.5-fold increase in the B-50 level as measured by radioimmunoassay. Immunofluorescence microscopy shows that B-50 is detectable in fixed permeabilized PC12 cells, as intensified membrane-associated staining in the neurites, especially in the growth cones, of the NGF-differentiated cells and as diffuse staining in the cell bodies of the controls and the NGF-differentiated cells. In contrast, when living, non-permeabilized PC12 cells are incubated with B-50 antibodies and then fixed and probed with a fluorescein-conjugated secondary antibody, no immunofluorescence is detectable, suggesting that B-50 is inside the cells.

With the aim to learn more about the putative growth-associated function of B-50, we have compared its ultrastructural localization in control-proliferating PC12 cells with its distribution in PC12 cells induced to differentiate by various agents (50 ng/ml NGF, 1-mM dibutyryl cyclic-AMP, and substratum). The studies were performed on cells fixed in 2% paraformaldehyde/0.1% acrolein in PBS, embedded in gelatin, cryoprotected, and sectioned on an ultracryomicrotome at −90°C. Grids holding 70- to 100-nm-thick sections were incubated with B-50 antibodies, and the antigen–antibody complexes were detected by protein-A gold (10 nm) conjugates (26). To our surprise we found that in the cryosections of untreated control PC12 cells, the BIR is mainly associated with intracellular membrane-rich and vesicular structures, including organelles of the lysosome family and Golgi apparatus. The plasma membrane is virtually devoid of label. In contrast, after 48 hr of treatment with NGF or cyclic-AMP, BIR is most pronounced on the plasma membrane. Highest BIR is observed on plasma membrane surrounding sprouting microvilli, lamellipodia, and filopodia. In addition, extending neurites and growth cones contain cytosolic BIR, which is partially associated with chromaffin granules. In the

NGF-differentiated PC12 cells, the cytosolic location of B-50 is similar to untreated cells. Although the induction of neurite formation in PC12 cells by NGF and cyclicAMP is reported to occur by different pathways, B-50 distribution in dibutyryl cyclicAMP–differentiated cells closely resembles that observed in the NGF-treated cells. Of interest is that these findings illustrate that various differentiating agents induce in PC12 cells a changed ultrastructural B-50 distribution, shifting the B-50 protein to the plasma membrane (26).

Recent further ultrastructural studies of the time course of the NGF effect on the B-50 distribution indicate that after approximately 4 hr the beginning of the shift of B-50 to the plasma membrane can be observed and after 8 hr the translocation appears to be fully established. When PC12 cells are grown for the same time (48 hr) in the presence of epidermal growth factor (EGF, 50 ng/ml), a growth factor inducing proliferation in PC12 cells, the cell numbers increase, the B-50 levels increase by 50%, but few neuritic protrusions are formed. The ultrastructural distribution of B-50 in the case of EGF is rather similar to that in the untreated control cells (*unpublished results*). This indicates that the translocation of B-50 appears to be linked to the formation of neuritic protrusions. Therefore, the function of B-50 may reside in membrane-associated processes, such as membrane addition, vesicle fusion, and signal transduction.

Subcellular Localization of B-50/GAP43 in Isolated Neuronal Growth Cones

We studied the subcellular distribution of B-50 in growth cones by immuno-gold labeling of B-50 antibodies in ultrathin cryosections of isolated neuronal growth cones (10). Ultrastructure of isolated neuronal growth cones clearly shows a dense matrix of smooth endoplasmic reticulum (SER), round and oval vesicles of various sizes, and small mitochondria. Eighty percent of the B-50 immunoreactivity is located at the plasma membrane, whereas 20% is present in the cytoplasm of the growth cone, occasionally in the proximity of vesicles (27).

Developing Rat Pyramidal Tract

In the rat, the outgrowth of pyramidal tract (PT) fibers occurs mainly during the postnatal development. The pioneer fibers arriving from neurons located in layer V of the sensorimotor cortex enter the cervical spinal cord around the time of birth. Two days after birth (P2), still a great number of axons grow into upper cervical segments of the spinal cord, where they occupy the most ventral part of the dorsal funiculus. The light microscopic immunocytochemical distribution of B-50 during development of the rat PT has been reported, showing that at P2 and P7 these fibers display intense BIR in contrast to the earlier developing ascending fiber tracts of the cuneatus and gracilis. By immuno-electron microscopy, Gorgels and co-workers (28) studied the localization of B-50 in the third cervical segment. At P2, cross-sectioned growth cones (asterisks, Fig. 1) in the PT are recognized by their large

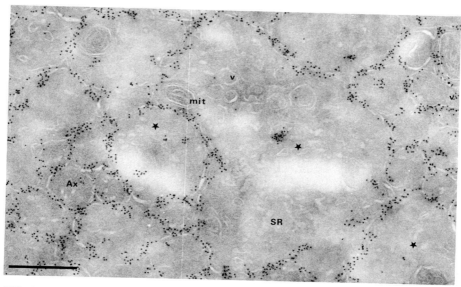

FIG. 1. Immuno-gold labeling of cryosections of pyramidal tract of a 2-day-old rat, using goat antirabbit immunoglobulins coated on gold particles (10 nm) after incubation with affinity-purified rabbit antibodies to B-50. Gold particles are mainly located at the axolemma of axons (Ax) and at the plasma membrane of growth cones (*asterisks*). SR, smooth endoplasmic reticulum; mit, mitochondrion; v, vesicles, Scale bar, 0.5 μm.

diameter, the presence of vesicles, and a meshwork of SER in distinction to axon profiles (Ax). Some of the sectioned growth cones taper distally into filopodia (28). Similarly to the isolated growth cones, the majority of the gold particles indicating BIR are located at the cytoplasmic side of the plasma membrane. Occasionally, some label is encountered in the cytoplasm of growth cones, probably attached to vesicles. Noteworthy, all axon profiles carry also BIR at the axolemma (28).

Developing Rat Hippocampus

Electron microscopic immunocytochemical studies of the developing rat hippocampus were carried out to examine the subcellular distribution of B-50 in developing axons and dendrites. At postnatal day one (P1), the pyramidal cells of the CA1 area are in the process of migrating to form a pyramidal cell layer. At this stage the prominent apical dendrites that eventually grow into the stratum radiatum are not yet formed. In the area of stratum radiatum, bundles of cross-sectioned axons are found, as well as extensions of irregular-shaped plasma membranes. With their content of SER and vesicles, these structures resemble very well growth cones in the neonatal PT (28). Few growth cones contain clusters of 10- to 20-nm vesicles apposed to the growth cone plasma membrane, which are immunoreactive for the vesicle-specific protein synaptophysin (p38). High BIR is observed at the plasma membranes of the axons and growth cones, whereas the plasma membranes of pyramidal cells show a low but detectable immunolabeling.

Hippocampal Pyramidal Cells in Culture

The localization of B-50 in various growth cone elements (lamellipodia, filopodia) can be adequately studied in growth cones of cultured cells, because these can be sectioned parallel to the substratum of adhesion. Thus, it is possible to section the cell body, neurites, and the growth cones simultaneously in one plane. This yields some information about the localization in the connecting neurite extending from the cell body. Similar to their *in situ* counterparts, cultured hippocampal pyramidal cells form morphologically distinct axonal and dendritic processes, providing the basis for functional polarization of neurons. The sequence of events leading to the development of a polarized mature neuron has been documented by Dotti and colleagues (29). Goslin and co-workers (30–32) showed by immunofluorescence that after morphological polarization of the pyramidal neurons B-50

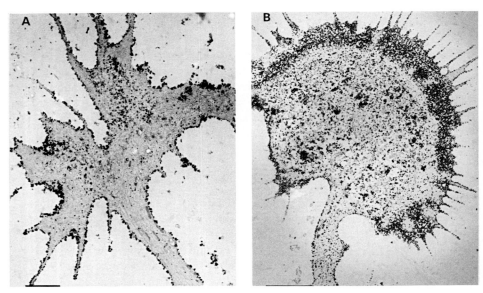

FIG. 2. Growth cones of 2-day-old hippocampal pyramidal cells, incubated with rabbit antibodies to B-50 and 1-nm gold particles conjugated to goat antirabbit antibodies. After silver enhancement, the cells were embedded in Lowicryl HM20 (**A**) or Epon (**B**). Note intense staining of the growth cone plasma membrane. In the central domain some vesicles are stained. In the lamellipodial growth cone (**B**) intense B-50 staining is found in the periphery. Scale bars: **A**, 5 μm; **B**, 12 μm.

becomes selectively located in the axonal growth cone. We studied the cultures of pyramidal cells to relate the subcellular distribution of B-50 in growth cones and neurites to the developmental stage of the neurons.

Cultures of several developmental stages were incubated with B-50 antibodies and thereafter with ultrasmall gold conjugates. Subsequently, the gold particle diameter was increased by silver enhancement, and the immunoincubated cells were embedded in Epon resin or Lowicryl HM20. Shortly after the cells have attached to the substratum, lamellipodia develop at the periphery of the cells. Intense BIR is found at the surrounding membrane, as well as in the lamellipodial region of the cell body. Some membranes of vacuoles in the cytoplasm display BIR as well. Electron micrographs of growth cones in 2-day-old cultures of hippocampal cells show neurofilaments and microtubuli, SER, mitochondria, and vesicles in the central domain. We distinguished two types of growth cones at this developmental stage. The smaller type (Fig. 2A) has an irregular contour formed by lamellipodia and filopodia. The majority of these growth cones are attached to elongated neurites. The large type (Fig. 2B) forms a half-circular contour displaying lamellipodia. The growth cones are either directly attached to the cell body or to short neurites. The plasma membrane of the neurites and the growth cones display intense BIR, as shown by silver-enhanced gold particles. The large circular lamellipodial growth cones in addition show intense BIR in the periphery. In both growth cones, the

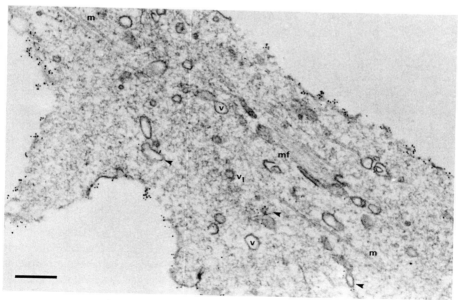

FIG. 3. Part of a dendritic growth cone immunoreacted with B-50 antibodies and 5-nm gold particles conjugated to goat-antirabbit immunoglobulins. B-50 immunoreactivity is found at the plasma membrane and at some vesicles in the growth cone cytosol (*arrowheads*). mf, microfilaments; v_1, dense core vesicle; v, electron lucent vesicle; m, microtubules. Scale bar, 0.2 μm.

vesicles in the central domain contain BIR. The localization of B-50 at the plasma membrane and vesicular structures in the central region of the growth cone suggests that B-50 is involved in the addition of new material to protruding edges of the growth cone.

Microtubule-associated protein-2 (MAP2) is a component of the microtubular cytoskeleton. At the end of the first week in culture, molecular polarization of hippocampal neurons in culture becomes evident by the preferential association of MAP2 with cell somata and dendrites (33). Goslin and co-workers (30) showed in their studies that the selective expression of B-50/GAP43 in axons is correlated with reduced staining for MAP2. In 8-day-old cultures, we investigated at the electron microscopic level the localization of B-50 in growth cones of MAP2-positive neurites. These growth cones are either club-shaped (Fig. 3 shows detail of club-shaped growth cone) or extend long filopodia. The growth cones contain large amounts of vesicles with electron-lucent (v) or electron-dense (v1) content. BIR was clearly evident at the plasma membranes of the growth cones and occasionally at the membranes of vesicles (*arrowheads*). Noteworthy, the amount of BIR at the plasma membrane varies among the growth cones of the same neuron. Studies are in progress to investigate the issue whether polarized expression of B-50 is temporally correlated with polarized expression of MAP2 and functional differentiation of outgrowing processes.

DISCUSSION

Our localization studies in neuronal cell cultures demonstrate that the location of B-50 can be distinguished in two regions of the growth cone, namely, the central region and the cortical, marginal region (cf. ref. 34). Immunofluorescence studies (6,16) suggest that B-50 may be broadly distributed in the submembranous cortical region of the growth cone, in addition to spotty attachment to the plasma membrane. As yet there is little evidence that B-50 binds to specific cytoskeletal components, except for CAM as a Ca^{2+} carrier. However, the intracellular localization in the growth cone (Fig. 2B) suggests that in the cortical region, B-50 is co-localized with actin filaments and in the central region with various vesicles. B-50 localization in the actin-rich membrane cytoskeleton of growth cones is described in chick embryo brains (35) and in growth cones isolated from neonatal rat forebrain (36).

Apart from this cytosolic B-50, our ultrastructural studies in which various procedures of post- and preembedding labeling are applied show that BIR is predominantly located at the inner face of the plasma membrane. This is in accordance with biochemical studies that describe B-50 as an intrinsic membrane protein because of its resistance to extraction by high-salt or non-ionic detergents. Labeling studies by Skene and Virag (37) in neonatal rat cortex indicate that newly synthesized B-50 is found at first (within 20 min) in the cytosol and decreases as more B-50 molecules become posttranslationally associated with membranes. Their two-dimensional gel analyses suggest that B-50 is first attached to the membrane and subsequently is phosphorylated, displaying microheterogeneity of the adult isoforms. Using cultures from embryonic cerebral cortex and isolated growth cones, Skene and Virag (37) showed that B-50 is linked to palmitic acid, which is associated with B-50 in the membrane fraction. The linkage occurs probably by a thioester to the unique cysteine residues 3 and 4 in the molecule. This N-terminal domain of B-50 determines the anchoring to the membrane.

The prominent membrane localization indicates a local function of B-50 at the plasma membrane. The involvement of B-50 in signal transduction is suggested by our findings that in isolated intact growth cones, increases in intracellular Ca^{2+} levels induced either by chemical depolarization or by muscarinic receptor activation enhance the B-50 phosphorylation. Because concurrent exposure to the cholinergic agonist carbachol and depolarization induces increases in B-50 phosphorylation that are additive, we assume that these signals meet in a common pathway.

A specific function of GAP43 in the growth cones has been suggested recently. Strittmatter and colleagues (38) showed that a growth cone membrane fraction of neonatal rat is enriched, among other proteins (GAP43 and actin) in the α-subunit (p38) and the β-subunit (p34) of the GTP binding protein G_o. Tests with purified G_o and GAP43 reveal that GAP43 promotes the binding of GTP-γ-S to the G_o. If this interaction is shown to occur in the growth cone membrane, the growth cone would have a mechanism by which intracellular regulation of G_o-dependent pathways are independent of activation or the presence of certain receptors.

It is of interest to note that until now, using different biochemical approaches, we have found that B-50 in growth cones and growth cone membranes behaves qualitatively very similar to the mature system (e.g., the synaptosome and SPM). For instance, looking at the physiological significance of the binding of CAM to B-50, we detected that the B-50 attached to the membrane of both growth cones and SPM forms with CAM a complex of apparent M_r of 70 kDa, only at Ca^{2+} levels similar to basal intraterminal levels. Increasing the Ca^{2+} levels prevents complex formation. These findings are in line with the *in vitro* studies performed with the purified proteins (11). The concept is that because of a rise in intracellular free-Ca^{2+} levels, caused by opening Ca^{2+} channels or mobilization of Ca^{2+} from intracellular stores, CAM will dissociate from B-50 at the plasma membrane. So B-50 may locally provide CAM for various CAM/Ca^{2+}-dependent reactions. Once free, B-50 can be phosphorylated by PKC, influencing the Ca^{2+}-sensitive polyphosphoinositide response at the membrane (9). Dephosphorylation of B-50 by protein phosphatases (calcineurin) will lead to recruitment of CAM back in the complex and attenuate the Ca^{2+}-stimulated state (6). This B-50 function is in line with the crucial control of intracellular Ca^{2+} levels in growth cone motility and axon outgrowth (39). Especially notable is that our immunoelectron microscopy demonstrates that B-50 is located at the plasma membrane of growth cones, independent of their morphology, stage of differentiation, and the system in which the growth cone is studied (*in situ* or in cell cultures). Thus, enhanced B-50 expression appears to be necessary for neurite outgrowth and successful axonal regeneration (4,5). The expression of B-50 decreases as synaptogenesis and myelination start. Before differentiation sets in (e.g., in control PC12 cells), very little B-50 is detected at the plasma membrane.

This changes as soon as neuronal cells become committed to elaborate fibers (15), as we have illustrated here by NGF-induced neuronal differentiation of PC12 cells in which already after 4 hr, translocation of B-50 from intracellular compartments to the plasma membrane occurs. It is not known if B-50 plays a role in membrane fusion processes during neurite outgrowth, but there is evidence that antibodies to B-50 inhibit the Ca^{2+}-dependent release of neurotransmitter in permeabilized adult nerve terminals (40). B-50 at the axonal plasma membrane may serve the neuron by its function in membrane signal transduction involving CAM and PKC, allowing initiation of sprouting and membrane plasticity.

ACKNOWLEDGMENT

We wish to thank Carlos G. Dotti for culturing the hippocampal cells and Ruud J. Bloemen for affinity purification of B-50 antibodies.

REFERENCES

1. Kater SB, Letourneau PC. *Biology of the nerve growth cone*. New York: Alan Liss, 1985.
2. Lockerbie RO. The neuronal growth cone: a review of its locomotory, navigational and target recognition capabilities. *Neuroscience* 1987;20:719–729.
3. Letourneau PC. Nerve cell shape. In: Stein WD, Bronner F, eds. *Cell shape, determinants, regulation and regulatory role*. New York: Academic Press, 1989;247–289.
4. Skene JHP. Axonal growth-associated proteins. *Annu Rev Neurosci* 1989;12:127–156.
5. Zuber MX, Goodman DW, Karns LR, Fishman MC. The neuronal growth-associated protein GAP43 induces filopodia in non-neuronal cells. *Science* 1989;244:1193–1195.
6. Van Hooff COM, Oestreicher AB, De Graan PNE, Gispen WH. Role of the growth cone in neuronal differentiation. *Mol Neurobiol* 1989;3:101–133.
7. Zwiers H, Schotman, P, Gispen WH. Purification and some characteristics of an ACTH-sensitive protein kinase and its substrate protein in rat brain membranes. *J Neurochem* 1980;34:1689–1699.
8. Kristjansson GI, Zwiers H, Oestreicher AB, Gispen WH. Evidence that the synaptic phosphoprotein B-50 is localized exclusively in nerve tissue. *J Neurochem* 1982;39:371–378.
9. Gispen WH, Boonstra J, De Graan PNE, et al. B-50/GAP43 in neuronal development and repair. *Rest Neurol Neurosci* 1990;1:237–244.
10. Pfenninger KH. Of nerve growth cones, leukocytes and memory: second messenger systems and growth-related proteins. *Trends Neurosci* 1986;9:562–565.
11. Liu Y, Storm DR. Regulation of free calmodulin levels by neuromodulin: neuron growth and regeneration. *Trends Pharmacol Sci* 1990;11:107–111.
12. Benowitz LI, Routtenberg A. A membrane phosphoprotein associated with neural development, axonal regeneration, phospholipid metabolism and synaptic plasticity. *Trends Neurosci* 1987;12: 527–532.
13. Gispen WH, Van Dongen CJ, De Graan PNE, Oestreicher AB, Zwiers H. The role of phosphoprotein B-50 in phosphoinositide metabolism in brain synaptic membranes. In: Bleasdale JE, Hauser G, Eichberg J, eds. *Inositol and phosphoinositides*. New York: Humana Press, 1985;399–413.
14. Coggins PJ, Zwiers H. Evidence for a single protein kinase C–mediated phosphorylation site in rat brain protein B-50. *J Neurochem* 1989;53:1895–1901.
15. Biffo S, Verhaagen J, Schrama LH, Schotman P, Danho W, Margolis FL. B-50/GAP43 expression correlates with process outgrowth in the embryonic mouse nervous system. *Eur J Neurosci* 1990;2: 487–499.
16. Ramakers GJA, Oestreicher AB, Wolters PS, Van Leeuwen FW, De Graan PNE, Gispen WH. Developmental changes in B-50 (GAP43) in primary cultures of cerebral cortex: B-50 immunolocalization, axonal elongation rate and growth cone morphology. *Int J Dev Neurosci* 1991;9:215–230.
17. Ramakers GJA, De Graan PNE, Oestreicher AB, Boer GJ, Corner MA, Gispen WH. Develop-

glycerol gradients (K. Pfenninger and V. Miller, *in preparation*). This fractionation methodology will be particularly useful for studying vesicle contents, their membrane proteins, and the relationships between the various membrane compartments. Overall, quasi-complete subfractionation of growth cones is within reach and should revolutionize growth cone research further in the near future.

PLASMALEMMAL EXPANSION

Measuring Membrane Expansion

It has been known for some time that most newly synthesized lipid and a series of proteins are transported into the distal tips of growing nerve fibers (12,23–27). Surface-labeling studies have identified the growth cone as a major site of plasmalemmal expansion (4,28,29). To study this phenomenon in greater detail and to approach it at a molecular level, we designed a cell-free membrane expansion assay using intact GCPs. A radiolabeled ligand (wheat-germ agglutinin, WGA) is used to quantify binding sites exposed on the plasmalemmal surface after different incubations. Total binding sites are measured after permeabilization to calculate the size of the internal pool and as a bias (17,30). The results of such experiments can be expressed as the ratios of exposed over total binding sites. Examples are shown in Fig. 3: Potassium depolarization, calcium-ionophore treatment (A23187), or veratridine incubation (which leads to membrane depolarization by sodium influx) cause significant increases in exposed WGA binding sites within minutes. The effect is dependent on extracellular calcium, indicating that calcium influx is the trigger of the insertion event. Morphometric analysis of the same experimental system identifies the large, clear vesicles characteristic of nerve growth cones (cf. Fig. 2B) as the only internal membrane compartment that decreases concomitant with the increase in surface label. Therefore, the increase in ligand binding on the plasmalemma (i.e., plasmalemmal expansion) is a *regulated* phenomenon in the growth cone, triggered like exocytosis by calcium influx, and the source of the new membrane is the clear "growth cone vesicles." This identifies these vesicles as the *plasmalemmal precursor*.

Radiolabeled serotonin and γ-aminobutyric acid are taken up into live GCPs (31) by a sodium- and temperature-dependent mechanism. However, these transmitters are not released on potassium depolarization or ionophore-induced calcium influx (i.e., the conditions that lead to plasmalemmal expansion) (17,30). These observations indicate that membrane fusion events for plasmalemmal expansion and for transmitter exocytosis are regulated independently and emerge sequentially in development. Furthermore, the plasmalemmal precursor vesicles are not the stores of the neurotransmitters taken up into the GCPs. The lack of transmitter release from these fetal GCPs is consistent with other reports (31–34) and may be explained by storage of the transmitter in a nonreleasable, perhaps nonvesicular compartment (35). Indeed, the small vesicles typical of mature synaptic endings are very sparse in

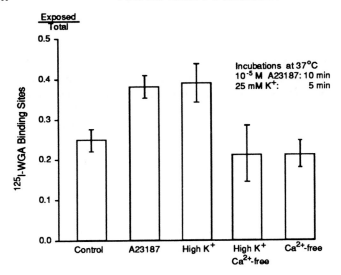

A. A23187 and K⁺ Stimulation

^{125}I-WGA Binding Sites / $\frac{\text{Exposed}}{\text{Total}}$

Incubations at 37°C
10^{-5} M A23187: 10 min
25 mM K⁺:   5 min

Control   A23187   High K⁺   High K⁺ Ca²⁺-free   Ca²⁺-free

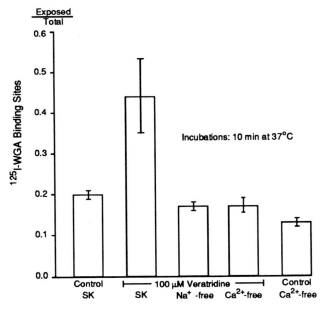

B. Veratridine Stimulation

^{125}I-WGA Binding Sites / $\frac{\text{Exposed}}{\text{Total}}$

Incubations: 10 min at 37°C

Control SK   SK   ├── 100 µM Veratridine ──┤   Control Ca²⁺-free
          Na⁺-free   Ca²⁺-free

FIG. 3. Cell-free assay of plasmalemmal expansion using labeling of exposed vs. total WGA binding sites after different incubations. Increase in exposed/total sites indicates externalization of membrane receptors. Note increases in exposed sites caused by calcium inonophore A23187, by potassium depolarization (25 mM), and by veratridine in calcium-dependent manner. The veratridine effect also requires extracellular sodium. SK, sucrose-modified Krebs buffer. Control experiments have been carried out to establish that there is no change in affinity of the WGA binding sites and that the label does not enter the GCPs under the various conditions. (From ref. 30, with permission.)

nerve growth cones and GCPs (9). The developmental regulation of the synaptic-vesicle-associated phosphoprotein synapsin I, which has been implicated in the regulation of transmitter release (36), offers a particularly intriguing correlation: Synapsin I is present in GCPs but, compared with synaptosomes, only in very small quantities (37). Transmitter vesicles may depend on the presence of synapsin I for their interaction with the plasmalemma before an exocytotic fusion event can occur, whereas plasmalemmal precursor vesicles do not. Thus, calcium-regulated membrane fusion seems dedicated to plasmalemmal expansion during neurite outgrowth. It appears that only during synaptogenesis when synapsin I levels rise does calcium influx assume the role of a trigger mechanism for transmitter release.

Possible Mechanisms of Membrane Fusion

Fusion of vesicles with the plasmalemma must result from a complex set of mechanisms. At least conceptually, the fusion process can be thought of at three different levels. Coalescence of membranes may proceed as soon as a vesicle comes close enough to the plasmalemma, as seen in *constitutive secretion*, which does not require a regulating trigger mechanism. In many cases, however, coalescence (most likely by a very similar mechanism) may proceed only in the presence of an appropriate trigger (e.g., a rise in intracellular calcium)—as in *regulated secretion*. In most cells, fusion is selective (e.g., only a specific type of vesicle will fuse with a particular plasmalemmal domain). This necessitates a specific docking or *membrane–membrane recognition* mechanism (5,38). It is conceivable that synapsin I is involved in the regulation of synaptic vesicle exocytosis at this level. Overall, we need to look for at least three different steps leading to plasmalemmal membrane expansion. Operationally, the simplest question at this time is what mechanisms are activated by the influx of calcium.

Perhaps the most obvious possibility is that calcium influx activates a calcium-dependent protein kinase. However, B- and C-kinase inhibition by trifluoperazine or phorbol ester activation of protein kinase C did not have any effect on the externalization of WGA binding sites (R. Lockerbie and K. Pfenninger, *unpublished*). These results, although somewhat preliminary, almost certainly rule out an involvement of the two kinases in the calcium trigger mechanism. In a number of secretory systems, both constitutive and regulated, the function of a metalloendoprotease was found to be essential for exocytosis (39,40). Indeed, studies on plasmalemmal insertion of saxitoxin (STX) binding sites (i.e., sodium channels) demonstrated that the activity of such an enzyme is required there, too (41,42). The metalloendoprotease involvement in both constitutive and regulated exocytosis mechanisms would suggest that the enzyme operates at the most basic level of the fusion mechanism.

The membrane-destabilizing properties of lysolipids have been known for a long time, and lysophospholipid generation has been proposed to trigger fusion of adjacent membranes (43). Of particular interest in this context is the calcium-dependent enzyme phospholipase A_2 (PLA_2), which removes from phospholipids the fatty acid

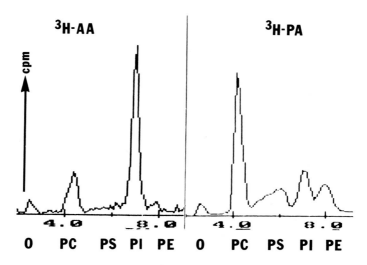

FIG. 4. Incorporation of two fatty acids, ^{3}H-arachidonate and ^{3}H-palmitate, into growth cone phospholipids (radioscan of thin-layer chromatogram). Intact GCPs were incubated for 45 min at 36° with either fatty acid, their lipids extracted and chromatographed. Note the high level of incorporation of ^{3}H-arachidonate into phosphatidylinositol (PI), a sparse phospholipid. ^{3}H-palmitate, in contrast, is incorporated primarily into the abundant phosphatidylcholine (PC), but much less so into PI. The rapid turnover of arachidonate in PI is diagnostic of a high level of phospholipase A_2 activity with a preference for IP as substrate. O, origin; PS, phosphatidyl serine; PE, phosphatidyl ethanolamine. Note that the cpm scales of the two scans are different.

in the sn-2 position, usually arachidonic acid. Analyses of fatty acids and fatty acid metabolism in GCPs reveal a high level of free arachidonic acid (3% of total endogenous arachidonic acid) and rapid turnover of this fatty acid—as opposed to, for example, palmitic acid (Fig. 4). The highest turnover of arachidonic acid is found in inositol lipids (which, however, account for only a small proportion of membrane phospholipids), and inositol lipids appear to be the primary substrates of GCP PLA_2 (44). PLA_2 activity appears to generate what we tentatively identify as a lyso-poly-phosphoinositide. It is conceivable that this compound may act as a detergent-like initiator of membrane fusion for plasmalemmal expansion. The other PLA_2 cleavage product, arachidonic acid, or one of its derivatives have to be considered as candidate fusogens as well (45). In any case, the metabolism of inositol lipids by PLA_2 appears to be a major, novel signaling pathway in GCPs.

Functional Conversion of Membrane Proteins During Plasmalemmal Insertion

Plasmalemmal insertion of membrane components has also been studied using STX as a probe for sodium channels (41,42). Like WGA receptors, STX binding

The Nerve Growth Cone, edited by P. C. Letourneau,
S. B. Kater, and E. R. Macagno, Raven Press, Ltd.,
New York © 1992.

11

Introduction

Lloyd A. Greene

*Department of Pathology, Columbia University College of Physicians and Surgeons, New
York, New York 10032*

In contrast to the chapters in Section 1 which dealt largely with the intrinsic components that compose the functional machinery of growth cones, those in this section focus primarily on how growth cones are influenced by extrinsic factors. In his wisdom, Cajal realized that the ordered development of a nonsyncytial nervous system requires the intervention of environmental signals. That is, although growth cones may possess an independent capacity for motility, they are not and cannot be endowed with a predestined and autonomous ability to find their correct targets. For this, they must respond to and depend on cues produced by their surroundings. As reviewed here in the chapter by Lumsden, Cajal advanced a "neurotropic" hypothesis for growth cone guidance by external factors. Cajal himself (1) averred that this theory was "premature and inadequate" and that more could be learned about the "deeper causes of development." The chapters to follow summarize various current points of view regarding our progress in understanding the means and mechanisms by which growth cone behavior is regulated by environmental cues. I believe that one will be impressed both by how far we have come as well as by how much farther we have yet to go.

In reading this group of contributions, one is in some ways reminded of the fable about the blind men and the elephant. Each chapter, partly because of the nature of the problem and partly because of the requirements for brevity and focus, presents a different perspective of growth cone regulation. However, the juxtaposition of these various views also provides an excellent opportunity to identify and sharpen unifying concepts. What follows is an idiosyncratic weaving together of some of the many exciting issues presented in these chapters.

EXPERIMENTAL ADVANCES IN STUDYING GROWTH CONE REGULATION

One notable common feature here is the introduction of increasingly sophisticated experimental means to manipulate the external environment of the growth cone and to monitor its responses thereto. For instance, these chapters relate the exploitation of an array of primary and transformed cell culture systems. Although often in the background, such systems represent the culmination of many years of development. To these cultures, both soluble and bound substances can be presented at will and can even be applied focally or in the form of gradients. Moreover, there is (or soon will be) available for such delivery an increasing armamentarium of purified and defined reagents. This includes many of the biologically active molecules described in these chapters, neutralizing antibodies prepared against them and/or their receptors, and drugs that specifically modify second-messenger pathways. Also emerging is the use of molecular genetics to alter the ability of growth cones to respond to such influences. Additionally described here are important advances in imaging. These permit high-resolution, real-time observation of both the macroscopic motility and intracellular ionic makeup of growth cones that are responding to various signals. These and additional new techniques included in this set of contributions will no doubt continue to drive progress in understanding how growth cones interact with their milieu.

MULTIPLE INFLUENCES ON GROWTH CONES

Among the common aims of the work described in these chapters is to define the classes as well as identities of the environmental components that influence growth cone behavior. Not surprisingly, there is a broad range of both soluble and bound molecules with such activity. These include neurotransmitters (chapter by Davies et al.), neurotrophic (chapter by Phelan et al.) and neurotropic (chapter by Lumsden) factors, matrix components (chapters by Letourneau and Schachner), cell surface or matrix components with adhesive or repulsive activities (chapters by Baier and Bonhoeffer, Raper et al., Schachner, and Letourneau), and specific proteases (chapter by Seeds et al.). In addition, as stressed in a number of the contributions, the environment is likely to confront the growth cone with a variety of simultaneous influences, some of which may be in opposition. The growth cone must therefore interpret and integrate inputs and choose an appropriate final response. Moreover, this may not be a simple additive procedure because, as noted in the chapter by Davies and colleagues, each signal may well alter the response to others. Finally, individual growth cones may react differently to the same set of signals. Detection will occur only when there is an appropriate match between the signals and the specific complement of receptor or recognition molecules with which each growth cone is endowed (chapters by Letourneau, Schachner, and Raper et al.). Furthermore, the same input may in different growth cones lead to generation of alternative second messengers and, consequently, different functional responses.

The existence of multiple extrinsic influences on growth cones leads to an additional theme, namely, that environmental influences on a given growth cone may not be constant but may change over time and position during development. The biological relevance of this important point is further developed in the following set of chapters relating to growth cones in intact systems.

GROWTH CONE GUIDANCE

A major unifying goal of the work presented in this set of contributions is to understand how environmental cues direct growth cones to their targets. A recurrent conclusion expressed here is that Nature has devised a variety of strategies for pathfinding and that this is reflected in the multiplicity of signals to which growth cones respond. Several key themes on this topic within these chapters seem especially noteworthy.

Extracellular Substrate: Opposing Influences of Permissive Versus Nonpermissive Adhesion and of Stimulation Versus Repulsion

A major guidance mechanism presented in several chapters here (chapters by Letourneau, Schachner, Raper et al., and Baier and Bonhoeffer) as well as in many of those in the following sections is based on the observations that growth cones locomote on cellular and extracellular substrates to which they favorably adhere and do not advance on substrates to which they poorly adhere. The consequence of this is that pathways may be specified by their content of appropriate adhesion molecules. A related theme that has been developed during the past several years is that substrates are also endowed with molecules (apart from those involved in adhesion) that either stimulate or inhibit/repulse growth cone advancement (chapters by Raper et al. and Baier and Bonhoeffer). Thus, the extracellular substrate may present the growth cone with several opposing types of cues. As noted above and emphasized in chapters by Letourneau and Raper and co-workers, this permits differential guidance in that one growth cone's meat may be another's poison. Furthermore, this opposition of activities permits the fine control afforded by a "push–pull" mechanism. Finally, these chapters review for us the impressive and exciting advances in identification and characterization of the molecules that underlie these activities.

Soluble Trophic Signals

Another principle found in these chapters is that growth cones may be steered by responding in an all-or-nothing manner to the local presence or absence of soluble trophic factors. As reviewed here in the chapter by Phelan and colleagues, at least in some cases, growth cones persist and function only when provided with appropriate trophic factors such as NGF. Thus guidance could occur when growth cone activity is permitted in zones containing a threshold level of factor but not in zones lacking the factor.

Gradients and Boundaries: Tropic Signals

Though Cajal's chemotropic hypothesis may not explain all aspects of neural specificity, several chapters here serve to reinforce the potential importance of gradients in guiding growth cones. For example, experiments presented in the chapters by Poo and Quillan and by Baier and Bonhoeffer convincingly demonstrate that growth cones can sense and respond to astonishingly small gradients, at least under experimental conditions. This is complemented by Lumsden's chapter, which provides several compelling examples of "chemotactic" guidance. It is of further significance that experiments in these chapters encompass gradients generated over both short and relatively long distances and of both soluble and bound molecules. Another aspect of the potential importance of gradients and boundaries is embodied in the observation reported in the chapter by Baier and Bonhoeffer that a molecule may be repulsive to growth cones when presented at a boundary but permissive to neurite outgrowth when no other choice is presented.

Effects of Growth Cones on Their Environment

Although most of these chapters concentrate on regulation of growth cones by external signals, several instances are provided in which growth cones release substances (proteases—chapter by Seeds et al.; neurotransmitters—chapter by Poo and Quillan), which in turn may affect their surroundings. This raises the prospect that guidance may involve mutual and perhaps interactive communication between growth cones and their environment.

MOLECULAR MECHANISMS OF RESPONSE TO ENVIRONMENTAL CUES

Another major concern in this section is to understand how external signals lead to intracellular events that in turn modulate growth cone behavior. The chapter by Davies and colleagues considers how Ca^{2+} may mediate growth cone responses to neurotransmitters and other agents, and the chapter by Poo and Quillan points to a potential role for cyclic AMP, a second messenger for certain neurotransmitters and hormones, in directing growth cone navigation. Although there has been much study of the signaling pathways used by growth factors and neurotransmitters, relatively little has been known about mediation of responses to cell–cell and cell–substrate interactions. Model studies related in the chapter by Schachner point to a variety of second-messenger pathways that may be activated via cell recognition molecules. One additional important mechanistic aspect touched on in several of the chapters is how changes in second messengers lead to functional alteration of growth cone properties. Presumably, elements of the growth cone such as those considered in the previous section must ultimately be affected, but the means and consequences of this are unclear. Suggestions raised here include changes in function brought about by regulation of local kinase activities and/or by alterations in intracelluar Ca^{2+} levels. Clearly, this emerging topic will be an important subject for future investigation.

The reader will no doubt appreciate that this group of chapters revolves around experiments performed primarily with *in vitro* models. It will thus be illuminating to consider them in the context of the following sections, which deal with growth cones in developing and adult organisms. For instance, do the activities and mechanisms described here seem appropriate to explain growth cone behavior *in vivo*? In several cases, it is gratifying to note that there is, in fact, a good correspondence between the principles suggested by observations with intact systems and those worked out *in vitro*. Do the *in vivo* observations indicate that additional types of environmental cues must be considered? Most important, what additional types of experiments can be performed with intact organisms to verify the hypotheses developed from *in vitro* experiments and vice versa? Cajal offered the opinion that the mechanisms responsible for specific neural connectivity constituted one of the deep mysteries of life. Perhaps they are now somewhat less mysterious for us, but they are certainly no less deep.

REFERENCE

1. Ramón y Cajal, S. *Recollections of my life*. Cambridge, Massachusetts: M.I.T. Press, 1937.

The Nerve Growth Cone, edited by P. C. Letourneau,
S. B. Kater, and E. R. Macagno, Raven Press, Ltd.,
New York © 1992.

12

Autonomous Activities of the Neuronal Growth Cone

Lauren Davis, Vincent Rehder, and Stanley B. Kater

*Program in Neuronal Growth and Development,
Department of Anatomy and Neurobiology, Colorado State University,
Fort Collins, Colorado 80523*

Each unique environment and developmental state presents the neuronal growth cone with a complex set of information. We have studied how different neurons at various developmental states can integrate selected signals into information that guides the generation of neuronal form. One of our primary questions concerns the degree of autonomy that the growth cone has from other components of the nerve cell. Our working hypothesis is that individual growth cones are largely independent from their cell body in their formulation of appropriate responses to environmental cues.

In experimental situations, information may be presented to the entire cell, as for example, when a cultured neuron is bathed in neurotransmitter. *In vivo*, however, complex cues undoubtedly impinge simultaneously to spatially separated parts of a developing neuron. We have asked how regions remote from the cell body use both local environmental information as well as information describing the developmental state of the cell as a whole. A schematic diagram illustrating some of the problems encountered by a growth cone integrating both local and global information is shown in Fig. 1. Neurites from a single cell extend into different environments, exposing each growth cone to a particular set of signals. A local signal may elicit responses within only a small subset of the growth cones of a given neuron. Additionally, a growth cone may be able to relay information about a local signal to the cell body. Such information may be disseminated throughout the cell, and thus a local environmental cue could have effects throughout the neuron.

The strongest support for the postulated ability of a growth cone to detect and respond to local signals would be if a growth cone could function in the complete absence of input from the cell body. Indeed, experimentally isolated growth cones can survive (8,11,25). The survival of an isolated growth cone indicates the presence of at least some of the machinery necessary for independent function and suggests that some growth cone events within intact cells may be accomplished

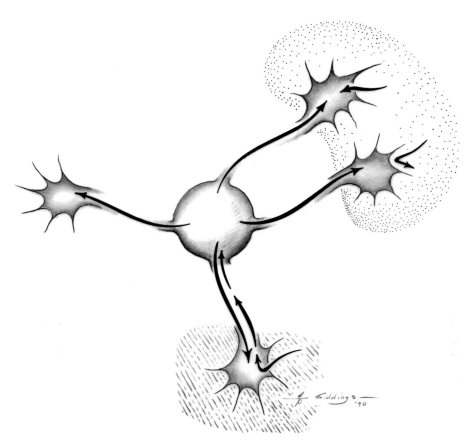

FIG. 1. Growth cones respond independently to environmental cues. This schematic diagram depicts a neuron whose neurites extend into different environments (i.e., cross-hatched, speckled, or plain). Cues in each environment affect only those growth cones that are exposed and receptive to a given signal; thus, information from a particular environment may be detected by some growth cones (arrow entering growth cones in speckled or cross-hatched environments), but the same information may not be detected by another growth cone (arrow from speckled environment deflected away from the growth cone). When information is detected by a growth cone, a local response may be elicited within the growth cone. In addition, information may be relayed from the growth cone into the cell body (arrows pointing from the cross-hatched environment toward the cell body via the neurite). Information may also be relayed from the cell body throughout the neuron (arrows from the cell body pointing toward the periphery).

through autonomous activities of individual growth cones. The focus of recent studies in our laboratory has been to determine the functional capabilities of isolated growth cones. The aim of this chapter is to present information from our *in vitro* experiments that bear on the degree of autonomy that the growth cone may employ *in situ*.

The first evidence that remote cellular regions can function independently was reported by Levi (15) in 1926, who demonstrated that nerve tips that had been severed from explants of chick spinal ganglia grown in plasma clots survive for up to a few hours. In 1953, Hughes (12) observed and measured the advance of nerve tips severed from neuronal explants and provided the first evidence that isolated neurites grow at the same rate as attached neurites. Both of these studies demonstrated that some activities of neurites are not dependent on input from the cell body. However, the clearest evidence that growth cones have the capacity for independent survival was presented by Shaw and Bray in 1977, who showed that single growth cones isolated from cultured dissociated chick sensory ganglion cells survive and remain motile in culture for up to 5 hr. The *in vitro* experiments by Shaw and Bray (25) demonstrated clearly that growth cones can function, to at least some extent, without any input from the cell body. More recently, Harris and colleages (9) have shown that retinal axons that were isolated from their cell bodies would continue to grow for up to 3 hr *in vivo* and were capable of recognizing and arborizing within the tectum. Taken together, these experiments using both *in vivo* and *in vitro* preparations provided the impetus for our current investigations on the independence of growth cone function.

We have studied the large growth cones of cultured identified neurons of the snail *Helisoma* and further extended these studies to the growth cones of cultured embryonic rat hippocampal neurons. The advantage to using *Helisoma* neurons is that different neurons can be individually identified, and the morphological, behavioral, and physiological properties of the growth cones of these identified neurons have been well-characterized. The hippocampal neurons offer the additional possibility of examining two very different classes of growth cones, those of axons and dendrites, on the same neuron.

The large growth cones (up to 50 μm across) of cultured *Helisoma* neurons can be readily isolated from the rest of the cell by transecting the neurite immediately proximal to the growth cone with the tip of a micromanipulator-controlled glass micropipette. *Helisoma* neuronal growth cones can survive for at least 3 days in culture (8). Isolated growth cones remain motile and either maintain a flattened morphology with a ruffling membrane, or thin out considerably and resemble fine, branched neurites tipped with flattened, ruffled areas (see Fig. 2).

Helisoma neurons in cell culture undergo a transition that may mimic that in development: At a given time (e.g., after 3–5 days in culture) all the growth cones on a neuron change from their characteristic motile form to a distinct nonmotile form with a club-shaped, phase-bright appearance. One of the major differences between isolated and attached growth cones is that only attached growth cones will

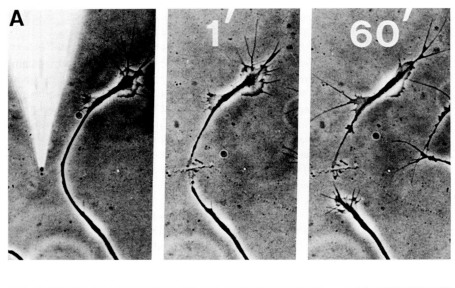

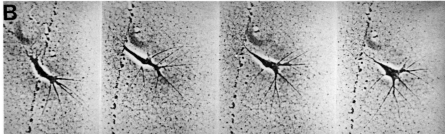

FIG. 2. Isolated growth cones are viable and motile. **A:** Growth cones can be physically isolated by transecting the neurite with the tip of a micropipette attached to a micromanipulator. The pipette tip is shown in close proximity to the neurite before transection (*left panel*). *Middle* and *right panel* show the isolated growth cone 1 and 60 min after transection. **B:** Isolated growth cones are motile. This series of photomicrographs shows a previously isolated growth cone moving over the growth substrate. The *scratch* can be used as a point of reference to demonstrate growth cone advance.

attain a stable state, whereas isolated growth cones continue to grow and never convert to a stable morphology (P. Guthrie and S. Kater, *unpublished observations*). This observation suggests that in an intact neuron, global signals that are likely to have emanated from the cell body instruct all the distant growth cones to initiate transformation to the stable state. This kind of centrifugal signaling is characteristic of the already well-defined processes of intracellular transport and, to some degree electrical information flow, that are now well-defined for neuronal cell biology.

GROWTH CONE AS AN INTEGRATOR OF COMPLEX
ENVIRONMENTAL CUES

One of our first examples that growth cones could respond to local stimuli came from the focal application of serotonin to individual growth cones; *Helisoma* neurons B19 exhibit reduced filopodial probing, a decrease in filopodial number, a reduction in the surface area of the growth cone, and inhibited neuritic elongation (10). This effect was neuron-specific, with growth cones from neurons such as B5 completely unaffected by serotonin. It is noteworthy that experiments *in situ* on *Helisoma* embryos demonstrate that serotonin represents a stimulus that a growth cone would normally encounter in its natural environment (7).

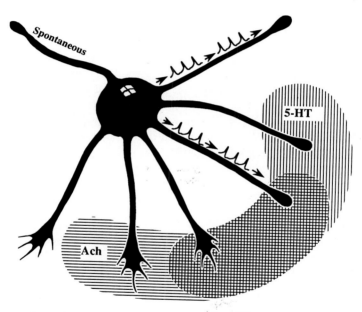

FIG. 3. Neuronal growth can be regulated by the integration of information from multiple stimuli. In the absence of stimuli, growth cones advance at a characteristic speed, exhibiting typical lamellipodial and filopodial behavior (growth cone at *bottom left*). After several days in culture, growth cones spontaneously assume a "stable state," club-shaped morphology, evidenced by loss of lamellipodia and filopodia (growth cone at *top left*). Termination of outgrowth can also be achieved by eliciting action potentials (growth cone at *top right*) or by application of serotonin (second growth cone from top). Although application of ACh alone does not affect growth cone behavior (bottom growth cone), when applied together with serotonin, ACh can negate the serotonin-induced inhibition of outgrowth (bottom right growth cone). If action potentials are elicited as a third stimulus, outgrowth is immediately terminated (third growth cone from top), demonstrating that different classes of stimuli are integrated and subsequently transduced into appropriate growth cone behavior.

In a subsequent study we expanded on these observations from the snail and found that the excitatory neurotransmitter glutamate also produces highly specific effects on the growth cones of cultured rat hippocampal neurons. The motility of dendritic growth cones is completely inhibited by low concentrations of glutamate, whereas growth cones on the axons of the same neurons are unaffected (16). Such findings have reinforced the idea that neurotransmitters may well act as signals to growth cones *in situ*. Furthermore, these findings suggest two key aspects of environmental growth cone signals: (a) local environmental signals may be presented to only a subset of growth cones, and (b) the capability for a growth cone to detect a signal is dependent on whether receptive devices, such as receptors and channels, are functional within a particular growth cone.

In situ, several cues may impinge simultaneously on the growth cone. We have gained some insight into the integrative capacity of growth cones through the simultaneous exposure of growth cones *in vitro* to pairs of neurotransmitters (Fig. 3). For example, acetylcholine (ACh) has no obvious effect when presented alone to a *Helisoma* B19 growth cone. However, in combination with serotonin application, ACh can completely negate the usual outgrowth-inhibiting effects of serotonin; motility continues as if no environmental information had been present (19). The inhibitory transmitter for rat hippocampal neurons, GABA, has essentially identical effects in that system; GABA applied with its potentiator diazepam will block the glutamate-induced inhibition of dendritic growth (17).

Neurotransmitters probably act on growth cones through changes in membrane potential. Both ACh and GABA are regarded as inhibitory neurotransmitters in their respective systems. Furthermore, clamping the membrane potential of *Helisoma* neurons near rest by electrophysiological methods negates the growth-retarding effects of serotonin (20). Thus, the effects of this class of environmental cues may well be exclusively expressed by alterations on membrane potential.

INTRACELLULAR CALCIUM LEVELS AND CONTROL OF GROWTH CONE BEHAVIOR

Several lines of evidence have led to the conclusion that environmental cues can inhibit growth cone behaviors by inducing rises in intracellular calcium. For example, direct observation of calcium levels has demonstrated that serotonin causes a calcium rise in the growth cones of neurons B19 but not B5 (4,22). Additionally, action potentials inhibit outgrowth in all the neurons that we have investigated (3,5,20), and action potentials also produce a rise in calcium in each cell type (4). Finally, the transmitter ACh, which negates the serotonin-induced inhibition of B19 growth cone motility, also inhibits the calcium rise induced by serotonin (19). Essentially identical results are observed in hippocampal neurons on exposure to glutamate and glutamate plus GABA (17); these experiments have provided an additional basis for suggesting a major role for intracellular calcium in the transduction of specific environmental cues into changes in growth cone behavior.

We have begun to examine additional links in the chain of intracellular messengers that lead to changes in growth cone behavior. In particular, our recent results indicate a role for calpains in transducing the effects of rises in intracellular calcium evoked by agents such as glutamate. Application of the calpain inhibitor EST completely negates the effects of raised calcium levels on the growth cones of hippocampal neurons (26). Dendrites continue to elongate despite rises in intracellular calcium when EST is present. In a similar set of experiments, Cohan and colleagues found that pharmacological inhibition of calmodulin in *Helisoma* neurons completely blocked the effects of serotonin on these growth cones (23). These findings on potential roles for calpains and calmodulin suggest that the intracellular path for calcium-mediated control in neurons may well have several bifurcations, as well as several different effects on growth cone behavior.

OBSERVATIONS ON AUTONOMOUS GROWTH CONE FUNCTION

Isolated Growth Cones Resemble Intact Growth Cones

Many aspects of isolated growth cone behavior are apparently equivalent to intact growth cones. Freeze-fracture analyses of the membranes of isolated growth cones and growth cones still attached to the parent neuron revealed that the density and size distributions of intramembrane particles are similar in both. (8). Furthermore, isolated growth cones exhibit many electrophysiological properties that are typical of intact growth cones (Fig. 4). Individual identified *Helisoma* neurons display a characteristic action potential waveform that serves as a unique "fingerprint" of the identified neuron. Growth cones that have been isolated from identified neurons display the same characteristic action potential waveform as the parent cell body, suggesting that the relative densities of ionic channels contributing to the action potential are the same in isolated growth cones as in the parent neuron (8; and see Fig. 4). The voltage-clamp currents of isolated growth cones are similar to the voltage-clamp currents of parent neurons, with the exception that an identifiable A-current is absent in isolated growth cones. Because intact growth cones were not analyzed, it is impossible to determine whether the absence of the A current is a characteristic of all growth cones or only isolated growth cones. Nevertheless, these studies do demonstrate that there are many similarities in the electrophysiological properties of isolated growth cones and their parent neurons.

Isolated Growth Cones Respond to Serotonin

The isolated growth cone preparation provides the most direct information on autonomous function. Isolated B19 growth cones respond to serotonin in a manner similar to intact B19 growth cones; filopodia and lamellipodia retract and growth cone motility ceases (11; and see Fig. 5). After serotonin application is halted, isolated growth cones flatten out to regain their previous morphology and resume

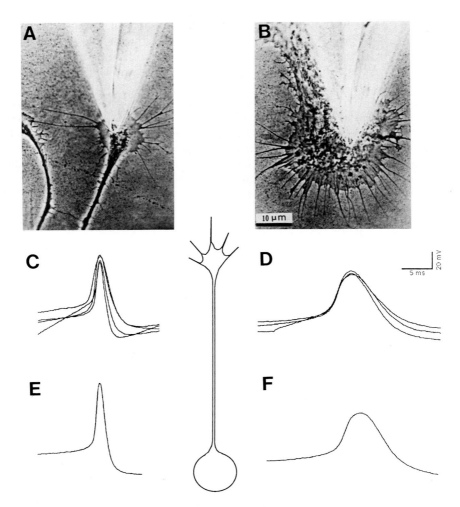

FIG. 4. Growth cones from different identified *Helisoma* neurons have characteristic properties. Photomicrographs of growth cones of a neuron B19 (**A**) and a neuron B5 (**B**). Patch-
clamp recordings can be made from attached and isolated growth cones (note the patch electrode on the central region of each growth cone). B5 growth cones are significantly larger than
those of B19 and have more filopodia. B19 growth cone filopodia are significantly longer than
those of B5. Action potentials can be evoked and recorded in growth cones (*upper traces*) and
cell bodies (*lower traces*) of cells B19 (**C** and **E**) and B5 (**D** and **F**). Action potentials of cell
bodies and growth cones are similar for each neuron type, indicating that isolated growth
cones retain membrane properties of the parent neuron. Different cell types, however, can be
characterized by cell-specific action potential forms.

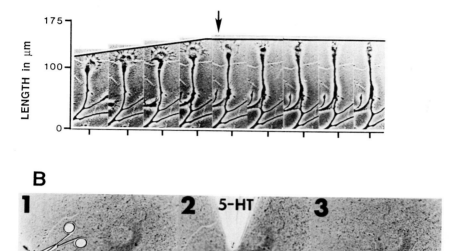

FIG. 5. Serotonin inhibits outgrowth in neuron B19 growth cones. **A:** Growth cones, connected via their neurites to the cell body (out of field of view), advance at a characteristic rate (note constant slope). On application of serotonin (*arrow*), outgrowth ceases (note decrease in slope). Previously motile growth cones lose lamellipodia and filopodia and become phase-bright, assuming a club-shaped morphology. Photomicrographs are displayed at frame intervals of 40 min. **B:** After isolation (indicated by scissors), growth cones remain motile and have lamellipodia and filopodia indistinguishable from attached growth cones (1). On focal pipette application of serotonin, growth cone motility is inhibited and filopodial number decreases (2). This inhibition is reversible, because filopodia reappear and growth cone motility resumes after the removal of the serotonin containing micropipette (3). The effect of serotonin on isolated growth cones indicates that serotonin is a signal detected and processed by the growth cone proper. Calibration bar: 10 μm.

their formerly active behavior. Because isolated growth cones respond reversibly to serotonin application for at least 2 days after isolation and because this response is indistinguishable from responses of intact growth cones, it is clear that both the mechanisms responsible for detecting this stimulus and the machinery necessary for producing the behavioral responses are present within the growth cone.

CURRENT RESEARCH DIRECTIONS

Our current research focuses on the growth cone's intrinsic capability to (a) regulate $[Ca]_i$ and (b) independently synthesize proteins.

Calcium Homeostasis Within Isolated and Attached Growth Cones

We have tested the ability of growth cones to maintain normal levels of free intracellular calcium ($[Ca]_i$) in the face of experimentally changing calcium influx and efflux rates (24). For changes in calcium levels to provide information, deviations from a constant baseline level must occur. Intracellular calcium levels must be restored to terminate a signal and to make cells responsive to subsequent stimuli. $[Ca]_i$ is controlled by several mechanisms. It can be lowered by the combined actions of Ca-ATPases located in the plasma membrane and in the membrane of the endoplasmic reticulum, by the Na/Ca exchanger, and the mitochondria. $[Ca]_i$ is increased by influx through Ca channels in the plasma membrane, as well as by release from intracellular stores (1,2,18).

When an intact neuron is experimentally challenged, the changes in calcium levels seen in growth cones represent the sum of the regulatory mechanisms of the whole neuron. To gain insight into the calcium homeostatic properties of the growth cone itself, we have examined isolated growth cones and compared these with their intact counterparts. To perturb the $[Ca]_i$, the calcium influx into the growth cone was either continuously decreased or increased experimentally, and the compensatory changes in the $[Ca]_i$ monitored using the flourescent calcium indicator fura-2.

Elimination of Calcium Influx

Influx of calcium may be negated by changing the extracellular medium to calcium-free conditions (see Fig. 6). In calcium-free medium, $[Ca]_i$ decreases immediately in both intact and isolated growth cones, demonstrating the existence of a "leak" calcium current under basal conditions. However, this decrease is transient and $[Ca]_i$ is restored within 45 to 60 min in the continued absence of extracellular calcium. The restoration is most likely due to release from intracellular stores because influx is not possible under these conditions. The use of 10-mM $CoCl_2$ to block Ca channels leads to a comparable time course of changes in $[Ca]_i$. Because attached and isolated growth cones perform almost equally well when challenged by

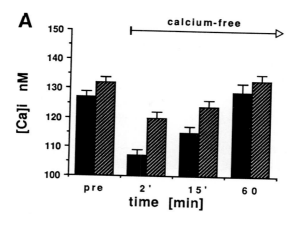

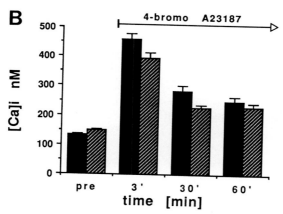

FIG. 6. Compensatory responses of attached and isolated growth cones to perturbations of their $[Ca]_i$. Ability of growth cones to homeostatically regulate their $[Ca]_i$ was tested by experimentally decreasing (**A**) or increasing (**B**) the calcium influx into growth cones. Isolated growth cones compensated for changes in influx in a similar manner to attached growth cones. The duration of stimulus presentation is indicated by the *horizontal bar* above each graph. $[Ca]_i$ was monitored using the fluorescent calcium indicator, fura 2. **A:** Under normal conditions there is a calcium influx into the growth cone. This calcium influx can be halted by changing the medium (4.1-mM Ca) to calcium-free conditions (nominally zero calcium with 0.5-mM EGTA added). Note rapid decrease in both attached (*solid bars*) and isolated growth cones (*hatched bars*). Subsequent restoration to pretreatment levels is most likely caused by calcium release from intracellular stores. **B:** Calcium influx is increased by application of the calcium ionophore 4-bromo A23187 (0.75 μM) to attached (*solid bars*) and isolated growth cones (*hatched bars*). Because of steep calcium gradient across the plasma membrane, $[Ca]_i$ rapidly rises to peak values about 3 min after application. However, after about 30 min in the continuous presence of ionophore (i.e., continuously elevated calcium influx), $[Ca]_i$ is reduced significantly from its peak value, indicating an increase in cellular calcium clearance mechanisms. Data shown are means ± SEM.

this treatment, three conclusions can be drawn: (a) A "leak" calcium current exists in both attached and isolated growth cones; (b) intracellular stores are capable of a compensatory release of calcium for the restoration process; (c) growth cones have the equivalent of a "calcium sensor" and effectively monitor the deviation of $[Ca]_i$ from its "setpoint."

Increases in Calcium Influx

Our experiments testing the growth cone's ability to compensate for a continuous increase in calcium employ the calcium ionophore 4-bromo A23187 (see Fig. 6). Both attached and isolated growth cones show a large, initial peak in $[Ca]_i$. Despite the high values reached, $[Ca]_i$ is subsequently reduced, with clearance mechanisms for calcium overcoming the influx produced by the ionophore. Restoration under these circumstances is incomplete, however, because $[Ca]_i$ remains on a plateau significantly above pretreatment levels. Isolated and attached growth cones perform about equally well, again indicating that important extrusion and sequestering mechanisms are present and functional in the isolated growth cone.

Taken together, these experiments demonstrate that isolated growth cones maintain many features of calcium homeostasis observed in attached growth cones, despite the fact that antero- and retrograde transport of information and material is impossible. Although important questions remain, such as how energy and material is provided, it is clear that growth cones should be viewed as at least partially autonomous structures, being able to maintain their functional integrity for long periods after isolation.

Protein Synthesis Within Isolated Growth Cones

In neurons, as in other cells, the components of most cellular machinery are synthesized in the cell body and transported to destinations throughout the cell. In neurons, the task of selective transport is likely to be more difficult than in other cell types because of the inherent structural and functional complexity of their discrete axonal and dendritic compartments. In addition, the materials necessary to construct presynaptic and postsynaptic specializations must be distributed to the appropriate sites. Moreover, many components of the synaptic machinery undoubtedly need to be replaced or modified, thus necessitating the selective delivery of materials during the course of a neuron's lifetime.

The capacity for synthesis of relevant molecules near the site of utilization would allow an efficient method of production of new components in response to an appropriate local stimulus. An intriguing suggestion that proteins are synthesized in remote regions is provided by the demonstration that polyribosomes are selectively localized beneath synaptic sites in CNS neurons and that RNA is transported into dendrites by a highly regulated active transport mechanism (see ref. 27). The most direct demonstration of protein synthesis in remote cellular regions would be if protein synthesis could occur in isolation from the cell body.

We have examined the incorporation of radiolabeled amino acids into proteins in isolated *Helisoma* growth cones (6). Cultures of *Helisoma* neurons were briefly pulse-labeled with ^{3}H-leucine after growth cones were isolated by transection from the cell body. After pulse-labeling, cultures were fixed with paraformaldehyde to remove the free ^{3}H-leucine, leaving the bound ^{3}H-proteins in the cell, and then processed for autoradiography. Autoradiographs reveal labeling over isolated growth cones, suggesting that amino acids are taken up and incorporated in isolated growth cones (see Fig. 7). Because the growth cones were transected before pulse-labeling, it is impossible that labeled proteins could have been synthesized in the cell body and transported into the growth cone. Labeling is inhibited when cultures are pulse-labeled in the presence of inhibitors of protein synthesis in eukaryotic systems.

These data suggest that proteins are synthesized within growth cones via a eukaryotic ribosomal mechanism. At this point one can only speculate on the role of protein synthesis within growth cones. Perhaps such proteins are destined for use within the growth cone. This would imply that the structural or functional components of the growth cone can be modified independently of components in other

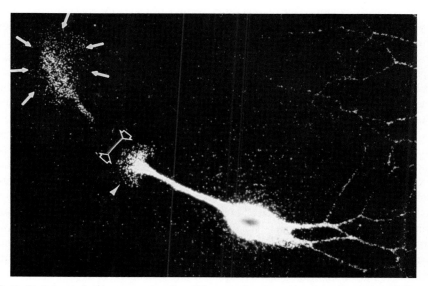

FIG. 7. Protein synthesis occurs locally within growth cones. Neurites of cultured *Helisoma* neurons were transected (*between open arrows*) several hours before pulse-labeling with ^{3}H-leucine (30 min) to yield cultures containing isolated growth cones. Autoradiographs prepared from pulse-labeled cultures reveal the site of synthesis of ^{3}H-proteins. Silver grains, which appear white in this darkfield photomicrograph, are located over the isolated growth cone (surrounded by *arrows*) as well as over the parent neuron. Because the growth cone was isolated before pulse-labeling, ^{3}H-proteins result from protein synthesis locally in the growth cone. In contrast, ^{3}H-proteins throughout the rest of the cell and in the attached growth cone (*arrowhead*) could result from locally synthesized proteins or from ^{3}H-proteins that were transported from the cell body.

parts of the neuron. This raises the further possibility that protein synthesis in remote regions may be regulated by events occurring specific to that region of the neuron.

In the context of the scenario presented in Fig. 1, a local signal could regulate protein synthesis within a single, independent growth cone. The materials that are synthesized in response to a local signal might enable that growth cone to modify its response to further signals. Additionally, synthesized materials might be retrogradely transported to the cell body as a way of signaling the cell body of events within the distant growth cone.

FUTURE DIRECTIONS

Many laboratories have recognized the need to define more precisely the molecular terrain over which neurons must grow (e.g., see chapters in this volume by Baier and Bonhoeffer, Letourneau, Raper et al., and Schachner). Our laboratory has investigated the role of second messengers in transducing the effects of environmental cues into meaningful changes in growth cone behavior (see Fig. 8). Clearly, intracellular calcium levels play a prominent role in governing the behavior of neuronal growth cones. Equally clear is that other secondary (e.g., cyclicAMP; see chapter by Poo and Quillan in this volume) and even tertiary molecules (e.g., the calpains) are in the chain of information between an environmental stimulus and a particular growth cone response. A major task for the future will be to link the effects of specific messengers into a comprehensive picture of the control of growth cone behavior. An understanding of how environmental information affects particular intracellular pathways will be critical to our understanding of the complex responses that are characteristic of growth cones.

There are many steps between the initiation of neuritic outgrowth and the formation of a functional connection. As elongation proceeds, the growth cone becomes more distant from the cell body and the response time for information flow grows longer. It has therefore seemed likely to us that the growth cone is endowed with a considerable potential for autonomous function. Indeed, in isolation it is!

One major new finding reviewed in this chapter is that protein synthesis can occur within the growth cone proper. We currently have no information on the control of protein synthesis within growth cones. Each growth cone may be capable of reacting individually to discrete environmental stimuli with the synthesis of unique proteins. We plan to investigate the potential for regulation of remote protein synthesis. A major area for future research will be to determine precisely how specific environmental cues are transduced through particular second messengers and, thus, affect protein synthesis. Equally important is the specification of the protein subspecies that are affected and how these, in fact, contribute to (a) the behavior of the growth cone and (b) to the behavior of the neuron as a whole.

Another major new finding is that growth cones contain the homeostatic machinery necessary to regulate $[Ca]_i$. This autonomous capability could enable a growth

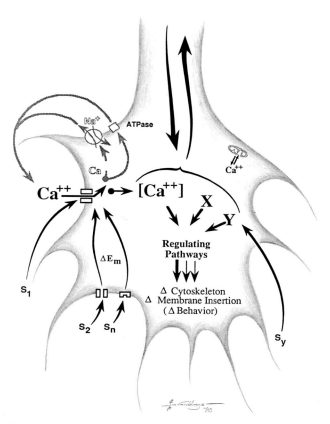

FIG. 8. Control of neuronal growth cone behavior. Local and global signals may affect known (intracellular calcium) and as yet unknown other second-messenger systems (X,Y). $[Ca^{2+}]$ plays an important role in the regulation of neuronal growth, because many aspects of cytoskeletal dynamics are sensitive to changes in intracellular calcium. A variety of different stimuli (S_1-S_y) impinge onto the neuronal growth cone. Stimuli may modulate $[Ca]_i$ directly by affecting voltage-dependent calcium channels (S_1) or indirectly by depolarizing the growth cone via voltage- (S_2) or ligand-gated channels (S_n); other stimuli (S_y) may affect alternative regulating pathways yet to be determined. Intracellular calcium concentration within the growth cone is under homeostatic control of several other mechanisms, of which only the Na^+/Ca^{2+} exchanger of plasma membrane, Ca^{2+}-ATPase, and mitochondria are shown. Information flow may be bidirectional between the cell body and growth cone (*long arrows* in neurite); information that is locally received or integrated by the growth cone can be relayed to the cell body, and information can be centrifugally disseminated.

cone to initiate mechanisms that are sensitive to $[Ca]_i$, and may indicate that the regulation of other second messengers is also independently controlled by the growth cone. Future experiments will explore the type of local signals that can alter the $[Ca]_i$ in isolated growth cones, as well as determine the interplay of mechanisms regulating $[Ca]_i$. We have also begun to ask which of the several different subsystems that contribute to regulating calcium levels within the growth cone can themselves be developmentally regulated (21).

Probably the hardest task for the future will be to link information from a variety of experimental designs and perturbations to understand how specific components of the growth cone *interact* with one another. One cannot fail to appreciate that each growth cone is probably integrating multiple internal and external cues. Although individual growth cones are capable of autonomous activities, the neuron as a whole must be apprised of such activity in remote growth cones. A likely area for future research will focus on the coupling of autonomous and coordinate functions of growth cones with the parent neuron. Finally, we must investigate how each neuron integrates information from all its growth cones into a functional unit and ultimately becomes incorporated into a neuronal circuit.

In addition to developmental processes, we must also keep in mind the potential roles of the growth cone in neural plasticity and in readapting neural circuitry to new functions. It seems very likely that the processes we unravel in looking at the behavior of growth cones in development will bear significantly on the potential of adult circuitry to react to events in the mature nervous system. For example, are there discrete transformations between the growth cone and the synaptic terminal into which it develops? Can such transformations be reversed and the synaptic terminal revert to a motile growth cone? Surely such questions will occupy at least one more generation of neuroscientists.

REFERENCES

1. Blaustein MP. Calcium transport and buffering in neurons. *Trends Neurosci* 1988;11:438–443.
2. Carafoli E. Intracellular calcium homeostasis. *Annu Rev Biochem* 1987;56:395–433.
3. Cohan CS. Frequency-dependent and cell-specific effects of electrical activity on growth cone movements of cultured *Helisoma* neurons. *J Neurobiol* 1990;21:400–413.
4. Cohan CS, Conner JA, Kater SB. Electrically and chemically mediated increases in intracellular calcium in neuronal growth cones. *J Neurosci* 1987;7:3588–3599.
5. Cohan CS, Kater SB. Suppression of neurite elongation and growth cone motility by electrical activity. *Science* 1986;232:1638–1640.
6. Davis L, Kater SB. Local protein synthesis within isolated growth cones of cultured snail neurons (*Abstr*). *Soc Neurosci Abstr* 1990;16:961.
7. Goldberg JI, Kater SB. Expression and function of the neurotransmitter serotonin during development of the *Helisoma* nervous system. *Dev Biol* 1989;131:483–495.
8. Guthrie PB, Lee RE, Kater SB. A comparison of neuronal growth cone and cell body membrane: electrophysiological and ultrastructural properties. *J Neurosci* 1989;9:3596–3605.
9. Harris WA, Holt CE, Bonhoeffer F. Retinal axons with and without their somata, growing to and arborizing in the tectum of *Xenopus* embryos: a time-lapse video study of single fibres *in vivo*. *Development* 1987;101:123–133.
10. Haydon PG, Cohan CS, McCobb DP, Miller HR, Kater SB. Neuron-specific growth cone properties as seen in identified neurons of *Helisoma*. *J Neurosci Res* 1985;13:135–147.

11. Haydon PG, McCobb DP, Kater SB. Serotonin selectively inhibits growth cone motility and synaptogenesis of specific identified neurons. *Science* 1984;226:561–564.

12. Hughes A. The growth of embryonic neurites: a study on cultures of chick neural tissues. *J Anat* 1953;87:150–162.

13. Kater SB, Guthrie PB. The neuronal growth cone: calcium regulation of presecretory structure. In: Armstrong CM, Oxford GS, eds. *Secretion and its control*. New York: Rockefeller Univ. Press, 1989; 111–122.

14. Kater SB, Guthrie PB, Mills LR. Integration by the neuronal growth cone: a continuum from neuroplasticity to neuropathology. In: P. Colman et al., eds. *Progress in brain research. Molecular and cellular mechanisms of neural plasticity in aging and Alzheimer's disease*. 1990.

15. Levi G. Richerche sperimentali sovra elementi nervosi sviluppati "in vitro." *Arch Exp Zellforsch* 1926;2:244–272.

16. Mattson MP, Dou P, Kater SB. Outgrowth regulating actions of glutamate in isolated hippocampal pyramidal neurons. *J Neurosci* 1988;8:2087–2100.

17. Mattson MP, Kater SB. Excitatory and inhibitory neurotransmitters in the generation and degeneration of hippocampal neuroarchitecture. *Brain Res* 1989;478:337–348.

18. McBurney RN, Neering IR. Neuronal calcium homeostasis. *Trends Neurosci* 1987;10:164–169.

19. McCobb DP, Cohan CS, Connor JA, Kater SB. Interactive effects of serotonin and acetylcholine on neurite elongation. *Neuron* 1988;1:377–385.

20. McCobb DP, Kater SB. Membrane voltage and neurotransmitter regulation of neuronal growth cone motility. *Dev Biol* 1988;130:599–609.

21. Mills LR, Kater SB. Neuron-specific and state-specific differences in calcium homeostasis regulate the generation and degeneration of neuronal architecture. *Neuron* 1990;4:149–163.

22. Murrain M, Murphy AD, Mills LR, Kater SB. Neuron-specific modulation by serotonin of regenerative outgrowth and intracellular calcium within the CNS of *Helisoma trivolvis*. *J Neurobiol* 1990; 21:611–618.

23. Polak KA, Edelman AM, Wasley JWF, Cohan CS. A novel calmodulin antagonist, CGS9343B, modulates calcium dependent changes in neurite outgrowth and growth cone movements. *J Neurosci* 1991;11:534–542.

24. Rehder V, Jensen JR, Dou P, Kater SB. Calcium homeostasis in an identified neuronal growth cone (*Abstr*). *Soc Neurosci Abstr* 1990;16:457.

25. Shaw G, Bray D. Movement and extension of isolated growth cones. *Exp Cell Res* 1977;104:55–62.

26. Song DK, Mykles DL, Kater SB. Effects of a calpain inhibitor, EST, on calcium ionophore A23187-induced changes in neurite outgrowth in isolated hippocampal pyramidal neurons (*Abstr*). *J Cell Biol Abstr* 1990;3:244a.

27. Steward O, Davis L, Dotti C, Phillips LL, Rao A, Banker G. Protein synthesis and processing in cytoplasmic microdomains beneath postsynaptic sites on CNS neurons: a mechanism for establishing and maintaining a mosaic postsynaptic receptive surface. *J Mol Neurobiol* 1988;2:227–261.

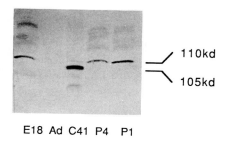

110kd

105kd

E18 Ad C41 P4 P1

FIG. 1. Immunoblot detection of myosin I–cross-reactive species in extracts of embryonic (E) and postnatal (P) rat brain and PC12-C41 cells but not in adult (Ad) rat brain. Immunoreaction employed monoclonal antibody 2.18 (26).

MW of 105 and 110 kDa as candidates for mammalian myosin I. The level of the 105-kDa species significantly increases with NGF treatment, and it is enriched in growth cone fractions prepared by the method of Sobue and Kanda (16). In contrast, the 110-kDa protein is enriched in cell body fractions, and its levels are not increased on NGF treatment. As is characteristic of myosins, these species cosediment with F-actin in the absence but not presence of ATP. Furthermore, the 105- and 110-kDa molecules are also recognized by other antibodies directed to the conserved portion of the myosin head. These features suggest that these are novel forms of vertebrate myosin I. Also consistent with a role for these species in nervous system development is their detectability in embryonic and early postnatal rat brain, where they appear to be more abundant than in adult brain (Fig. 1). These findings thus provide evidence for the presence of NGF-regulatable myosin I isoforms in the mammalian nervous system and reinforce the attractiveness of this species as a participant in growth cone function.

Assessment of Growth Cone–Enriched Preparations

Studies of additional trophic factor–regulated growth cone molecules will be significantly aided by the availability of enriched growth cone fractions. As illustrated above, the Sobue and Kanda preparation appears to be quite promising, at least for PC12 cells. These can potentially provide information that is complementary to that provided by growth cone particles prepared from developing brain (see chapters by Pfenninger et al. and by Gordon-Weeks and Mansfield), particularly because of the homogeneity of the starting population and its responsiveness to NGF.

Because of the potential of this preparation, we have extended its characterization. Both the cell body and growth cone–enriched fractions from PC12 cells were examined by AVEC-DIC microscopy (see below and chapters by Goldberg et al. and by Smith and Jahr). The former consisted of clustered 10-μm cell bodies with distinct nuclei and nucleoli (Fig. 2A). The latter contained mainly very small (<2 μm) particles (Fig. 2B–D). Membranous shafts resembling severed neurites were extremely rare in this fraction, but numerous elaborate particles were seen that bore plasmalemmal spikes and that were morphologically active in the presence of NGF. Biochemical characterization has further confirmed the efficacy of the fractionation and the presence of metabolically active material. SDS-PAGE analysis revealed that nuclear histone proteins are localized to the cell body fraction and that the growth cone fraction is highly enriched in several species. When the growth cone particles were incubated in the presence of ^{32}P-orthophosphate and glucose, radioactivity was incorporated into proteins. This labeling was inhibited by azide, thus indicating that it is accomplished through the metabolic production of ^{32}P-ATP.

The NGF-untreated PC12 cells provide a useful negative control for the growth cone particle isolation procedure. If this technique is valid, very little growth cone material should be obtained from such cells. On a protein basis, the "growth cone" preparation from untreated cells provided a yield that was only 20% of that obtained with treated cells. Moreover, when the preparations were adjusted to contain equal protein levels, the fraction from untreated cells incorporated only 20% as much labeled phosphate. In summary, further experiments support the characterization of the Sobue and Kanda fraction as an enriched source of active NGF-induced growth cone particles. These should be amenable not only to further compositional analysis, but also for studies of acute responses to NGF as discussed below.

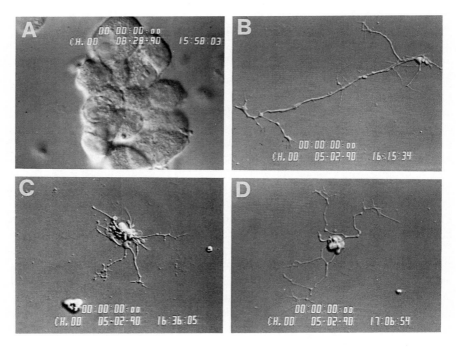

FIG. 2. Examination of PC12 cell body and growth cone particle fractions using AVEC-DIC microscopy. **A:** Cell body fraction, containing clusters of PC12 cell somatas. **B–D:** Examples of growth cone particles that have attached and spread on the substrate.

Future Directions

Current studies of the means by which trophic factors influence growth cone formation are clearly at an initial stage. A major issue for the future is to extend present *in vitro* studies to demonstrate that growth factors also affect growth cone formation during development *in vivo*. If we assume this does occur, questions arise: Which neurotrophic factor(s) regulates growth cone formation by specific neuron types; what is the source of the neurotrophic agents and how do they reach neuroblasts; is growth cone formation by a developing neuron influenced by more than one neurotrophic factor, and if so, are there temporal and spatial differences in presentation of such factors; do different neurotrophic factors exert the same effects on the synthesis/distribution of growth cone components, or does each factor have distinct effects? The past several years have seen a dramatic increase in the types of tools that we have to address these questions. A number of defined factors with neurotrophic activity have been identified, and these are becoming increasingly available from recombinant sources. In addition, antibodies and cDNA probes for many of the factors have been or soon will be produced, and one may look forward to comparable reagents for localizing and interfering with specific growth factor receptors. Despite these advances, there is one major problem that must be dealt with in defining the role of neurotrophic factors in regulating growth cones *in vivo*. That is, it may be difficult to separate trophic factor effects on survival from those on growth cone generation. This may require the identification of agents that maintain neuronal survival but that do not promote the formation of growth cones.

A number of additional important issues remain that can be addressed at least in part with model *in vitro* systems such as the PC12 cell. For instance, what additional growth cone–related molecules are there that undergo regulation of expression/distribution by neurotrophic agents? What are the mechanisms whereby growth factors exert these actions? What are the functions of each of the regulated growth cone species? How are they targeted to the growth cone? Is there a rate-limiting component for growth cone formation, and is it regulated by neurotrophic factors?

LOCAL ACTIONS OF NGF ON GROWTH CONES

Aside from synthetic actions on components that are required for the formation of growth cones, as will be considered in this section, neurotrophic factors exert a second, very different type of role in regulating growth cone function.

Background Review

Among the first demonstrations that neurotrophic agents have local actions on growth cones was the work of Campenot (27,28), in which sympathetic neurons were cultured in a device where cell bodies and distal portions of neurites were exposed to dissimilar media. It was observed that neurites would neither grow nor be retained within a local environment lacking NGF, irrespective of whether the cell body or proximal neurites were provided with the factor. Gundersen and Barrett (29) exposed the tips of cultured sensory neurons to a locally supplied NGF gradient and observed rapid turning of the growth cones toward the highest concentration of NGF. Letourneau (30) plated dissociated neurons on culture dishes possessing a concentration gradient of NGF. The newly formed processes preferentially oriented toward the direction of highest concentration. Gundersen (31) demonstrated a haptotactic action of NGF. The factor was applied along specific "trails" on substrata. Neurons cultured on this substrata extended their neurites only along the areas that were coated with the NGF. Menesini-Chen and colleagues (32) performed an *in vivo* homologue of such experiments by injecting high levels of NGF into the brain. It was observed that under these conditions, peripheral sympathetic axons would turn to, enter, and grow for significant distances within the CNS, toward the site of NGF administration.

The above experiments have been widely interpreted with respect to the possibility that NGF and other trophic factors may provide directional guidance for growing axons. Irrespective of the validity of this view, such findings clearly indicate that in addition to its synthetic influence at the cell body, NGF also exerts local actions on the growth cone. As described below, work from our laboratory has extended and further analyzed these effects.

NGF Withdrawal/Readdition Paradigm

Our initial studies revealed that addition of NGF and other trophic factors to PC12 cells elicits a rapid, transient ruffling response on the cell body (33). To extend these experiments to NGF-pretreated PC12 cells and NGF-requiring cultured sympathetic neurons, the following protocol was developed (34). The cells were grown with NGF to permit establishment of growth cone–tipped neurites. NGF was then withdrawn from the cultures for about 5 hr and thereafter re-added. This short period of NGF deprivation did not compromise neuronal survival. Initial observations by scanning electron microscopy (34) showed that the cell bodies were relatively free of ruffles in the continuous presence of NGF as well as after its withdrawal. However, numerous ruffles were generated on the soma and along neurites within 30 sec of NGF readdition. As on "naive" PC12 cells, the ruffling was transient and disappeared within 15 to 30 min after introduction of NGF.

Growth Cone Responses to NGF Withdrawal/Readdition

Given the resemblance of the cell body and neurite ruffles to growth cone lamellipodia, the removal/readdition paradigm was subsequently extended to the study of growth cones. Initial examination by SEM (35,36) revealed that growth cones of sympathetic neurons and PC12 cells responded morphologically to each phase of growth factor manipulation. Whereas the control, NGF-treated growth

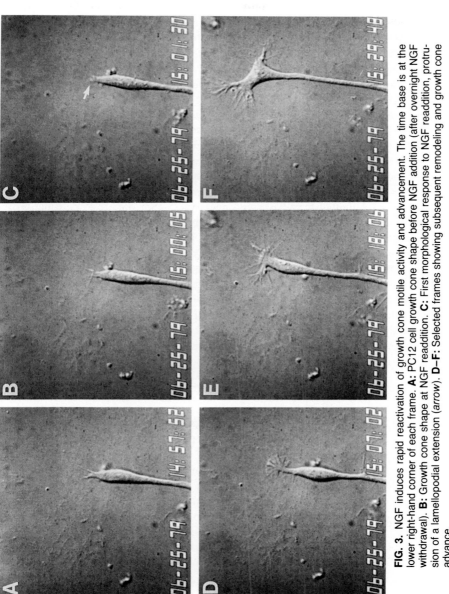

FIG. 3. NGF induces rapid reactivation of growth cone motile activity and advancement. The time base is at the lower right-hand corner of each frame. **A:** growth cone shape before NGF addition (after overnight NGF withdrawal). **B:** Growth cone shape at NGF readdition. **C:** First morphological response to NGF readdition, protrusion of a lamellopodial extension (*arrow*). **D–F:** Selected frames showing subsequent remodeling and growth cone advance.

cones were well spread and possessed filopodia and extensive lamellipodial-like ruffles, those deprived of the factor were rounded and had few filopodia or ruffles. Within 30 sec of NGF readdition, the ruffles reappeared, and shortly thereafter, the beginning of respreading and reformation of filopodia was evident. However, in contrast to the cell bodies and neurites, these responses were not transient but lasted for the duration of NGF readdition.

The morphological responses of growth cones to NGF withdrawal/readdition suggested that these might be associated with changes in function. To assess this, growth cones were observed by time-lapse phase-contrast cinematography (37) and, more recently, by Allen's video-enhanced contrast-differential interference contrast (AVEC-DIC) video recording (38). As anticipated, growth cones of cells maintained in the continuous presence of NGF are flattened, possess highly motile lamellipodia and filopodia, and advance with time. In contrast, those deprived of the factor are round and blunt-ended, show few, if any, motile extensions, and do not advance. Although they have not degenerated, they appear to be functionally inactive. Readdition of NGF rapidly (commencing within 50 sec) re-initiates return to the prewithdrawal state. The first response is the appearance of microspikes and the extension/retraction of lamellipodia (ruffles, as seen by SEM). This occurs along neurites, as well as at growth cones, but is transitory on the neuritic shaft. These changes are followed by general spreading of the growth cone body and appearance of filopodia and, after a lag, by the return of advancement. An illustration of such events is given in Fig. 3. Similar responses occur even at the ends of neurites that have been severed from their cell bodies. Such findings have led to the conclusion that NGF, and presumably other neurotrophic agents, regulate the form, motility, and locomotion of growth cones and do so by means of rapid, local actions.

Possible Role of Protein Kinases in Mediating Local Neurotrophic Factor Actions at the Growth Cone

To probe the mechanisms by which NGF and other agents regulate growth cone function, we have coupled a cell superfusion assembly to the AVEC-DIC microscopy system. This allows us to rapidly administer and exchange compounds of interest, such as growth factors and a variety of pharmacological compounds, while observing their morphological effects on growth cones in real-time. The NGF withdrawal/readdition paradigm elicits and defines the basic growth cone response of our motility studies. We have used this reliable and robust response to test the ability of various pharmacological agents to interfere with growth cone reactivation and motility.

Among the agents studied have been purine analogues. This class of compounds inhibits an NGF-regulated serine protein kinase designated PKN (39). One analogue, 6-thioguanine (6-TG), appears to be quite specific for PKN; in contrast, the analogue 2-aminopurine (2-AP), although not a general kinase inhibitor, appears to block protein kinase activities in addition to PKN. When applied to PC12 cells, both compounds suppress NGF-promoted neurite regeneration and induction of ornithine decarboxylase activity. However, 2-AP blocks NGF-dependent c-*fos* mRNA induction, whereas 6-TG does not. This differential inhibition of the PC12 cell responses indicates the presence of multiple pathways in the NGF mechanism and shows the utility of the inhibitors in dissecting these. Such findings also suggest required roles for PKN and other kinases in the NGF mechanism.

Experiments with our system demonstrated that the purine analogues 2-AP and 6-TG differentially affect the NGF-induced reactivation of PC12 cell growth cones (40). After a short pretreatment with 2-AP, growth cones failed to respond to NGF. This occurred at doses similar to those that inhibit PKN activity and that block neurite outgrowth. In contrast, 6-TG failed to inhibit the rapid reactivation of growth cones, even at doses far above those that suppress PKN and the above-mentioned responses to the factor. These findings indicate that PKN may not play a role in triggering the rapid motility events that are elicited by the addition of NGF. Because 6-TG reversibly inhibits neurite regeneration but not NGF-induced growth cone reactivation, this purine analogue may exert its effect at a step of neurite outgrowth subsequent to initiation of growth cone motility. Consistent with this, differentiated PC12 cells treated with 6-TG and NGF for 18 hr display neurite retraction. However, the efficacy of 2-AP in blocking growth cone reactivation implicates the required action of another kinase that is sensitive to this compound.

The implication of trophic factor–modulated phosphorylation in local growth cone regulation raises an attractive prospect. Growth factors, including NGF, control both tyrosine and serine/threonine kinases. Moreover, at least several of the molecules present in growth cones (such as GAP-43, integrins, vinculin, and CAMs) are phosphoproteins. Phosphorylation, in turn, represents a rapid means for altering function. For instance, the ATPase activity of *Acanthamoeba* myosin I is

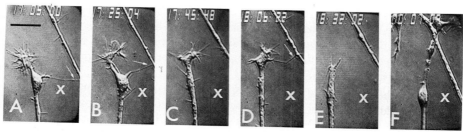

FIG. 4. Potential role of varicosities in NGF-promoted growth cone behavior. Advancement of PC12 cell neurites, like that of neurons, is episodic. In these frames from an overnight sequence of video recordings, a large varicosity was present during a period of motility and active remodeling of the growth cone (**A, B**). Over time, as the girth of the varicosity was reduced, motility and advance were likewise diminished (**C, D**), until a point at which an immobile club-shaped ending was evident (**E**). By the next morning, when growth and motility had resumed, varicosities were once again present. Bar = 14μm.

present only when the molecule is phosphorylated (41). It may therefore be hypothesized that the rapid, local actions of trophic factors are mediated by changes in the phosphorylation, and thereby functional activities, of growth cone–associated molecules. This model is testable, and experiments are underway. Finally, as detailed in other chapters here (Davis, et al.), growth cone activity is modulated by extrinsic agents that lead to changes in $[Ca^{2+}]_i$. Among its other actions, $[Ca^{2+}]_i$ modulates kinase activities. This suggests a potential symmetry between the mechanisms whereby trophic factors and other agents regulate growth cone function.

Possible Role of Varicosities in Growth Cone Function and Local Responses to Neurotrophic Factors

An evident feature of NGF-induced neurites in PC12 cells are focal swellings along the shaft, which have been called *varicosities* (38). They occur in two broad categories: one type is relatively larger and located within 20 μm of the leading edge of the growth cone, whereas the other is smaller in dimension and located all along the length of the neurite. Similar structures in chick embryonic neurons have been termed *neuronal parcels* (42). These features are not unique to neurons in culture but have also been documented in brain tissue by various means (43,44). One intriguing early study with cerebellar Purkinje cell axons described an age-dependent developmental regulation of the appearance of focal axonal swellings (45). In the PC12 cell system there is a correlation between the presence of one or more large varicosities near the growth cone and active elongation (Fig. 4). An additionally interesting characteristic of such varicosities is their ability to alter size and shape during growth cone advance, including bulk movement of the entire structure along the neurite.

Although the specific biochemical composition of these swellings is completely unexplored in PC12 cells, neuronal parcels are known to contain tubulin and neurofilaments, and Koenig and collaborators (46) found spectrin, actin, and calmodulin in analogous structures in regenerating axons of goldfish retinal ganglion cells in culture. The accumulations of membranous vesicles in varicosities of PC12 cells (Aletta and Brown, *unpublished observations*) and retinal ganglion cell axons (46) resemble components of the growth cone LIRB described by Burmeister and co-workers (47) in *Aplysia*.

The function of such growth cone–associated varicosities has not been defined, but one possibility is that they contribute material for axonal growth. Although growth cone motility can be re-activated within seconds by re-adding NGF to previously NGF-withdrawn cultures, there is a delay of several minutes between this response and stable elongation of the neurite. Perhaps mobilization of components from storage sites in the varicosity accounts for this delay. Further studies on the effects of NGF withdrawal and NGF readdition on the structure and composition of varicosities should help to test this notion.

Possible Consequences of Growth Factor Actions on Both Formation and Function of Growth Cones

We have argued here that factors such as NGF influence both the synthesis and the functional utilization of growth cone components. Why both types of action, and what are the consequences of this dual control? On the one hand, neurotrophic factors may regulate the synthesis of components that are rate-limiting for growth cone production. In this way, they may signal developing neurons to commence growth cone formation and neurite outgrowth. Moreover, growth factors may also provide modulatory feedback from the periphery; altered demand for growth could lead to changed neurotrophic factor levels, which in turn elicit appropriate changes in expression of growth cone constituents and consequently modified neurite growth.

Neurotrophic factor actions on synthesis do have biologically relevant limitations. For instance, they are relatively slow. Not only is there a time lag for synthetic events, but particularly when neurites are involved, there is an additional time delay required for the growth factor to be retrogradely transported from the periphery and for the newly synthesized products to be conveyed out to the growth cone from the cell body. In addition, actions limited to synthesis alone would lack spatial specificity. All growing tips of a given neuron might be indiscriminately affected by altered synthesis of growth cone molecules. Local control of function by neurotrophic factors, however, would permit the local environment to communicate rapidly with and influence the growth cone. Localized changes in growth factor levels would translate into rapid effects on growth cone shape, motility, and locomotion, thereby altering the rate and possibly direction of neurite growth as well as extent of innervation (see, for instance, chapters by Mason and Godement and by Lumsden). Locally induced neuritic microspiking, as observed in our cultures after NGF reintroduction, could furthermore have relevance to the phenomenon of axonal back-branching seen *in vivo* (48). Localized secretion of an exogenous factor by the secondary axonal target could elicit growth from the axonal shaft leading to branch formation. Such local actions might be important not only during development, but also for growth associated with neuronal repair and plasticity.

Future Directions

Many of the types of questions raised above for neurotrophic factor effects on formation of growth cones can also be posed for local regulation of growth cone function. Do growth factors exert local actions on growth cones *in vivo*? What is the relative importance of these actions as compared with other external influences? Are there neurotrophic factors that exert inhibitory influences on growth cones? Where do growth cones encounter neurotrophic agents; where are the latter synthesized, and how are they presented? Is a given growth cone exposed to different growth factors at different times and in different places along its route? Do different growth factors have different effects on growth cones of the same neuron; does the same growth factor have different effects on different neurons? Is a growth factor merely permissive for growth cone function, or does it also have "instructive" actions? Do neurotrophic agents play a role in growth cone guidance *in vivo*? What are the molecular mechanisms whereby growth cone function is affected by trophic factors? Finally, what are the relative roles of neurotrophic factors and other extrinsic agents on growth cone behavior? Are they complementary, redundant, or antagonistic?

With the types of model systems described above as well as the present/projected availability of reagents such as purified neurotrophic agents and associated antibodies and probes, one may with some degree of hopeful expectation look forward to resolution of these and related issues.

ACKNOWLEDGMENTS

This work was supported in part by grants from the National Institutes of Health and March of Dimes Birth Defects Foundation. We are indebted to Dr. Mary E. Hatten for providing the use of her AVEC-DIC system, to Kenneth Teng for providing PC12-C41 cells, and to Drs. Hatten, Carol Mason, Cinzia Volonté, Mark Mooseker, and Thomas Pollard for their helpful discussions.

REFERENCES

1. Levi-Montalcini R. The nerve growth factor: 35 years later. *EMBO J* 1987;6:1145–1154.
2. Greene LA, Tischler AS. Establishment of a noradrenergic clonal line of rat adrenal pheochromocytoma cells which respond to nerve growth factor. *Proc Natl Acad Sci USA* 1976;73:2424–2428.
3. Togari A, Baker D, Dickens G, Guroff G. The neurite-promoting effect of fibroblast growth factor on PC12 cells. *Biochem Biophys Res Commun* 1983;114:1189–1193.
4. Satoh T, Nakamura S, Taga T, et al. Induction of neuronal differentiation in PC12 cells by B-cell stimulatory factor 2/interleukin 6. *Mol Cell Biol* 1988;8:3546–3549.
5. Burstein DE, Greene LA. Evidence for both RNA-synthesis-dependent and -independent pathways in stimulation of neurite outgrowth by nerve growth factor. *Proc Natl Acad Sci USA* 1978;75:6059–6063.
6. Van Hooff CO, De Graan PN, Boonstra J, Oestreicher AB, Schmidt-Michels MH, Gispen WH. Nerve growth factor enhances the level of the protein kinase C substrate B-50 in pheochromocytoma PC12 cells. *Biochem Biophys Res Commun* 1986;139:644–651.
7. Costello B, Meymandi A, Freeman JA. Factors influencing GAP-43 gene expression in PC12 pheochromocytoma cells. *J Neurosci* 1990;10:1398–1406.
8. Perrone-Bizzozero NI, Irwin N, Lewis SE, Fischer I, Neve RL, Benowitz LI. Posttranslational regulation of GAP-43 mRNA levels during process outgrowth (*Abstr*). *Soc Neurosci Abstr* 1990; 16(2):814.
9. Van Hooff CO, Holthuis JC, Oestreicher AB, Boonstra J, De Graan PN, Gispen WH. Nerve growth factor–induced changes in the intracellular localization of the protein kinase C substrate B-50 in pheochromocytoma PC12 cells. *J Cell Biol* 1989;108:1115–1125.
10. Zuber MX, Goodman DW, Karns LR, Fishman MC. The neuronal growth-associated protein GAP-43 induces filopodia in non-neuronal cells. *Science* 1989;244:1193–1195.
11. Salton SR, Richter-Landsberg C, Greene LA, Shelanski ML. The NGF-inducible large external (NILE) glycoprotein: studies of a central and peripheral marker. *J Neurosci* 1983;3:441–454.
12. Prentice HM, Moore SE, Dickson JG, Doherty P, Walsh FS. Nerve growth factor–induced changes in neural cell adhesion molecule (N-CAM) in PC12 cells. *EMBO J* 1987;6:1859–1863.

13. Rossino P, Gavazzi I, Timpl R, et al. Nerve growth factor induces increased expression of a laminin-binding integrin in rat pheochromocytoma PC12 cells. *Exp Cell Res* 1990;189:100–108.
14. Halegoua S. Changes in the phosphorylation and distribution of vinculin during nerve growth factor induced neurite outgrowth. *Dev Biol* 1987;121:97–104.
15. Sobue K, Kanda K. Localization of pp60^{c-src} in growth cone of PC12 cell. *Biochem Biophys Res Commun* 1988;157:1383–1389.
16. Sobue K, Kanda, K. α-Actinins, calspectin (brain spectrin or fodrin) and actin participate in adhesion and movement of growth cones. *Neuron* 1989;3:311–319.
17. Knecht DA, Loomis WF. Antisense RNA inactivation of myosin heavy chain gene expression in *Dictyostelium discoideum*. *Science* 1987;236:1081–1086.
18. De Lozanne A, Spudich JA. Disruption of the *Dictyostelium* myosin heavy chain gene by homologous recombination. *Science* 1987;236:1086–1091.
19. Korn ED, Hammer JA III. Myosins of nonmuscle cells. *Annu Rev Biophys Biophys Chem* 1988; 17:23–45.
20. Pollard TD, Doberstein SK, Zot HG. Myosin-I. *Annu Rev Physiol* 1991;53:653–667.
21. Pollard TD, Korn ED. Acanthamoeba myosin. I. Isolation from *Acanthamoeba castellanii* of an enzyme similar to muscle myosin. *J Biol Chem* 1973;248:4682–4690.
22. Fukui Y, Lynch TJ, Brzeska H, Korn ED. Myosin I is located at the leading edges of locomoting *Dictyostelium* amoebae. *Nature* 1989;341:328–331.
23. Adams RJ, Pollard TD. Binding of myosin I to membrane lipids. *Nature* 1989;340:565–568.
24. Mitchison T, Kirschner M. Cytoskeletal dynamics and nerve growth. *Neuron* 1988;1:761–772.
25. Sherr EH, Greene LA. Detection of an NGF regulated 105 kd protein displaying myosin I-like properties in PC12 cells. *J Cell Biol* 1990;111:167a.
26. Kiehart DP, Kaiser DA, Pollard TD. Monoclonal antibodies demonstrate limited structural homology between myosin isozymes from *Acanthamoeba*. *J Cell Biol* 1984;99:1002–1014.
27. Campenot RB. Local control of neurite development by nerve growth factor. *Proc Natl Acad Sci USA* 1977;75:6059–6063.
28. Campenot RB. Development of sympathetic neurons in compartmentalized cultures. I. Local control of neurite outgrowth by nerve growth factor. *Dev Biol* 1982;93:1–12.
29. Gundersen RW, Barrett JN. Characterization of the turning response of dorsal root neurites toward nerve growth factor. *J Cell Biol* 1980;87:546–554.
30. Letourneau PC. Chemotactic response of nerve fiber elongation to nerve growth factor. *Dev Biol* 1978;66:183–196.
31. Gundersen RW. Sensory neurite growth cone guidance by substrate absorbed nerve growth factor. *J Neurosci Res* 1985;13:199–212.
32. Menesini-Chen MG, Chen JS, Levi-Montalcini R. Sympathetic nerve fibers ingrowth in the central nervous system of neonatal rodent upon intracerebral NGF injections. *Arch Ital Biol* 1978;116:53–84.
33. Connolly JL, Greene LA, Viscarello RR, Riley WD. Rapid, sequential changes in surface morphology of PC12 pheochromocytoma cells in response to nerve growth factor. *J Cell Biol* 1979;82:820–827.
34. Connolly JL, Green S, Greene LA. Pit formation and rapid changes in surface morphology of sympathetic neurons in response to nerve growth factor. *J Cell Biol* 1981;90:176–180.
35. Connolly JL, Seeley PJ, Greene LA. Regulation of growth cone morphology by nerve growth factor: a comparative study by scanning electron microscopy. *J Neurosci Res* 1985;13:183–198.
36. Connolly JL, Seeley PJ, Greene LA. Rapid regulation of neuronal growth cone shape and surface morphology by nerve growth factor. *Neurochem Res* 1987;12:861–868.
37. Seeley PJ, Greene LA. Short latency, local actions of nerve growth factor on growth cones. *Proc Natl Acad Sci USA* 1983;80:2789–2793.
38. Aletta JM, Greene LA. Growth cone configuration and advance: a time-lapse study using video-enhanced differential interference contrast microscopy. *J Neurosci* 1988;8:1425–1435.
39. Volonté C, Rukenstein A, Loeb D, Greene LA. Differential inhibition of NGF responses by purine analogues: correlation with inhibition of an NGF-activated protein kinase. *J Cell Biol* 1989;109: 2395–2403.
40. Phelan KA, Volonté C, Greene LA. NGF-induced PC12 cell growth cone motility and its differential inhibition by purine analogues (*Abstr*). *Soc Neurosci Abstr* 1990;16:417.6.
41. Albanesi JP, Fujisaki H, Hammer JA, et al. Monomeric *Acanthamoeba* myosins I support movement *in vitro*. *J Biol Chem* 1985;260:8649–8652.

42. Hollenbeck PJ, Bray D. Rapidly transported organelles containing membrane and cytoskeletal components: their relation to axonal growth. *J Cell Biol* 1986;105:2827–2835.
43. Murray M. Regeneration of retinal axons into goldfish optic tectum. *J Comp Neurol* 1976;168:175–196.
44. Godement P, Vanselow J, Thanos S, Bonhoeffer F. A study in developing visual systems with a new method of staining neurones and their processes in fixed tissue. *Development* 1987;101:697–713.
45. Gravel C, Leclerc N, Plioplys A, Hawkes RB. Focal axonal swellings in rat cerebellar Purkinje cells during normal development. *Brain Res* 1986;363:325–332.
46. Koenig E, Kinsman S, Repasky E, Sultz L. Rapid mobility of motile varicosities and inclusions containing a-spectrin, actin and calmodulin in regenerating axons *in vitro. J Neurosci* 1985;5:715–729.
47. Burmeister DW, Chen M, Bailey CH, Goldberg DJ. The distribution and movement of organelles in maturing growth cones: correlated video-enhanced and electron microscopic studies. *J Neurocytol* 1988;17:783–795.
48. O'Leary DDM, Terashima T. Cortical axons branch to multiple subcortical targets by interstitial axon budding: implications for target recognition and "waiting periods." *Neuron* 1988;1:901–910.

The Nerve Growth Cone, edited by P. C. Letourneau, S. B. Kater, and E. R. Macagno, Raven Press, Ltd., New York © 1992.

14

Chemotaxis in the Developing Nervous Systems of Vertebrates

Andrew Lumsden

Division of Anatomy and Cell Biology, United Medical and Dental Schools, Guy's Hospital, London SE1 9RT, England

The idea that growth cones could be guided by attractants diffusing from their targets belongs to Cajal (1,2). Inspired by the observations of chemotaxis by fern sperm (3) and leucocytes (4), Cajal conceived a universal mechanism whereby the precise specificity and vast complexity of neural connections could develop.

> If one admits that neuroblasts are bestowed with chemotactic sensitivity, one can imagine that they are capable of amoeboid movement elicited by substances secreted by epithelial, mesodermal or nervous elements. Consequently their extensions will orient themselves along the chemical currents and will bring them to meet the secreting cells [2, p. 658].

Chemical attraction, acting within the mechanical guides and constraints imposed by tissue spaces and planes provided the earliest and simplest solution to the problem of directed growth cone navigation.

Growth cone chemotaxis, however, lacked experimental verification and waned in popularity, whereas the tissue culture demonstrations by Harrison (5), Weiss (6), and others of the power of contact guidance led to an increasing fixation with the substratum, culminating in the contemporary view, expressed by Hamburger (7) that "the growth cone is guided by signals encoded in the structures with which it is in direct contact." This is an extreme opinion, however, and one that conflates the requirements for growth and those for guidance. It is assumed that the molecules that make axons grow will be employed, by temporally or spatially restricted expression, in guiding their growth. The most plausible example is fasciculation, in which axons are guided by the surfaces of preexisting axons. Preformed pathways of growth-promoting molecules such as laminin (8) have also been demonstrated. But guidance cues expressed by pathway cells and specific for the earliest axons of a system are yet to be discovered in vertebrates. Despite 100 years of research, it is still not known what makes a growth cone turn toward its target. It is reasonable, therefore, to reexamine Cajal's "neurotropic" hypothesis and consider what evidence can now be adduced in its favor.

Circumstantial yet compelling evidence comes from the observation that in normal development, axons grow directly and accurately to their targets (9). Experimental findings in the chick (10) have revealed that when specific segments of spinal cord are shifted in relation to the limb bud, motor neurons still connect with specific muscles by extending their axons along aberrant pathways. The visual projection of *Xenopus* provides a further example of such "homing behavior," in which the retinal ganglion cell axons of ectopically replaced eyes grow directly to their target, the optic tectum, by novel routes (11). These demonstrations of normal and abnormal axon trajectories are entirely consistent with the possibility of target attraction and, in some cases, may also reveal the redundancy of specific preformed pathways.

Growth cone chemotaxis during normal development has yet to be demonstrated directly, but some expectations of such a mechanism have been met by studies of the effects of nerve growth factor. Menesini-Chen and colleagues (12) injected NGF into the brainstems of newborn rodents and found that postganglionic sympathetic axons abnormally entered the spinal cord by way of the dorsal roots and grew up the dorsal funiculus toward the injection site. Thus, diffusible molecules with neurite-promoting activities can establish effective gradients over appreciable distances, in this case well beyond those required during embryonic development. Gundersen and Barrett (13) showed that the growth cones of dorsal root ganglion neurons *in vitro* can respond to a point source of a diffusible factor by turning and growing

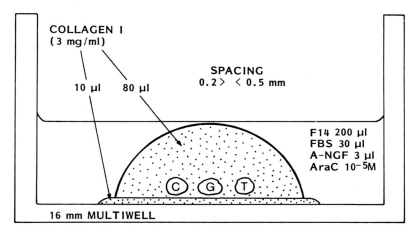

FIG. 1. Method for collagen gel co-cultures. A platform of soluble rat tail collagen is gelled in a 16-mm well; explants (C, control; G, ganglion; T, target) are added and embedded in a larger drop of collagen. Once gelled, liquid tissue culture medium is added (for further details, see ref. 14).

strongly suggest that the epidermal ectoderm, which itself receives sparse innervation in birds, plays a role in attracting sensory axons from deep-lying trunks. The ectoderm of bird skin also releases a short-range repulsion factor that inhibits nerves from approaching closer than about 70 μm to the surface (24).

COMMISSURAL AXONS OF THE SPINAL CORD

During the early stages of spinal cord development in higher vertebrates, different subsets of secondary afferent relay neurons extend their axons in stereotyped directions. Neurons in the dorsal and lateral mantle zone grow first ventral and then longitudinal (Fig. 5); some make their orthogonal turn on the ipsilateral side (association neurons) and others on the contralateral side (commissural neurons). Commissural growth cones initially grow down the neuroepithelial endfeet of the marginal zone (25) but at about the mid-dorsoventral level they leave the margin and head on an oblique course directly for the midline, which they cross on the endfeet of specialized glial cells in the ventral floor plate (2,25). Cajal noted that

> the production of attractive substances at the level of the ventral epithelial rim, more intense than those emitted by the rest of the epithelium, explains the oblique direction.

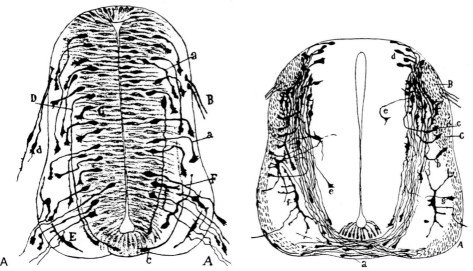

FIG. 5. Chick embryo spinal cord in transverse section. Golgi method. Drawings from Cajal (ref. 2). **A:** at 3 days. A, ventral root; a, association neuron; B, dorsal root; C, young commissural neuron; c, growth cone of commissural neuron entering the floor plate; D, commissural neuron; d, dorsal root ganglion neuron; E,F, motor neurons. **B:** at 4 days. A, ventral funiculus; a, commissure; B, dorsal funiculus; b, c, association neurons; C, lateral funiculus; d, commissural neurons; e, growth cones within matrix layer; f,g, motor neurons.

. . . It is more difficult to understand the subsequent growth of the axon cylinder upon the external limiting membrane of the ventral cord on the opposite side, where it becomes longitudinal. Maybe one can explain this by invoking influences from the extremities of the cord, or even an attractive influence from the motor neurons which are in more distant medullary segments [2, p. 661].

Thus Cajal expounded the idea of serial chemotaxis, axons being lured in turn by intermediate targets along a pathway. In his account of errors made by growth cones (2), he described "cones arrested and enprisoned" beneath the external limiting membrane of the floor plate glia (Fig. 6), apparently unable to switch to the next attractant.

The chemotactic lure of the floor plate was first demonstrated experimentally by Weber (26). He roughly transected the spinal cords of 2-day chick embryos and later observed a variety of abnormal routes taken by commissural axons in the repaired region. In one case (Fig. 7a), commissural neurons isolated in a rosette of traumatized neuroepithelium perforated the external limiting membrane and traveled through mesenchyme before reentering the ventral cord region and decussating. Despite the grossly deformed morphology of the cord, these axons had pursued a virtually direct course toward the floor plate. In another case (Fig. 7b), commissural axons reached the floor plate by growing through a large blood clot, seeming to have preferred this presumably cueless substratum to their normal pathway cells.

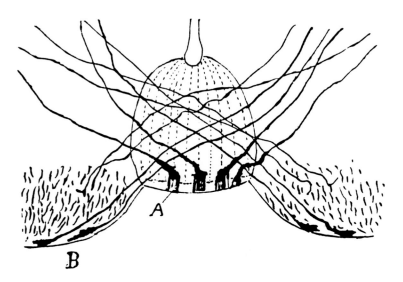

FIG. 6. Commissural region of the spinal cord, 4-day chick embryo. A, commissural growth cones arrested in the floor plate; B, growth cones beneath the external limiting membrane. (From ref. 2.)

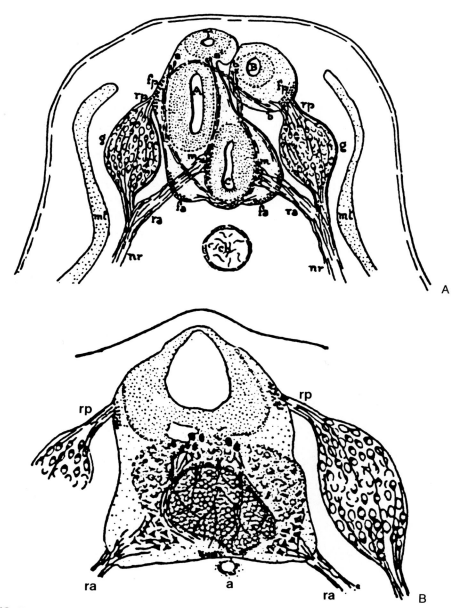

FIG. 7. Transverse sections through 4-day chick embryo spinal cord, which had been cut across at 2 to 3 days. Szepsenwol's method. **A:** Commissural neurons (b, b′) in an isolated dorsal cord vesicle (B) leave the cord, cross mesenchyme, reenter the main cord vesicle (A) and decussate at the floor plate (C). Other commissurals remaining in the main vesicle (a, a′) also reach the floor plate. **B:** Commissural axons have grown directly through a blood clot to reach the floor plate. cb, notochord; fa, ventral funiculus; fp, dorsal funiculus; g, dorsal root ganglion; mt, myotome; nr, spinal nerve; ra, ventral root; rp, dorsal root (ref. 26).

If commissural neurons can extend axons toward their intermediate target through what amounts to a fibrillar tissue culture medium *in vivo*, a floor plate–derived diffusible activity is indicated, and floor plate explants should be able to attract commissural neuron outgrowth across a 3-D collagen gel *in vitro*. This potency has since been confirmed using explants from rat embryo spinal cord (27,28).

Further studies of the floor plate–commissural axon interaction have suggested the possibility of redundancy among axon guidance mechanisms. When the floor plate is congenitally absent in mice, as in the Danforth's short-tail (Sd) mutant (29), or ablated in chick embryos by UV-irradiation of its precursor cells (A.G.S. Lumsden & A. Hornbruch, *unpublished results*), commissural axons are still able to reach the ventral midline. But in both cases, they do so by following the external limiting membrane for their entire trajectory. The oblique arcuate pathway, by which they normally cut inside the motor column, is not formed. The significance of this is difficult to evaluate because motor neurons also appear to be absent in these notochord and floor plate–deficient animals. Once at the midline, the commissural axons fail to decussate but leave the spinal cord and form a large median fascicle in the submedullary mesenchyme (Fig. 8). The tendency of commissural

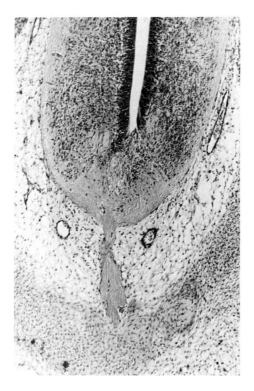

FIG. 8. Transverse section through the medulla of stage 24 chick embryo, after UV-irradiation of Hensen's node and prenodal epiblast at stage 4. Both notochord and floor plate are absent, and secondary afferent axons follow a circumferential path to the ventral side of the neural tube where they leave in a novel peripheral nerve. (From Lumsden and Hornbruch, *unpublished results*.)

axons to leave spinal cord when deprived of a floor plate had been noted by Weber (26).

The role of the floor plate in the normal development of axon pathways is not simply that of attracting growth cones to the ventral midline by the shortest path. Its specialized properties seem also to influence the subsequent behavior of these axons in forming the commissure and maintaining their projections within the spinal cord. In addition, it is conceivable that the floor plate exerts a repulsive effect on association neurons, countering their inherent tendency toward ventral growth and forcing them to turn into the ipsilateral longitudinal funiculi, where they become subject to the stronger guiding influence of fasciculation.

RAT CORTICOPONTINE PROJECTION

Individual neurons in the mammalian neocortex project branched axons over considerable distances to multiple subcortical targets (30), the parent axon producing collaterals successively in association with each target. An insight into how this multiple-branched projection pattern develops has come from studies of layer 5 cortical neurons in the rat by O'Leary and colleagues (31). Most cortical areas make connections with the basilar pons, establishing a major pathway that is essential for the control of motor behavior, yet primary axons from layer 5 do not grow into this target nor do branches to it form by bifurcation of their growth cones. Rather, the corticopontine projection develops by the process of delayed interstitial budding of collateral branches from primary axons that have already grown past the basilar pons down the corticospinal tract (31). This mechanism of collateralization is used regardless of whether the parent axon's postpontine segment is retained (motor cortex) or subsequently eliminated (visual cortex) (32). Thus, the target appears not to be recognized by the growth cone as it passes over it, yet within 2 days it becomes recognized by the axon cylinder.

What controls the formation of collateral buds at stereotyped positions directly over the basilar pons? One possibility would be an intrinsic neuronal program that times extension and measures distance behind the growth cone. Less unlikely would be the maturation of cues in the specific local environment of the corticospinal tract. Alternatively, the basilar pons could control its own innervation by producing a long-range signal that induces budding and lures collateral growth from overlying corticospinal axons. That the process is linked to the target is suggested by the striking correlation between the timing of collateral budding and differentiation of the constituent neurons of the basilar pons after their immigration from the medullary rhombic lip (33).

When explants of neonatal rat cortex are co-cultured in 3-D collagen gels with basilar pons, the pontine target tissue elicits an increase in the number of axons emerging from the proximal face of the cortical explant (when compared with control explants of brain regions that do not receive a cortical input) and also has a measurable influence on their turning behavior (34). These effects could be observed in phase contrast, but they increase in prominence when axons are traced by injecting the lipophilic membrance probe DiI either into the pontine and control explants or directly into the collagen matrix (Fig. 9). Retrograde labeling of cortical axons contacting the pontine explant reveals that they grow by one of two means. Some primary axons turn from their initial ventricular surface-directed course to emerge on the lateral pons-facing surface and enter the pontine explant without branching. More commonly, however, they maintain their straight trajectory toward the ventricular surface but give off collaterals into the pons (Fig. 9a). Most of the cell bodies labeled by this route lie within the cortical explant in a position that corresponds with the layer 5 location of corticospinal-corticopontine neurons. Pons-directed collaterals of varying extents are also demonstrated by retrograde labeling of the neurons whose axons grew out the ventricular surface into the matrix (Fig. 9b).

Not only does the pontine explant affect the directional growth of cortical axons, but it can affect at a distance the extension and directed growth of axon collaterals. This inductive and chemotactic effect appears to be specific for the class of cortical neurons that innervates the basilar pons *in vivo*. We suggested that the corticopontine projection develops by a two-stage process (34). First, the primary axons of a subset of layer 5 neurons grow down a defined path that leads them over the basilar pons into the spinal cord. Second, coincident with its maturation, the basilar pons induces the formation of collateral buds and attracts their ingrowth through the release of a diffusible molecule. The fact that primary axons turn toward and enter the pontine explants *in vitro* shows that their growth cones do respond to the attractant. Their failure to recognize the pons as a target *in vivo* may be because either the

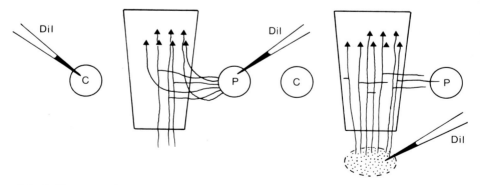

FIG. 9. Diagrammatic representation of co-cultured cortical explants. Full radial thickness explant of cortex (ventricular side facing down in the figure) is flanked by basilar pons (P) and control (C) explants. Layer 5 neurons are shown as triangles. **Left:** DiI injected into the pons explant traces axons and collaterals from layer 5 cell bodies. **Right:** Depot injection of DiI into the collagen matrix traces collaterals directed toward, but not necessarily contacting, the pons explant.

attractant is not produced by the immature pons at the time they pass or because the guiding influences of the corticospinal tract are dominant. In accord with these possibilities, normally late-arriving layer 5 axons will grow directly into the basilar pons when the early axons of the corticospinal tract are removed *in vivo* (35).

Further *in vivo* experiments support this chemotactic mechanism (36). When fetal rats are X-irradiated during the generation and migration of basilar pontine neurons, a substantial reduction or absence of the basilar pons results. When absent, anterograde DiI labeling of corticospinal axons reveals that no collaterals form at positions that would normally overlie the pons. When remnants of the neuronal population persist, they form small islands on the inferior surface of the medulla. The corticospinal axons form collaterals directly above each of these ectopic islands of basilar pontine neurons.

CONCLUSIONS

Chemotaxis has the merit of being a simple mechanism, and in those systems where its action is known and well understood (such as leucocyte migration), it is a most efficient way of giving directionality to moving cells (37). Conceptually also it would allow greater plasticity in the guidance of axons, both ontogenetically and phylogenetically, than would be allowed by a system that relied on the precise placement of both the target and pathway cues. Although ignored for many years and still dismissed as speculation (7), Cajal's chemotactic hypothesis of growth cone guidance now finds support from three developing systems in the CNS and the PNS. In each of these systems, the crucial demonstration has been that normal target tissue can attract outgrowth from specific neurons across neutral matrix, strongly suggesting that a similar target effect could be involved, possibly in conjunction with other guiding influences, in the establishment of normal axonal projections. In particular, evidence that a signal derived from the basilar pons can operate over a distance and affect the elaboration of a crucial neural connection in the mammalian brain suggests an important role for diffusible molecules.

REFERENCES

1. Cajal SR. La Retine des Vertebres. *La Cellule* 1893;9:119–258.
2. Cajal SR. *Histologie du Systeme Nerveux de l'Homme et des Vertegres*, Madrid:CSIC, 1909.
3. Pfeffer W. Locomotorische Richtungsbewegungen durch chemische Reize. *Untersuch a d bot Inst zu Tubingen* 1884;1:363–482.
4. Massart J, Bordet C. Le chimiotaxisme des leucocytes et l'infection microbienne. *Ann de l'Inst Pasteur, Paris* 1891;5:417–444.
5. Harrison RG. The outgrowth of the nerve fiber as a mode of protoplasmic movement. *J Exp Zool* 1910;9:787–848.
6. Weiss P. Nerve patterns: the mechanics of nerve growth. *Growth (Suppl.)* 1941;5:163–203.
7. Hamburger V. The ontogeny of neuroembryology. *J Neurosci* 1988;8:3535–3540.
8. Cohen J, Burne JF, McKinlay C, Winter J. The role of laminin and the laminin/fibronectin receptor complex in the outgrowth of retinal ganglion cell axons. *Dev Biol* 1987;122:407–418.
9. Jacobson M, Huang S. Neurite outgrowth traced by means of horseradish peroxidase inherited from neuronal ancestral cells in frog embryos. *Dev Biol* 1985;110:102–113.

10. Landmesser L. The development of specific motor pathways in the chick embryo. *Trends Neurosci* 1984;7:336–339.
11. Harris WA. Homing behaviour of axons in the embryonic vertebrate brain. *Nature* 1986;320:266–269.
12. Menesini-Chen MG, Chen JS, Levi-Montalcini R. Sympathetic nerve fibre ingrowth in the central nervous system of neonatal rodents upon intracerebral NFG injections. *Arch Ital Biol* 1978;116:53–84.
13. Gundersen RW, Barrett JN. Neuronal chemotaxis: chick dorsal root axons turn towards high concentrations of nerve growth factor. *Science* 1979;206:1079–1080.
14. Lumsden AGS, Davies AM. Earliest sensory nerve fibres are guided to peripheral targets by attractants other than nerve growth factor. *Nature* 1983;306:786–788.
15. Davies AM, Lumsden AGS. Relation of target encounter and neuronal death to nerve growth factor responsiveness in the developing mouse trigeminal ganglion. *J Comp Neurol* 1984;223:124–137.
16. Davies AM, Bandtlow C, Heumann R, Korsching S, Rohrer H, Thoenen H. Timing and site of nerve growth factor synthesis in developing skin in relation to innervation and expression of the receptor. *Nature* 1987;326:353–358.
17. Elsdale T, Bard J. Collagen substrata for studies on cell behaviour. *J Cell Biol* 1972;54:626–637.
18. Ebendal T, Jordell-Kylberg A, Soderstrom S. Stimulation by tissue explants on nerve fibre outgrowth in culture. *Zoon* 1978;6:235–243.
19. Cajal SR. *Studies on vertebrate neurogenesis.* Springfield, Illinois: Charles C. Thomas, 1960.
20. Lumsden AGS, Davies AM. Chemotropic effect of specific target epithelium in the development of the mammalian nervous system. *Nature* 1986;323:538–539.
21. Lumsden AGS. Diffusible factors and chemotropism in the development of the peripheral nervous system. In: Parnavelas JG, Stern CD, Stirling RV, eds. *The making of the nervous system.* Oxford University Press, 1988;166–187.
22. Bray D. Filopodial contraction and growth cone guidance. In: Bellairs R, Curtis A, Dunn G, eds. *Cell behaviour.* Cambridge University Press, 1982;299–317.
23. Martin P, Khan A, Lewis J. Cutaneous nerves of the embryonic chick wing do not develop in regions denuded of ectoderm. *Development* 1989;106:335–346.
24. Verna J-M, Saxod R. Differential growth of sensory neurons *in vitro* in presence of dermis and epidermis. *Cell Differentiation* 1986;18:183–188.
25. Holley JA. Early development of the circumferential axonal pathway in mouse and chick spinal cord. *J Comp Neurol* 1982;205:371–382.
26. Weber A. Croissance des fibres nerveuses commissurales lors de lesions de la moelle epiniere chez de jeunes embryons de Poulet. *Biomorphosis* 1938;1:30–35.
27. Tessier-Lavigne M, Placzek M, Lumsden AGS, Dodd J, Jessell TM. Chemotropic guidance of developing axons in the mammalian central nervous system. *Nature* 1988;336:775–778.
28. Placzek M, Tessier-Lavigne M, Jessell T, Dodd J. Orientation of commissural axons *in vitro* in response to a floor plate–derived chemoattractant. *Development* 1990;110:1930.
29. Bovolenta P, Jessell TM, Dodd J. Disruption of commissural axon guidance in the absence of the midline floor plate *(Abstr).* *Soc Neurosci Abstr* 1988;14:271.
30. Cajal SR. *Les Nouvelles Idees sur la Structure du Systeme Nerveux chez l'Homme et chez Vertebres,* Paris: Reinwald, 1894.
31. O'Leary DDM, Terashima T. Cortical axons branch to multiple subcortical targets by interstitial axon budding: implications for target recognition and "waiting periods." *Neuron* 1988;1:901–910.
32. O'Leary DDM, Stanfield BB. Occipital cortical neurons with transient pyramidal tract axons extend and maintain collaterals to subcortical but not intracortical targets. *Brain Res* 1985;336:326–333.
33. Altman J, Bayer SA. Prenatal development of the cerebellar system in the rat—cytogenesis and histogenesis of the inferior olive, pontine gray, and the precerebellar reticular nuclei. *J Comp Neurol* 1978;179:49–76.
34. Heffner CD, Lumsden AGS, O'Leary DDM. Target control of collateral extension and directional axon growth in the mammalian brain. *Science* 1990;247:217–220.
35. Missias A, Kutka LJ, Reinoso BS, O'Leary DDM. *In vivo* evidence for target control of collateral formation and directional axon growth in mammalian brain. *Soc Neurosci Abstr* 1990;16:139.
36. O'Leary DDM, Bicknese AR, De Carlos JA, et al. Target selection by cortical axons: alternative mechanisms to establish axonal connections in the developing brain. *Cold Spring Harbor Symp* 1991;55 *(in press).*
37. Trinkaus JP. Further thoughts on directional cell movement during morphogenesis. *J Neurosci Res* 1985;13:1–19.

The Nerve Growth Cone, edited by P. C. Letourneau,
S. B. Kater, and E. R. Macagno, Raven Press, Ltd.,
New York © 1992.

15

Integrins and *N*-Cadherin Are Adhesive Molecules Involved in Growth Cone Migration

Paul C. Letourneau

*Department of Cell Biology and Neuroanatomy, University of Minnesota,
Minneapolis, Minnesota 55455*

PROBLEM OF GROWTH CONE NAVIGATION

The elongation of a neurite from its cell body to a synaptic target has been described as a process of navigation by the motile nerve tip, or growth cone, through diverse environments in which the growth cone is sensitive to environmental features that influence the path of growth cone migration. An appropriate analogy is an automobile trip from your home to a distant location via the freeway system. Significant to this analogy is the idea that on the freeway, you take a route shared by many other drivers, but when deciding which is the correct off ramp to exit and where to turn on residential streets, you must recognize signs that make sense to only some drivers. Similarly, migrating growth cones may follow universally recognized environmental routes for large portions of their pathway, but subsets of growth cones diverge onto distinct paths that are marked by signals to which only some growth cones are sensitive.

Much research has been directed to the elucidation of positive directional cues for growth cone navigation. This includes differential adhesivity, haptotaxis, and chemotaxis (see chapters by Lumsden, Poo and Quillan, Baier and Bonhoeffer). In the context of our highway analogy, this would be the road signs that mark particular routes to take. However, evidence from several experimental systems indicates that growth cone guidance may also occur through negative signals that inhibit growth cones from migrating on certain paths or in certain directions (see chapters by Raper et al., Baier and Bonhoeffer, and Davis et al.). The highway analogy also includes freeway median strips, *Do not enter* signs, and road blocks that keep autos from driving on certain streets or in certain directions. This analogy is entertaining and instructive for presenting the study of growth cone navigation. However, real understanding of how growth cones navigate requires identification of the environmental molecules that influence growth cone navigation and how their expression is determined, characterization of the molecules that confer sensitivity to growth cones for particular environmental features, and elucidation of the mechanisms by which molecules interact at the growth cone to influence growth cone migration and neurite formation.

The role of adhesion to a substratum in growth cone migration was recognized long ago by Ross Harrison in studies of neurites elongating along threads of spider web (1). Subsequent studies of growth cone behavior *in vivo* and *in vitro* noted that filopodia could contact, adhere to, and even pull on other cells or extracellular features (2–6). However, how these contact interactions regulate growth cone migration was not investigated in depth. As cell locomotion became viewed as a stepwise process of extension, adhesion, and forward exertion of tension, growth cone migration was analyzed according to the same proposed mechanism. The role of actin filament networks and bundles in producing the motile behavior of growth cones was recognized, and growth cones were viewed as extending forward and making adhesive contacts to gain traction for the forward movement of the neuritic cytoskeleton and other cytoplasmic components (7–12).

In vitro studies of nonneuronal locomotory cells provided evidence that regional differences in adhesivity could regulate the rates and even patterns of cell movement (13–15), and when similar approaches were applied to neuronal cultures, it was dramatically clear that neurite elongation could be directed along substrata comprised of patterned regions of higher and lower adhesivity (16,17). Recognizing that a growth cone establishes the adhesive contacts of an elongating neurite, it was proposed that exploratory movements of a growth cone sample environmental surfaces, and stabilization of particular growth cone sites by strong growth cone–substratum adhesivity leads to forward transport of neuritic components and elongation toward that site. Studies by Bray (18–20) showed the significance of mechanical tensions exerted by the growth cone (see chapter by Bray). A combination of these concepts of stabilization by adhesion and growth cone pulling further strengthened the hypothesis that an important part of growth cone navigation involves crawling along pathways of high adhesivity. Of course, this work was *in vitro* and, thus, open to criticism as not relevant to *in vivo* events. However, elegant analyses of the pathfinding behavior of growth cones of identified neurons in insect embryos supported this proposal by revealing the characteristic (and necessary) interactions of migrating growth cones and their filopodia with specific cells and axon bundles (21–24; see chapters by Goodman et al. and Bentley and O'Conner). Although the adhesive contacts of growth cones and filopodia are not easily verified within intact tissues, the behavior of growth cones *in vivo* is consistent with *in vitro* studies in which adhesive interactions can be more easily shown.

Molecular dissection of the role of adhesive contacts in growth cone navigation has progressed with the identification of cell surface and extracellular glycoproteins that mediate adhesive interactions of growth cones. These classes of cell adhesion molecules are the immunoglobulin superfamily, which includes NCAM and L1 (25,26), the cadherins (27), which includes *N*-cadherin (28), the integrin family

(29,30), which includes several α/β heterodimers that recognize components of extracellular matrices, and extracellular molecules, such as fibronectin, laminin, collagens, and tenascin (31–34; see chapter by Schachner). Biochemical studies have characterized the adhesive activities of these molecules, and immunocytochemical studies have demonstrated the temporal and spatial distribution of these molecules in relationship to periods of growth cone navigation. Much direct evidence for the roles of these molecules in neurite elongation has been derived from *in vitro* studies involving treatment of substrata with purified adhesive molecules and from the use of antibodies or related molecules that specifically block the binding of particular adhesive molecules (29,35–42). Additional approaches that may demonstrate the role of adhesive molecules in growth cone navigation involve the application of antibodies, enzymes, or other molecules to intact embryos, developmental analysis of *Drosophila* embryos with genetic mutations for adhesion molecules, and transfection of cells with genes for adhesion molecules (see chapters by Goodman, et al., Bentley and O'Conner, Seeds, and Landmesser).

Despite the information now available about adhesive molecules and their distributions, understanding their interactions and their roles in growth cone navigation is difficult, because growth cones and the surfaces they encounter frequently express multiple adhesive components. Thus, it is a complex task to investigate which adhesive interactions occur and affect growth cone function in particular situations. Even more challenging may be the elucidation of how extremely diverse interactions of growth cones with environmental cues are integrated to produce characteristic patterns of growth cone migration.

ROLES FOR INTEGRINS AND *N*-CADHERIN IN GROWTH CONE MIGRATION

We have investigated the role of two cell surface adhesive molecules in the migration of growth cones extended by sensory neurons of chick embryos (43,44). These components are the integrins, which mediate cell adhesion to several extracellular macromolecules, and the calcium-dependent homophilic adhesion molecule, *N*-cadherin. The experiments were done *in vitro* to define the substratum for growth cone migration and to permit application of antibodies and other manipulations that may interfere with specific adhesive activities of integrins or *N*-cadherin. Our results indicate that integrins are involved in growth cone migration on substrata composed of laminin and fibronectin, but they are not necessary for growth cone migration on glioma cell surfaces, whereas *N*-cadherin is important in the migration of growth cones onto the surfaces of Schwann cells.

The neurons used in these studies were sensory neurons from dorsal root ganglia of 10-day chicken embryos. Immunocytochemical staining of these neurons indicated that at this developmental stage, sensory neurons express at least four different cell adhesion molecules (integrin, L1, *N*-cadherin, and NCAM) on their neurites, growth cones, and filopodial and lamellipodial extensions (45). This evidence is a minimal indication of their involvement in growth cone adhesions. Closer examination revealed variations in the local distribution of these molecules on growth cone surfaces. Staining for integrin was particularly intense on filopodia, including the tips of filopodia, and staining for L1 was also strong on growth cone filopodia (Figs. 1 and 2). Staining for N-cadherin and NCAM was more uniform, as filopodial staining did not seem greater than on more proximal growth cone regions (Fig. 3). The significance of these topographic differences in adhesive molecules is unclear and might be related to differences arising from fixation, extraction, or other technical details. Despite this uncertainty, the staining differences suggest the presence of differences in insertion at the cell surface and transmembrane associations with cytoplasmic components that may be related to the functions of these adhesive molecules. For example, an antibody that recognizes the cytoplasmic domain of the 180-kDa form of NCAM, but not the 120- or 140-kDa forms, stained neurites and growth cones but did not stain filopodia and lamellipodia (45). This distribution implicates this form of NCAM in more stable adhesive contacts of neurites, but not in the exploratory behavior of growth cones. Another consideration is that these adhesion molecules may exist in multiple forms, which have different specificities and functions. Integrins are comprised of different α and β subunits that combine to bind distinct adhesive domains of several extracellular glycoproteins (30). The antibody we used recognizes the β_1 integrin, which is present in some but not all integrins. Thus, these immunocytochemical studies provide static evidence that particular adhesive molecules are present on growth cones, but studies with living growth cones can implicate the adhesion molecules in actual behaviors of growth cones.

Growth cone behavior *in vitro* was recorded on videotape to assess the involvement of integrins in growth cone migration on substrata coated with purified laminin or fibronectin (43). Individual growth cones were located and their behavior was recorded for a period before and after the addition of molecules that might interfere

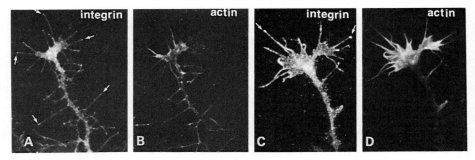

FIG. 1. **A** and **C:** Labeling of neurites and growth cones with anti-integrin. Note bright integrin staining at filopodial tips (*arrows*). This terminal staining was only seen with anti-integrin among cell adhesion molecules. **B** and **D:** Corresponding staining with fluorescent phalloidin shows the length of filopodia. ×945. (From ref. 45, with permission.)

other aspects of cytoplasmic organization and dynamics may be affected in ways that alter membrane protrusion or the forward transport of neuritic components (see chapters by Bridgman, Goldberg, et al., Phelan et al., and Pfenninger et al.). Adhesion molecules themselves may be modulated by cytoplasmic second messengers and exhibit variations in adhesive function. Analogues that inhibit or activate second messengers are useful experimental probes, as are techniques to monitor the fluctuations in concentration or location of second messengers in relation to specific growth cone behaviors (see chapters by Bentley and O'Conner, Davis et al., and Poo and Quillan). Elucidation of the biochemical and cellular consequences of the formation of each adhesive bond is necessary to understand fully how growth cones integrate the multiple adhesive interactions that may occur as they navigate complicated environments.

Information that is gained from molecular and biochemical approaches should be validated by studies that probe living growth cones and their behaviors. These studies require additional attention to the microscopic apparatus for viewing living growth cones and the methods used to present growth cones with experimental surfaces or substrata. However, with such creative approaches, detailed information about growth cone behavior in specific experimental contexts is acquired. These observations of growth cones can be as simple as confrontation with a boundary between two alternative substrata of purified adhesive molecules (see chapter by Baier and Bonhoeffer) or as complex as individual living growth cones within intact portions of nervous tissue (see chapters by Eisen and Pike, Smith and Jahr, and Mason and Godement). The future of research on growth cone navigation offers many exciting prospects.

ACKNOWLEDGMENTS

This research was supported by grants HD19950 and NS24403 from the National Institutes of Health and grants from the Minnesota Medical Foundation. The work of Terri Shattuck, Florence Roche, and Irene Pech is described here, and antibodies were generously supplied by Leo Furcht, Ben Geiger, Alan Horwitz, Vance Lemmon, James McCarthy, Melitta Schachner, and Masatoshi Takeichi.

REFERENCES

1. Harrison RG. The reactions of embryonic cells to solid structures. *J Exp Zool* 1914;17:521–531.
2. Nakai J. Studies on the mechanism determining the course of nerve fibers in tissue culture. II. The mechanism of fasciculation. *Zeit fur Zellforsch* 1960;52:427–449.
3. Nakai J, Kawasaki Y. Studies on the mechanism determining the course of nerve fibers in tissue culture. I. The reaction of the growth cone to various obstructions. *Zeit fur Zellforsch* 1959;51:108–122.
4. Speidel C. Studies of living nerves. II. Activities of ameboid growth cones, sheath cells and myelin segments, as revealed by prolonged observation of individual nerve fibers in frog tadpoles. *Am J Anat* 1933;52:1–79.
5. Speidel C. Adjustments of nerve endings. *Harvey Lect* 1941;36:126–158.

6. Godina G. The morphological and structural features of neurons *in vitro* studied by phase-contrast and time-lapse movies. In: Rose GG, ed. *Cinematography in cell biology*. New York: Academic Press, 1964;313–338.
7. *Locomotion of tissue cells. Ciba Found Symp 14 (new series)*. Amsterdam: Elsevier, 1973.
8. Wessells NK, Spooner BS, Luduena MA. Surface movements, microfilaments and cell locomotion. In: *Locomotion of tissue cells. Ciba Found Symp 14 (new series)*. Amsterdam: Elsevier, 1973;53–82.
9. Bray D, Bunge MB. The growth cone in neurite extension. In: *Locomotion of tissue cells, Ciba Found Symp 14 (new series)*. Amsterdam: Elsevier, 1973;195–209.
10. Bunge MB. Fine structure of nerve fibers and growth cones in isolated sympathetic neurons in culture. *J Cell Biol* 1973;56:713–735.
11. Luduena MA, Wessells NK. Cell locomotion, nerve elongation and microfilaments. *Dev Biol* 1973;30:427–440.
12. Yamada KM, Spooner BS, Wessells NK. Ultrastructure and function of growth cones and axons of cultured nerve cells. *J Cell Biol* 1971;49:614–635.
13. Carter SB. Principles of cell motility: the directionality of cell movement and cancer invasion. *Nature (Lond)* 1965;208:1183–1187.
14. Gail MH, Boone CW. Cell-substrate adhesivity. *Exp Cell Res* 1972;70:33–40.
15. Harris A. Behavior of cultured cells on substrata of variable adhesiveness. *Exp Cell Res* 1973;77:285–297.
16. Letourneau PC. Possible roles for cell-to-substratum adhesion in neuronal morphogenesis. *Dev Biol* 1975;44:77–91.
17. Letourneau PC. Cell-to-substratum adhesion and guidance of axonal elongation. *Dev Biol* 1975;44:92–101.
18. Bray D. Mechanical tension produced by nerve cells in tissue culture. *J Cell Sci* 1979;37:391–410.
19. Bray D. Filopodial contraction and growth cone guidance. In: Bellair R, Curtis A, Dunn G, eds. *Cell behavior*. Cambridge: Cambridge University Press, 1982;298–318.
20. Bray D. Axonal growth in response to experimentally applied mechanical tension. *Dev Biol* 1984;102:379–389.
21. Bentley D, Keshishian H. Pathfinding by peripheral pioneer neurons in grasshoppers. *Science* 1982;218:1082–1088.
22. O'Conner TP, Duerr JS, Bentley D. Pioneer growth cone steering decisions mediated by single filopodial contact *in situ*. *J Neurosci* 1990;10:3935–3946.
23. Bastiani MJ, Doe CQ, Helfand SL, Goodman CS. Neuronal specificity and growth cone guidance in grasshopper and *Drosophila* embryos. *Trends Neurosci* 1985;8:257–266.
24. Harrelson AL, Goodman CG. Growth cone guidance in insects: fasciclin II is a member of the immunoglobulin superfamily. *Science* 1988;242:700–708.
25. Rutishauser U, Jessell T. Cell adhesion molecules in vertebrate neural development. *Physiol Rev* 1988;68:819–857.
26. Edelman G. Morphoregulatory molecules. *Biochemistry* 1988;27:3343–3353.
27. Takeichi M. The cadherins: cell–cell adhesion molecules controlling animal morphogenesis. *Development* 1988;102:639–656.
28. Hatta K, Okada TS, Takeichi M. A monoclonal antibody disrupting calcium-dependent cell–cell adhesion of brain tissues. Possible role of its target antigen in animal pattern formation. *Proc Natl Acad Sci USA* 1985;82:2789–2793.
29. Bozyczko D, Horwitz AF. The participation of a putative cell surface receptor for laminin and fibronectin in peripheral neurite extension. *J Neurosci* 1986;6:1241–1251.
30. Hynes RO, DeSimone DW, Lawler JJ, et al. Nectins and integrins: versatility in cell adhesion. In: Edelman GM, Cunningham BA, Thiéry JP, eds. *Morphoregulatory molecules*. New York: John Wiley and Sons, 1990;173–200.
31. Rogers SL, Letourneau PC, Palm SL, McCarthy JB, Furcht LT. Neurite extension by peripheral and central nervous system neurons in response to substratum-bound fibronectin and laminin. *Dev Biol* 1983;98:212–220.
32. Carbonetto S, Gruver MM, Turner DC. Nerve fiber growth in culture on fibronectin, collagen, and glycosaminoglycan substrates. *J Neurosci* 1983;3:2324–2335.
33. Manthorpe M, Engvall E, Ruoslahti E, Longo FM, Davis GE, Varon S. Laminin promotes neuritic regeneration from cultured peripheral and central neurons. *J Cell Biol* 1983;97:1882–1890.
34. Wehrle B, Chiquet M. Tenascin is accumulated along developing peripheral nerves and allows neurite outgrowth *in vitro*. *Development* 1990;110:401–416.

35. Tomaselli K, Neugebauer KM, Bixby JL, Lilien J, Reichardt LF. N-cadherins and integrins: two receptor systems that mediate neuronal process outgrowth on astrocytic surfaces. Neuron 1988; 1:33–43.

36. Rogers SL, Letourneau PC, Peterson BA, Furcht LT, McCarthy JB. Selective interaction of peripheral and central nervous system neurons with two distinct cell-binding domains of fibronectin. J Cell Biol 1987;105:1435–1442.

37. Seilheimer B, Schachner M. Studies of adhesion molecules mediating interactions between cells of peripheral nervous system indicate a major role for L1 in mediating sensory neuron growth on Schwann cells. J Cell Biol 1988;107:341–351.

38. Lagenaur C, Lemmon V. An L1-like molecule, the 8D9 antigen, is a potent substrate for neurite extension. Proc Natl Acad Sci USA 1987;84:7753–7757.

39. Bixby JL, Lilien J, Reichardt LF. Identification of the major proteins that promote neuronal process outgrowth on Schwann cells in vitro. J Cell Biol 1988;107:353–361.

40. Chang S, Rathjen FG, Raper JA. Extension of neurites on axons is impaired by antibodies against specific neural cell surface glycoproteins. J Cell Biol 1987;104:355–362.

41. Grumet M, Hoffman S, Edelman GM. Two antigenically related neuronal CAMs of different specificities mediate neuron–neuron and neuron–glia adhesion. Proc Natl Acad Sci USA 1984;81:267–271.

42. Matsunaga M, Hatta K, Nagafuchi A, Takeichi M. Guidance of optic nerve fibers by N-cadherin adhesion molecules. Nature (Lond) 1988;334:62–64.

43. Letourneau PC, Pech IV, Rogers SL, Palm SL, McCarthy JB, Furcht LT. Growth cone migration across extracellular matrix components depends on integrin, but migration across glioma cells does not. J Neurosci Res 1988;21:286–297.

44. Letourneau PC, Shattuck TA, Roche FK, Takeichi M, Lemmon V. Nerve growth cone migration onto Schwann cells involves the calcium-dependent adhesion molecule, N-cadherin. Dev Biol 1990; 138:430–442.

45. Letourneau PC, Shattuck TA. Distribution and possible interactions of actin-associated proteins and cell adhesion molecules of nerve growth cones. Development 1989;105:505–519.

46. Ruoslahti E, Argraves WS, Gehlsen KR, Gailit J, Pierschbacher MD. The Arg-Gly-Asp sequence and its receptors: a versatile recognition system. In: Edelman GM, Cunningham BA, Thiery JP, eds. Morphoregulatory molecules. New York: John Wiley and Sons, 1990;201–216.

47. Volberg T, Geiger B, Kartenbeck J, Franke WW. Changes of membrane–microfilament interaction in intercellular adherens junctions upon removal of extracellular Ca^{++}. J Cell Biol 1986;102:1832–1842.

The Nerve Growth Cone, edited by P. C. Letourneau,
S. B. Kater, and E. R. Macagno, Raven Press, Ltd.,
New York © 1992.

16

Axon Guidance *in vitro* by a Target-Derived Cell Membrane Component

Herwig Baier and Friedrich Bonhoeffer

Max-Planck-Institut für Entwicklungsbiologie, W-7400 Tübingen, Germany

Many decades have passed since the phenomenon of axon guidance during the formation of topographic neuronal projections first attracted the attention of biologists (1). Very early on it was hypothesized that the target organ of the axons expresses directional cues on its surface and that such directional cues could be provided by concentration gradients of some cell surface molecules (2). For the formation of a topographic projection from the source to the target—in our discussion, from the retina to the optic tectum—a simple gradient model requires a set of two antagonistic gradients along each of the two spatial dimensions (anterior-posterior and dorsal-ventral) of the target (3). In addition, the axons coming from different positions of the source must differ in their abilities to read the gradients in the target field, otherwise all axons would be guided to the same position. In a gradient model, these reading properties of the axons must also depend on their position within the source organ in a graded fashion (4).

With the introduction of modern tracing methods for axonal trajectories, it became quite clear that in the retinotectal system the target tissue contains directional cues for both the anterior-posterior and the dorsal-ventral axes (5–7). The elucidation of the physical and chemical nature of such cues is the goal of some *in vitro* studies, which will briefly be summarized here.

REACTIONS OF TEMPORAL RETINAL AXONS TO SUDDEN SPATIAL OR TEMPORAL CHANGES OF A GUIDING MOLECULE (REVIEW)

We have investigated guidance of chick retinal axons by cell membranes derived from various positions of the target organ, the *tectum opticum*. We will mainly discuss the behavior of axons originating in the temporal retina. These axons terminate *in vivo* in the anterior and do not invade the posterior tectum. In the *in vitro* experiments, we use retinal explants and place them on carpets of cell membranes. These carpets consist of alternating narrow stripes of anterior and posterior tectal membranes. Axons extending from the explant may now show their ability to distinguish between these two membrane substrata (Fig. 1).

In accord with their behavior *in vivo*, the temporal retinal axons exhibit a strong preference for growth on stripes of anterior membranes (8). By inactivation studies it was possible to show that this preference is not due to the attractiveness of anterior membranes but rather to a repellent or inhibitory property of posterior membranes (9). This inhibitory property of posterior membranes is also found in fish (10) and mouse (11). It can only be detected during the period when the retinotectal projection is being formed, for example, between embryonic day 6 and 14 in chick. The repellent activity appears to have a graded distribution along the anterior-posterior tectal axis (12). Early experiments on the biochemical nature of the repellent or inhibitory activity of posterior membranes showed that it can be inactivated by antiserum that is directed against purified membranes of posterior tectum (13), by mild heat treatment (9), and by treatment of the posterior membranes with phosphatidylinositol-specific phospholipase C (PI-PLC) (14), an enzyme that removes those glycoproteins from the cell surface that are anchored in the plasma membrane by a glycosyl-phosphatidylinositol linkage (15). Inactivation by PI-PLC indicates that the protein responsible for the observed *in vitro* guidance is not a transmembrane protein.

Whereas we have found a gradient along the anterior-posterior axis of the tectum, we have been unable to detect a gradient along the nasal-temporal axis in the retina. In contrast, when retinal explants from various positions along the nasal-temporal

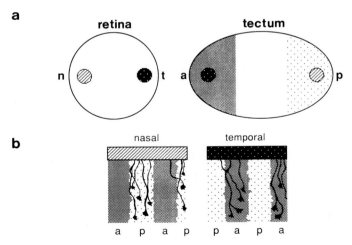

FIG. 1. Simplified schematic diagram of retinotopic projection (**a**) and the stripe assay (**b**). **a:** The figure indicates that temporal (t) retinal axons project to the anterior (a) and nasal (n) axons to the posterior (p) part of the optic tectum. **b:** When retinal explants are placed on a carpet consisting of alternating stripes of anterior (a) and posterior (p) tectal membranes, temporal and nasal axons grow preferentially on membranes of their target region (8,22).

axis are examined with respect to their ability to distinguish between anterior and posterior membranes, an abrupt transition becomes apparent. Within 0.2 mm the properties change from temporal (all axons detect the anterior-posterior difference) to nasal (the axons in general are unable to detect the anterior-posterior difference) (8). This is not expected according to the gradient model.

The experiments mentioned above show that temporal axons, when offered a choice between anterior and posterior membranes, will avoid the posterior membranes and grow on anterior membranes. Surprisingly, when presented with pure membranes of either kind, temporal axons grow about as well and as fast on posterior as they do on anterior membranes (16). This result indicates that posterior membranes are not simply inhibitory for growth of temporal axons. Instead, temporal axons seem to be repelled or deflected when they encounter the border at which the concentration of posterior membranes increases abruptly.

In addition to the guiding activity, posterior membranes exhibit another interesting property; they can induce the collapse of temporal growth cones (17). Growth cones of axons elongating on laminin *in vitro* are dynamic structures, which usually exhibit a number of filopodia and large flat and spread-out lamellipodia. Several

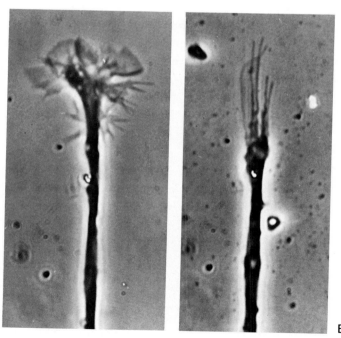

A   B

FIG. 2. Collapse of temporal growth cones induced by posterior membranes. **a:** Temporal growth cone on laminin; **b:** same growth cone 10 min after addition of membrane vesicles derived from posterior tectum (courtesy of B. Müller).

different treatments can cause the growth cones to collapse. During collapse, the growth cone thickens and the filopodia shorten unless they are fixed to the substratum at their tips. Lamellipodia lose contact to the substratum and become resorbed. As a consequence, axons retract within a few minutes (Fig. 2). Such growth cone collapse was originally observed by Kapfhammer and Raper (18), when growth cones encountered axons of heterotypic neurons. It can also be induced by cell membranes or membrane proteins incorporated into lipid vesicles. When growing retinal axons of temporal retinal origin are exposed to membranes of posterior tectal origin, rapid growth cone collapse is observed (17). As in the case for *in vitro* axon guidance, posterior tectal membranes affect temporal and not nasal retinal growth cones. Anterior tectal membranes do not cause collapse of temporal growth cones. The collapse-inducing activity of posterior membranes decreases with increasing developmental age (B. Müller, *personal communication*), as does the guiding activity (8).

The similarities between the guiding and the collapse-inducing activities led us to suspect that both phenomena may be caused by the same molecule. The collapse and the stripe assay were used to search for the responsible molecule in chick embryos. Biochemical fractionation of tectal membranes in combination with the use of an antiserum that abolishes the guiding activity of posterior membranes, led to the identification of a glycoprotein that is involved in growth cone collapse and in *in vitro* guidance of temporal axons (13) (Fig. 3). This molecule, which has a molecular weight of about 33 kDa, is removed from the membranes by PI-PLC, binds to

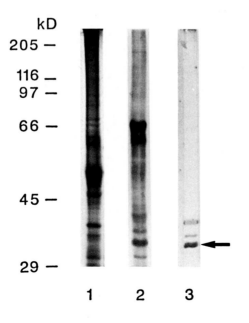

FIG. 3. Protein patttern of increasingly enriched fractions of collapse-inducing activity. Samples collected during enrichment of the 33-kDa component were fractionated by SDS-PAGE. Lanes from left to right show starting material (lane 1—brain membranes), the 1-M NaCl-eluted fraction (lane 2), and reconstituted vesicles from this fraction (lane 3). Gel is stained with silver.

increasing **p**-gradient served as preformed pathways for fiber outgrowth. Retinal fibers on these stripes can only grow straight ahead and cannot evade the gradient by turning to one side or the other. Whereas nasal axons grow seemingly undisturbed from pure **a**-substrate to **p**-rich regions and reach distances of about 3 to 4 mm (or even more), the response of temporal fibers to the **p**-gradients depends strongly on the steepness of the gradient.

At this point it is necessary to introduce some conventions in the description of gradient forms. The maximum **p**-concentration is declared to be 100%, pure **a**-material to be 0%. (As far as concentration differences are concerned it is not important how much of the repellent component is in anterior membranes.) A standard growth cone extends over about 30 μm. This is also the extreme distance between two sites of measurement for gradient detection within the growth cone at any one time. The slope of a **p**-gradient is then given as a difference in **p**-concentration per growth cone length. A gradient's maximum slope value appeared to be most useful to correlate it with axonal behavior.

The reactions of temporal axons to increasing **p**-gradients can roughly be grouped into three classes: no visible reaction, slowing down, and complete growth stop. These three responses were distinguished by comparing the growth of temporal and adjacent nasal fibers. Nasal fibers served in any case as a control for culture conditions.

No clearly visible reaction is seen in gradients of less than 1% per growth cone. In such experiments, temporal growth cones—like their nasal companions—can reach 100% **p**.

In gradients of more than 1% per growth cone and up to 5% per growth cone temporal fibers can also grow into regions of maximum p-concentration. But in these cases, there is a detectable difference (> 0.3 mm) in overall fiber length between nasal and temporal axons (Fig. 7). The difference seems likely to be due to a decreased mean growth rate by temporal growth cones. Whether this results from a continuously slower growth or from periods of growth rate reduction interrupting normal rates of growth cannot be deduced from studies on fixed material.

At gradients of more than 5% per growth cone, temporal fibers stop growing within the gradient field or at its bottom and do not reach 100% **p**. They form dense bundles that are morphologically distinct from fibers that were still growing at the time of fixation.

It is, however, still possible that axons held up by relatively steep gradients may—after a waiting or habituation period—grow further. The classification of gradients given above may critically depend on the experimental time; so far only 48 hr has been tested.

These results provide a glimpse of how shallow a gradient a growth cone can detect. The astonishing sensitivity is revealed only if the conditions are chosen properly. Whereas in the stripe assay, temporal growth cones can only respond to differences of 30% **p** or more, they are able to sense minute differences of less than one-tenth of 30% of **p**-material over their length, if it is presented to the growth cone continuously as a long-range gradient.

It is tempting to compare the dimensions of gradients such as these with those of

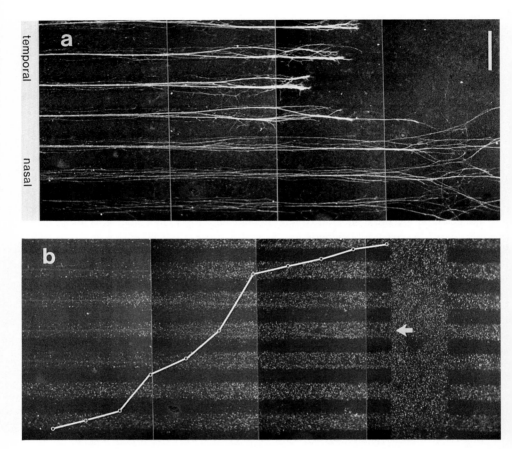

FIG. 7. Retinal axons (**a**) growing from left to right on narrow membrane lanes, each containing a gradient of posterior membranes indicated by the density of fluorescent beads (**b**). The gradient depicted in **b** is presented as in Fig. 6 and was measured in the middle lane (*arrow*). (Changes in light intensity are due to the photographic reproduction process and might be misleading.) The retina was stained with the fluorescent dye rhodamine-B-isothiocyanate. Temporal axons (indicated) obviously grew over a shorter distance than their nasal counterparts. The transition zone from nasal to temporal is small, extending over at most 200 μm. The maximum slope of the gradient shown here is 4.2% per growth cone. At the right margin of **b**, separate membrane lanes are joined by a perpendicular membrane stripe reached only by nasal fibers. This feature results from the design of the filtration device and indicates the edge of the membrane carpet. Scale bar, 0.2 mm.

the *in vivo* target, the tectum. A linear gradient with a slope that is effective in slowing down (and presumably also guiding) temporal axons would be in the millimeter range (e.g., a gradient with 1% per growth cone extends to 3 mm if it starts at 0 and ends at maximum concentration). This is about half the length of the tectum (in anterior-posterior dimension) when first innervated by retinal axons.

So, this conceptually rather simple *in vitro* assay reveals a sensitivity of growth cones toward gradients that is in the order of magnitude expected for the *in vivo* situation. This coincidence, however, has to be interpreted with care, as long as we have no information about the actual spatial distribution of the putative guiding factor found in tectal membranes.

CONCEIVABLE APPROACHES TO OPEN QUESTIONS ABOUT AXON GUIDANCE AND THE RETINOTECTAL SYSTEM

Questions concerning the formation of the retinotectal map by axon pathfinding and guidance can be addressed at three interdependent levels.

The purified 33-kDa glycoprotein offers opportunities to do molecular studies. Cloning and sequencing of the protein will provide insight into the molecular basis of axon repulsion and growth cone collapse. By raising antibodies against the purified protein, we should be able to determine the pattern of expression of this antigen on tectal cells. *In situ* hybridization studies would help to elucidate whether this expression pattern arises by transcriptional regulation. In a next step, one might search for the putative receptor expressed on retinal growth cones.

A second approach deals with the cellular events that take place before, during, and after guidance. Pharmacological studies to characterize the second-messenger pathways involved in axon guidance and growth cone collapse are under way. Inevitably, one will have to look in living cultures and observe growth cones and their responses to repulsive material using video-microscopic recordings. One project, for example, could be the measurement of changes in calcium concentrations within growth cones turning away from posterior membrane borders. This is done by applying a calcium-sensitive fluorescent dye (fura-2) to neurites growing *in vitro*.

Third, it is, of course, important not to lose sight of the biology of the retinotectal system. There are still a large number of unsolved problems. One of these is the topographic ordering of fibers along the dorsal-ventral axis, a phenomenon, that cannot be tackled using one of the existing *in vitro* assays. In addition, we have yet to demonstrate that the retinal fibers possess graded positional information as postulated by the model. In fact, the converse seems to be true: In each of the *in vitro* assays developed so far (8,17,21), just as in the gradient experiments presented here, a sharp transition within the retina from temporal to nasal properties has been observed. This is also seen with a monoclonal antibody that specifically stains the temporal half of the retina (McLoon, *unpublished*).

This, of course, cannot be a complete list of possible activities in this area. The retinotectal projection is a complex phenomenon at all levels, from growth cone biochemistry to embryonic pattern formation. But it is, hopefully, not too complex to be understood by the 200th birthday of the growth cone.

ACKNOWLEDGMENTS

We wish to thank Dr. Daniel St. Johnston, Dr. Jochen Walter, and Bernhard Müller for critically reading and improving the manuscript.

REFERENCES

1. Sperry RW. Visuomotor coordination in the newt (*Triturus vivescence*) after regeneration of the optic nerves. *J Comp Neurol* 1943;79:33–55.
2. Sperry RW. Chemoaffinity in the orderly growth of nerve fiber patterns and connections. *Proc Natl Acad Sci* 1963;5:703–710.
3. Gierer A. Development of projections between areas of the nervous system. *Biol Cybern* 1981; 42:69–78.
4. Bonhoeffer F, Gierer A. How do retinal axons find their targets on the tectum? *Trends Neurosci* 1984;7:378–381.
5. Fujisawa H, Watanabe K, Tani N, Ibata Y. Retinotopic analysis of fiber pathways in amphibians. II. The frog *Rana nigromaculata*. *Brain Res* 1981;206:21–26.
6. Thanos S, Bonhoeffer F. Investigations on the development and topographic order of retinotectal axons: anterograde and retrograde staining of axons and perikarya with rhodamine *in vivo*. *J Comp Neurol* 1983;219:420–430.
7. Stuermer CAO. Pathways of regenerated retinotectal axons in goldfish. *J Embryol Exp Morphol* 1986;93:1–28.
8. Walter J, Kern-Veits B, Huf J, Stolze B, Bonhoeffer F. Recognition of position-specific properties of tectal cell membranes by retinal axons *in vitro*. *Development* 1987;101:685–696.
9. Walter J, Henke-Fahle S, Bonhoeffer F. Avoidance of posterior tectal membranes by temporal retinal axons. *Development* 1987;101:909–913.
10. Vielmetter J, Stuermer CAO. Goldfish retinal axons respond to position-specific properties of tectal cell membranes *in vitro*. *Neuron* 1989;2:1331–1339.
11. Godement P, Bonhoeffer F. Cross-species recognition of tectal cues by retinal fibers *in vitro*. *Development* 1989;106:313–320.
12. Bonhoeffer F, Huf J. *In vitro* experiments on axon guidance demonstrating an anterior-posterior gradient on the tectum. *EMBO J* 1982;1:427–431.
13. Stahl B, Müller B, van Boxberg Y, Cox EC, Bonhoeffer F. Biochemical characterization of a putative axonal guidance molecule of the chick visual system. *Neuron* 1990;5:735–743.
14. Walter J, Müller B, Bonhoeffer F. Axonal guidance by an avoidance mechanism. *J Physiol (Paris)* 1990;84:104–110.
15. Low MG, Saltiel AR. Structural and functional roles of glycosyl-phosphatidylinositol in membranes. *Science* 1988;239:268–275.
16. Müller B, Stahl B, Bonhoeffer F. *In vitro* experiments on axonal guidance and growth-cone collapse. *J Exp Biol* 1990;153:29–46.
17. Cox EC, Müller B, Bonhoeffer F. Axonal guidance in the chick visual system: posterior tectal membranes induce collapse of growth cones from the temporal retina. *Neuron* 1990;4:31–37.
18. Kapfhammer JP, Raper JA. Collapse of growth cone structure on contact with specific neurites in culture. *J Neurosci* 1987;7:201–212.
19. Walter J, Allsopp TE, Bonhoeffer F. A common denominator of growth cone guidance and collapse. *Trends Neurosci* 1990;13:447–452.
20. Heacock AM, Agranoff BW. Clockwise growth of neurites from retinal explants. *Science* 1977; 198:64–66.
21. Halfter W, Claviez M, Schwarz U. Preferential adhesion of tectal membranes to anterior embryonic chick retina neurites. *Nature (Lond)* 1981;292:67–70.
22. Stahl B, van Boxberg Y, Müller B, Walter J, Schwarz U, Bonhoeffer F. Directional cues for retinal axons. *Cold Spring Harbor Symp Quant Biol* 1990.

The Nerve Growth Cone, edited by P. C. Letourneau,
S. B. Kater, and E. R. Macagno, Raven Press, Ltd.,
New York © 1992.

17

Interactions Between Growth Cones and Axons: Selectively Distributed Extension-Promoting and Extension-Inhibiting Components

Jonathan A. Raper, Susannah Chang, and David W. Raible

Department of Anatomy/Chemistry, University of Pennsylvania School of Medicine, Philadelphia, Pennsylvania 19104-6058

The growth cones of embryonic neurons extend along highly reproducible and specific routes (e.g., refs. 16,21). These specific trajectories are determined by the distributions of cues outside growth cones and by their cell-specific responses to those cues.

Historically, attractive and permissive interactions have been considered to be of primary importance in growth cone guidance. Since Cajal, it has been hypothesized that target tissues release diffusible molecules that lure appropriate innervating axons to them, and within the past few years, chemoattraction has been convincingly demonstrated in several systems (e.g., refs. 30,31). Yet growth cones extend very slowly, if at all, unless they are in direct contact with a permissive substratum. Thus far, a relatively small number of endogenous molecules have been identified that demonstrably promote neurite outgrowth. These include fibronectin (2), laminin (3), L1/G4/8D9/NgCAM (28), TAG-1 (19), and *N*-cadherin (5). Inhomogeneous distributions of neurite-promoting substrata can control growth cone trajectories. By analogy with laminin, discrete tracks of any one of these neurite-promoting molecules should be able to capture and direct the extension of growth cones on a nonpermissive background (e.g., ref. 22). It seems safe to assume that differentially distributed neurite promoting molecules could differentially influence the trajectories of growth cones expressing disparate subsets of receptors.

In contrast to these exclusively positive interactions, repulsive cues could be equally effective in directing growth cone extension. Perhaps the first hint that negative guidance cues are important was the finding by Tosney and Landmesser (39) that outgrowing peripheral axons in chick embryos are canalized into a narrow opening through the chondrocytes that form the pelvic girdle. Since then, repulsive cues have been implicated in several other systems. These include the avoidance of posterior half-somites by spinal axons in the chick (14,26), the avoidance of posterior tectum by temporal retinal ganglion cell axons in the chick (13,40), the avoidance of serotonin secreting neurons by the processes of particular snail neurons (20), and the avoidance of oligodendrocytes by growth cones (17). In some cases there has been some progress in identifying the molecules that appear to be responsible for repulsion (9,10,14).

Our focus has been to identify growth cone guidance cues associated with axons. Early-forming axonal pathways are thought to form a highway system of sorts that later growing axons navigate on. Evidence from invertebrates and vertebrates suggests that particular growth cones grow on specific axonal pathways and that the absence of these pathways leads to navigational errors by those growth cones (e.g., 4,15,27,33,34). It has been proposed that axons are not only permissive for growth cone extension but are differentially labeled one from another and that particular growth cones prefer to grow in association with some labels as opposed to others (21,33). We have recently identified a cell surface glycoprotein that is expressed on a subset of axonal surfaces and that is implicated in the promotion of growth cone extension by a functional assay. We have used another functional assay to identify differentially expressed axonal cues that interfere with growth cone motility. These findings are consistent with the idea that axons are differentially labeled, that the labels can either fasciculate or inhibit extension, and that growth cones distinguish between these labels.

GLYCOPROTEINS ON AXONS IMPLICATED IN NEURITE PROMOTION

One method for identifying axonal surface molecules of interest has been to raise monoclonal antibodies against brain glycoproteins. Monoclonals raised against the axonal surface glycoprotein G4 by Rathjen and co-workers (37) stain most or all axons in the white matter of the embryonic chick spinal cord (Fig. 1A). G4 is related or identical to 8D9, L1, NILE, and NgCAM (6,18,29). Its most prevalent molecular weight is 130 kDa. It has been shown to promote growth cone extension in two bioassays. In one, single, fluorescently labeled sympathetic neurons are forced to grow on fascicles of unlabeled sympathetic axons (11). The lengths of labeled axons were measured after growing approximately 20 h in the presence or absence of anti-G4 polyclonal or monoclonal antibodies (Fig. 2A). The lengths of labeled axons shifted toward shorter values in the presence of antibody as compared with its absence. Anti-G4 antibodies have no effect on axon lengths if the experiment is repeated on laminin instead of axonal substrata, implying that anti-G4 antibodies are not toxic and do not interfere in a general way with growth cone extension. In a second assay, purified G4 is shown to promote vigorous neurite outgrowth from a variety of neurons (12,28).

G4 therefore serves as an archetype for neurite-promoting molecules. It is present

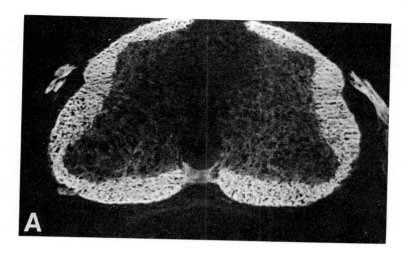

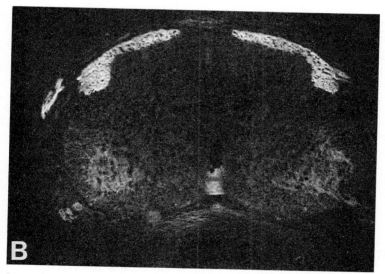

FIG. 1. Cross-sections of embryonic day 7 chick spinal cords stained with (**A**) anti-G4 and (**B**) anti-DM.

in quantity on the surfaces of nascent and embryonic axons, and it is a strong promoter of neurite outgrowth.

The same approach has led to the identification of another cell surface protein, DM, that is expressed on a subset of cell bodies and axons in the embryonic spinal cord (Fig. 1B). These are the dorsal funiculi, motor neurons and their axons, dorsal root ganglia and their axons, and cells within the floor plate. Sympathetic axons are

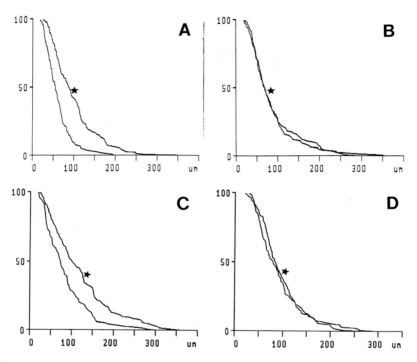

FIG. 2. Distributions of lengths of single sympathetic neurites growing (**A**) on sympathetic axons with and without (*) anti-G4, (**B**) on laminin with and without anti-G4, (**C**) on sympathetic axons with and without (*) anti-DM, and (**D**) on laminin with and without anti-DM.

labeled *in vivo*, and this labeling can be shown to be on sympathetic axon surfaces *in vitro*. By comparing the staining patterns of G4 and DM in the spinal cord, it is obvious that many axons do not express a significant amount of DM. A similar staining pattern has been described by other groups, and alternate names for the same protein may be SC1 or BEN (32,38). The molecular weight of DM is 95 kDa. A partial amino acid sequence of the amino-terminal end indicates that it is not related to any well-characterized protein. A monoclonal antibody against DM decreases the lengths of sympathetic neurites growing on other sympathetic axons (Fig. 2C) but does not affect the lengths of sympathetic neurites growing on laminin (Fig. 2D). DM therefore may be a substrate molecule or receptor involved in neurite promotion.

DM is expressed on a crisply defined subset of axons and may therefore represent a differentially expressed neurite-promoting molecule that allows growth cones to distinguish between axon types. Alternatively, it could be a differentially expressed receptor for a neurite-promoting molecule.

DM is a useful marker for motor neuron development. In wholemounts of the brainstem, cranial motor neurons can be visualized as they extend neurites from axonogenesis up through late stages. An example of anti-DM staining of the brain-

vivo (25). These studies and those above suggest that PAs have a role in neuronal cell migration in the developing cerebellum.

GROWTH CONE AND CELL SURFACE–ASSOCIATED PROTEASE

Most of the proteolysis seen in the fibrin overlay of granule neurons appears to be cell-associated, because a brief lowering of the pH (<4) or several rinses with a large volume of medium leads to a loss of fibrinolytic activity concomitant with the appearance of PA in the wash fluid (26). tPA accounts for about 90% of the PA secreted by granule neurons in culture and virtually all the cell-associated PA in the wash fluid (27). Because the fibrinolytic activity can be restored to the cells by a brief incubation with an exogenous source of tPA, granule neurons appear to possess a cell surface receptor for tPA (26).

Murine ^{125}I-tPA was used to characterize the properties of this presumed receptor. The binding is rapid, reaching completion within 20 min. tPA binding is specific, saturable, and of high affinity with a K_d of 50 pM (27). There are approximately 30,000 tPA binding sites per cell in these granule neuron cultures. The binding is reversible, and virtually all the bound tPA is released within minutes by washing, indicating that it is not internalized by an uptake site or surface-bound PA inhibitor (28). Even after several hours the released tPA is still intact single-chain tPA when examined by zymography (29).

Specificity of the ^{125}I-tPA binding was examined in the presence of an excess of different serine proteases or modified tPA molecules (Table 1). Both murine and recombinant human tPA compete for the binding, whereas neither mouse nor human uPA compete. Thrombin and plasminogen, two other serine proteases that bind to cells, also failed to compete for the binding. tPA binding to granule neurons does not involve its carbohydrate side chains nor the active site serine, because both

TABLE 1. ^{125}I-tPA binding to cerebellar neurons[a]

Competing protein	Molarity (nM)	% Binding
None	0	100
Murine tPA	11	0
Human tPA	11	0
Murine uPA	11	106
Human uPA	11	110
Human thrombin	11	94
Human plasminogen	11	78
Murine DFP-tPA	11	5
Deglycosylated tPA	11	0

[a]Cerebellar cells stripped of endogenous PA by pH 3 were washed and incubated for 30 min at 20°C with murine ^{125}I-tPA (0.23 nM) in absence or presence of a 50-fold molar excess of the competing protein. Percent specific binding was calculated relative to inhibition by a 50-fold molar excess of active nonlabeled tPA.

endoglycosidase H–treated tPA and diisopropylfluorophosphate–treated tPA were able to compete successfully for binding. The catalytic B chain alone does not bind to the neurons, suggesting that the cell binding domain of tPA resides in the amino-terminal portion of the molecule (29). Furthermore, using site-directed mutants of human tPA missing the finger, growth factor, finger + growth factor, kringle 1, or kringle 2 (30), in preliminary studies with Drs. M. Gething, R. Bassel-Duby, and J. Sambrook, we have found that tPA missing the growth factor domain fails to compete with native tPA for binding to neurons.

The tPA bound to granule neurons has been visualized at the electron microscope level with an antibody to murine tPA (28). Although tPA is bound over the entire surface of the granule neuron, it appears concentrated at the trailing edge of granule neurons migrating on neurite cables in culture, thereby being positioned at a critical site of cell detachment (25). tPA bound to the axon and growth cone of a granule neuron in culture is shown in Fig. 1. Interestingly, this growth cone possesses the laser-like path-cutting tPA molecule; however, its "boxing glove" appearance also lends support to the pugilistic theory (5) of growth cone advancement.

Our early studies with the fibrin overlay assay indicated that PA activity could be localized to neuronal growth cones (31). Therefore, the relationship between PA activity and axonal growth cone movement was explored with more readily observable neurons of the peripheral nervous system (32). Studies by Valinsky and LeDouarin (33) have shown that the migratory neural crest cells, precursors to these large neurons, actively secrete PA. The large and dynamic growth cones of dissociated sensory neurons in culture show a pronounced PA activity as indicated by the zone of fibrinolysis seen in Fig. 2. uPA is the major PA secreted into the medium by

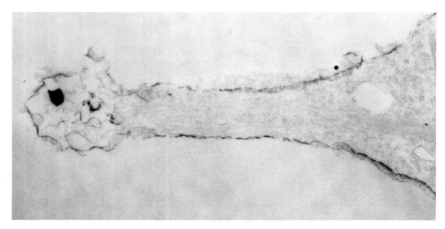

FIG. 1. EM immuno-localization of tPA bound to axonal surface and growth cone of cerebellar granule neuron. Indirect immunoperoxidase labeling with an antibody to murine tPA bound to live cerebellar cells in culture, followed by fixation and thin sectioning.

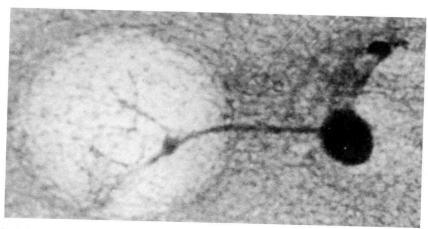

FIG. 2. Growth cone–associated plasminogen activator. Dissociated sensory neuron from 2-day mouse in culture for 3 days was overlayed with a fibrin clot containing plasminogen. Sites of plasminogen activator lead to fibrinolytic zones.

sensory neurons in culture, and the only form of PA released at the growth cone, as assessed by zymography (29). Similarly, Pittman (34) found that uPA is the major PA released at the growth cones of dissociated sympathetic neurons in culture. Furthermore, he (34,35) has also shown the secretion of a collagenase activity in his cultures.

Sensory and other peripheral neurons not only secrete PA but they deposit PA on the substratum underneath the advancing growth cone, where it may be strategically placed to participate in the local degradation of matrix or cell adhesion components (36). As much as one-fourth of the total PA activity in these sensory neuron cultures was associated with the substratum, where PA activity has a half-life of several hours and appears to be part of the substrate adhesion material (SAM) (37) normally deposited by growing neurites. The uPA may be bound to surface molecules and then deposited as a normal occurrence of membrane shedding or may be secreted by the neurons and then bind to SAM. There is evidence to favor the latter mechanism in nonneuronal systems in which PA binds *in vitro* to fibronectin and laminin in the extracellular matrix while retaining its proteolytic activity (18,38).

Axonal growth cones of sensory neurons clear a path in the underlying matrix when grown on a fibronectin substratum as seen in Fig. 3. This clearing is not a "snowplow" effect but a true degradation of the fibronectin matrix as indicated by the release of ^{125}I-fibronectin peptides into the culture medium (39). Although many small peptide fragments were seen when plasminogen was incorporated into the N2 culture medium, the clearing was independent of plasminogen in the medium, and several large 200,000 to 220,000 M_r fragments of fibronectin were seen on nonreducing SDS-PAGE. The plasminogen independence of this cleavage is confirmed by its insensitivity to plasmin inhibitors (Table 2).

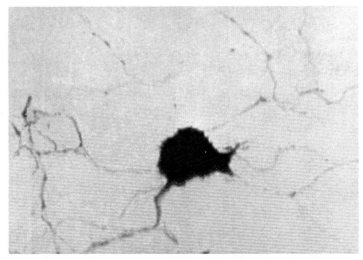

FIG. 3. Displacement of FITC-fibronectin from the substrata under a growing sensory neuron in a serum-free plasminogen-free medium for 16 hr as visualized by epi-fluorescence.

The fibronectin-degrading activity requires direct cell contact and does not readily diffuse into the culture medium, because a naked ^{125}I-fibronectin coverslip placed adjacent to an identical coverslip with neurons shows little release of radioactivity (39). This finding suggests that the protease(s) involved with fibronectin degradation is localized to the neuronal cell surface and/or its associated substratum; furthermore, protease(s) secreted into the medium may account for only a small part of matrix degradation. Isolation of integral membrane proteins and associated molecules by Triton X-114–phase separation shows that the only proteases identified in this material are uPA and tPA, and no other protease capable of cleaving either casein or fibronectin is detected by zymography of the detergent phase.

A series of protease inhibitors have been examined for their effect on ^{125}I-fi-

TABLE 2. *Inhibitor sensitivity of sensory neuron protease that cleaves fibronectin[a]*

Treatment	% of Total CPM released
None	12.9
Aprotinin (3,000 U/ml)	11.4
Aminocaproic acid (3 mM)	12.6
Hirudin (10 U/ml)	13.3
TIMP (10 μg/ml)	12.5
Protease nexin (human) (10 μg/ml)	3.2
Protease nexin (recombinant) (10 μg/ml)	4.4

[a]Percentage of ^{125}I-fibronectin CPM released from coated coverslips by growing sensory neurons within 16 hr is indicated. Cells were cultured in serum-free N2 medium in the absence of plasminogen.

bronectin degradation to help characterize the neuronal-associated protease responsible for the cleavage of fibronectin (Table 2). Although plasminogen was omitted from the culture medium, the possibility that cell-associated plasminogen (40) was providing a plasmin source was tested by the addition of a very high concentration of the plasmin inhibitor aprotinin. Cell-associated plasmin is not known to be protected from this low-molecular-weight inhibitor. Aprotinin at a concentration greater than 100 times that necessary to block any soluble plasmin was without effect on the fibronectin cleavage, as was aminocaproic acid, thus ruling out plasmin as the active enzyme. Similarly, inhibitors of thrombin (hirudin) and metalloproteases (TIMP) at high concentrations had no effect on the cleavage, thus eliminating these proteases from consideration. Of the inhibitors tested, only PN, an inhibitor of thrombin, plasmin, and uPA, significantly reduced the release of ^{125}I-fibronectin fragments (39). Also an antibody to mouse tPA had no effect on the cleavage event.

These findings suggest that cell-associated uPA (or an unidentified protease) may act directly to catalyze the limited cleavage of the fibronectin substratum. Quigley and co-workers (41) reported a similar limited cleavage of fibronectin in a "test tube" assay with uPA purified from an avian sarcoma. The formation of the 200,000 to 220,000 M_r fragments is consistent with cleavage at an Arg-Thr that occurs near the carboxyl terminal immediately before the interchain disulfide bonds, or at position 260–261 near the amino terminus. Cleavage near the carboxyl terminus would permit the conversion of the dimeric fibronectin into two monomeric chains, thereby breaking the cell–substratum attachment.

PROTEASE INHIBITORS AND AXONAL OUTGROWTH

Several years ago Monard and co-workers (42) characterized a glial-derived neurite promoting factor (43) as a serine protease inhibitor that was similar to PN I. Studies with sensory neurons and exogenously added protease inhibitors showed that a variety of these inhibitors would promote neurite outgrowth; however, high concentrations of inhibitor were often inhibitory to neurite outgrowth (44). These findings and those described above suggested that a balance between neuronal protease and protease inhibitors in the environment was critical for neurite outgrowth.

More recent studies showed that a diffusable source or immobilized protease or protease inhibitor can orient the direction of neurite outgrowth (45). Sensory neuron axons grow toward a region of protease inhibitor and away from a region of protease; however, high concentrations of protease inhibitor retard neurite growth. Inhibitors of PA activity including leupeptin, D-Phe-Pro-Arg-CH_2Cl, or L-lysine, immobilized by covalent coupling to the substratum under conditions in which they retain their biological activity, direct neurite outgrowth on to their surface. Whereas, uPA and thrombin-coupled surfaces direct neurite outgrowth away from the derivatized zone. Similarly, glial PN added to N2 culture medium at low concentrations (<100 ng/ml) promotes axonal outgrowth from sensory neurons; however, higher concentrations (>300 ng/ml) inhibit axonal growth (not shown). These studies provide further support for the hypothesis that a balance between extracellular protease and inhibitor activities is important in mediating the interaction between growth cones and the extracellular matrix.

CONCLUSIONS AND SPECULATIONS

Plasminogen activator activity is high in the developing nervous system at the time of active cell proliferation, migration, and axonal outgrowth. In the cerebellum and the CNS in general, the major PA is tPA, whose expression appears to be regulated at least in part at the transcriptional level. Important questions for the future focus on cellular and molecular regulators of tPA gene expression.

A high-affinity receptor for tPA exists on the surface of migrating granule neurons. This was one of the first of thus far only a few reports of cellular tPA receptors. The function of this tPA receptor on neurons is not clear, but it may serve one or more potential roles. These roles include a mechanism for preventing tPA diffusion away from the cell surface; a way to protect tPA from inactivation by protease inhibitors; an autocrine system that initiates a transmembrane signaling event; a mechanism for the cell to "arm itself" and to temporally and spatially concentrate functionally active protease on the surface at sites where it may act to disrupt cell–cell or cell–matrix interactions important in cell migration and axonal growth. Future studies must characterize this receptor and its regulation during neural development.

Axonal growth cones of sensory and other peripheral nerves secrete primarily uPA and deposit a significant portion on the underlying substratum. When grown on a fibronectin substratum, axonal growth cones of sensory neurons clear a path in the matrix. This clearing occurs by limited cleavage of fibronectin in the absence of plasminogen, apparently by the direct action of cell-associated uPA. Although this cleavage may facilitate growth cone–matrix detachment and hence movement, it may serve another function. Interesting studies by Werb and co-workers (46) suggested that partially degraded fibronectin may interact with integrin receptors in a manner distinct from native fibronectin to participate in a signal transduction event indicative of the extracellular environment.

Serine protease inhibitors promote neurite outgrowth by apparently increasing the adhesion between the growth cone and the substratum. A carefully regulated balance of protease and protease inhibitor would be required for net growth, and target tissues may prevent further growth or stabilize synapse formation by overproduction of protease inhibitors. Alternatively, proteases bound to neuronal cell surface receptors may interact with matrix-associated or glial-derived and -associated serpins through a lock-and-key mechanism. Such a mechanism could provide a preferred attachment surface and hence a guide for migrating growth cones as they proceed toward their target tissue.

A hypothetical model of the laser-like PA and its potential action at the growth

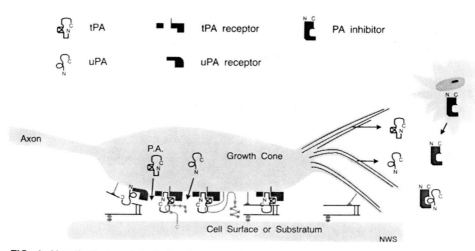

FIG. 4. Hypothetical model of plasminogen activator (PA) at the neuronal growth cone. PA release from the growth cone, its binding to cell surface receptors for uPA and tPA or its interaction with PA inhibitors, interaction of receptor-bound PA with extracellular matrix (fibronectin) and cell adhesion molecules that mediate growth cone attachment to other cells or substrata, and limited cleavage of fibronectin and the growth cone's detachment from the substratum at its trailing edge are shown.

cone is shown in Fig. 4. An excess of neuronal-secreted PA activity would be neutralized in part by soluble serpins, such as the glial-derived PN, thus permitting the attachment of filopodia to the substratum matrix molecules, thereby extending the forward edge of the growth cone. A concentration of PA (uPA and/or tPA) receptors on the under surface of the growth cone and possible concentration at the trailing edge may bring about the limited cleavage of substratum adhesion molecules or possibly cell adhesion molecules. This cleavage would promote the detachment of the trailing edge, an event apparently necessary for the continued forward movement of the growth cone, or alternatively the condensation of the axon shaft as described in the chapter by Goldberg et al.

ACKNOWLEDGMENTS

These studies were supported in part by grants from the National Institutes of Health (NS-09818), the National Science Foundation (BSN-86-07719), and the Muscular Dystrophy Association.

REFERENCES

1. Rakic P. Neuron–glia relationship during cell migration in developing cerebellar cortex. *J Comp Neurol* 1971;141:283–312.

2. Jacobs JR, Goodman CS. Embryonic development of axon pathways in the *Drosophila* CNS: a glial scaffold appears before the first growth cones. *J Neurosci* 1989;9:2402–2411.
3. Bate CM. Pioneer neurons in an insect embryo. *Nature* 1976;260:54–56.
4. Caudy M, Bentley D. Pioneer growth cone morphologies reveal proximal increases in substrate affinity within leg segments of grasshopper embryos. *J Neurosci* 1986;6:364–379.
5. Ramón j Cajal S. A quelle epoque apparaissent les expansions des cellules nerveuses de la moelle epinere du polet. *Anatomischer Anzeiger* 1890;21:1–13.
6. Ramón y Cajal S. Recollections of my life. (Craigie EH, transl). New York: Garland Pub, 1988.
7. Ramón y Cajal S. Algunas observaciones contrarias a la hipotesis syncytial de la regeneracion nerviosa y neurogenesis normal. *Trab del Lab de Inv Biol* 1921;18:4.
8. Krystosek A, Seeds NW. Plasminogen activator production by cultures of developing cerebellum. *Fed Proc* 1978;37:1702.
9. Unkeless JC, Gordon S, Reich E. Secretion of plasminogen activator by stimulated macrophages. *J Exp Med* 1974;139:834–850.
10. Dano K, Andreasen J, et al. Plasminogen activators, tissue degradation and cancer. *Adv Cancer Res* 1985;44:139–266.
11. Ossowski L, Reich E. Antibodies to plasminogen activator inhibit tumor metastasis. *Cancer Res* 1983;40:2300–2309.
12. Beers WH, Strickland S, Reich E. Follicular plasminogen activator and the effect of plasmin on ovarian cells. *Cell* 1975;6:387–394.
13. Strickland S, Reich E, Sherman MI. Plasminogen activator in early embryogenesis. *Cell* 1976; 9:231–240.
14. Saksela O, Rifkin DB. Cell-associated plasminogen activation. *Annu Rev Cell Biol* 1988;4:93–126.
15. Ny T, Elgh F, Lund B. The structure of the human tissue-type plasminogen activator gene. *Proc Natl Acad Sci USA* 1984;81:5355–5359.
16. van Zonneveld AJ, Veerman H, Pannekoek H. On the interactions of the finger and the kringle-2 domain of tissue-type plasminogen activator with fibrin. *J Biol Chem* 1986;261:14214–14218.
17. Silverstein RL, Nachman RL, et al. Activation of immobilized plasminogen by tissue activator. *J Biol Chem* 1985;260:10346–10352.
18. Salonen EM, Saksela O, et al. Plasminogen and tissue-type plasminogen activator bind to immobilized fibronectin. *J Biol Chem* 1985;260:12302–12307.
19. Loskutoff DJ, Edgington IS. Synthesis of fibrinolytic activator and inhibitor by endothelial cells. *Proc Natl Acad Sci USA* 1977;74:3903–3907.
20. Kawano T, Mormoto K, Uemura Y. Partial purification and properties of urokinase inhibitor from human placenta. *J Biol Chem* 1970;67:333–342.
21. Baker JB, Low DA, et al. Protease nexin: a cellular component that links thrombin and plasminogen activator and mediates their binding to cells. *Cell* 1980;21:37–45.
22. Krystosek A, Seeds NW. Plasminogen activator secretion by granule neurons in cultures of developing cerebellum. *Proc Natl Acad Sci USA* 1981;78:7810–7814.
23. Soreq H, Miskin R. Plasminogen activators in the rodent brain. *Brain Res* 1981;216:361–374.
24. Moonen G, Grau-Wagemans MP, Selak I. Plasminogen activator–plasmin system and neuronal migration. *Nature* 1982;298:753–755.
25. Seeds NW, Haffke S, et al. Cerebellar granule cell migration involves proteolysis. In: Lauder J, ed. *Molecular aspects of development and aging of the nervous system*. New York: Plenum Press, 1990;169–178.
26. Verrall S, Seeds NW. Tissue plasminogen activator binding to mouse cerebellar granule neurons. *J Neurosci Res* 1988;21:420–425.
27. Verrall, S, Seeds NW. Characterization of ^{125}I-tissue plasminogen activator binding to cerebellar granule neurons. *J Cell Biol* 1989;109:265–271.
28. Verrall S. *Characterization and purification of tissue plasminogen activator and its binding to the surface of cerebellar neurons*. Ph.D. Thesis. Denver: Univ Colorado HSC, 1989.
29. Seeds NW, Verrall S, et al. Plasminogen activator in the developing nervous system. In: Festoff B, ed. *Serine proteases and their serpin inhibitors in the nervous system*. New York: Plenum Press, 1990;173–184.
30. Gething MJ, Adler B, et al. Variants of human tissue plasminogen activator that lack specific structural domains of the heavy chains. *EMBO J* 1988;7:2731–2740.
31. Krystosek A, Seeds NW. Plasminogen activator release at the neuronal growth cone. *Science* 1981; 213:1532–1534.

32. Krystosek A, Seeds NW. Peripheral neurons and Schwann cells secrete plasminogen activator. *J Cell Biol* 1984;98:773–776.

33. Valinsky JE, LeDouarin NM. Production of plasminogen activator by migrating cephalic neural crest cells. *EMBO J* 1985;4:1403–1406.

34. Pittman RN. Release of plasminogen activator and a calcium dependent metalloprotease from cultured sympathetic and sensory neurons. *Dev Biol* 1985;110:91–101.

35. Pittman RN, Williams AG. Neurite penetration into collagen gels requires calcium dependent metalloprotease activity. *Dev Neurosci* 1989;11:41–47.

36. Krystosek A, Seeds NW. Normal and malignant cells, including neurons deposit plasminogen activator on the growth substrata. *Exp Cell Res* 1986;166:31–46.

37. Culp LA, Ansbacher R, Domen C. Substrate adhesion material of neuroblastoma cells. *Biochemistry* 1980;19:5899–5910.

38. McGuire PG, Seeds NW. Interaction of plasminogen activator with reconstituted basement membrane matrix and extracellular macromolecules produced by cultured epithelial cells. *J Cell Biochem* 1989;40:215–227.

39. McGuire PG, Seeds NW. Degradation of underlying extracellular matrix by sensory neurons during neurite outgrowth. *Neuron* 1990;4:633–642.

40. Plow EF, Freaney DE, et al. The plasminogen system and cell surfaces: evidence for plasminogen and urokinase receptors on the same cell type. *J Cell Biol* 1986;103:2411–2420.

41. Quigley JP, Gold L, et al. Limited cleavage of cellular fibronectin by plasminogen activator purified from transformed cells. *Proc Natl Acad Sci USA* 1987;84:2776–2780.

42. Guenther J, Nick H, Monard D. A glia derived neurite promoting factor with protease inhibitory activity. *EMBO J* 1985;4:1963–1966.

43. Monard D, Solomon F, et al. Glia induced morphological differentiation of neuroblastoma cells. *Proc Natl Acad Sci USA* 1973;70:1894–1897.

44. Hawkins RL, Seeds NW. Effect of proteases and their inhibitors on neurite outgrowth from neonatal mouse sensory ganglia in culture. *Brain Res* 1986;398:63–70.

45. Hawkins RL, Seeds NW. Protease inhibitors influence the direction of neurite outgrowth. *Dev Brain Res* 1989;45:203–209.

46. Werb Z, Tremble PM, et al. Signal transduction through the fibronectin receptor induces collagenase and stromelysin gene expression. *J Cell Biol* 1989;109:877–889.

The Nerve Growth Cone, edited by P. C. Letourneau,
S. B. Kater, and E. R. Macagno, Raven Press, Ltd.,
New York © 1992.

19

Growth Orientation and Transmitter Secretion by Nerve Growth Cones

Mu-ming Poo and Mark Quillan

Department of Biological Sciences, Columbia University, New York, New York 10027

Using isolated spinal cord neurons obtained from *Xenopus* embryos, we have examined a number of phenomena associated with the growth of nerve processes before and after its contact with the target muscle cell in culture. These include the turning response of growth cone in the presence of gradients of diffusible substances, ACh secretion from the growth cone induced by nerve impulse or muscle surface contact, and lateral mobility and localization of cell surface components before and after nerve–muscle contact. Results from these studies suggest possible existence of an array of complex interaction between the growth cone and its environment and between various cellular components within the growth cone induced by environmental cues. In this review, examples of experimental findings are illustrated and discussed with an emphasis on the relationship between these phenomena and membrane turnover at the growth cone.

CHEMOTAXIS OF GROWTH CONE: IS CYCLICAMP A SECOND MESSENGER?

The direction of growth cone extension can be influenced by a number of physical and chemical factors in the environment (1–3). It is likely that these factors, despite their different initial actions on the growth cone, trigger a common set of intracellular events, involving cytoplasmic second messengers, that eventually lead to the incorporation of new membrane material on one side of the growth cone. The internal cue for the turning response induced by these external factors may thus be determined by a gradient of second messengers within the growth cone. Cyclic adenosine monophosphate (cyclicAMP) is a likely candidate for such a second messenger. Agents that elevate cytoplasmic cyclicAMP in the growth cone markedly influence the transport of vesicles toward the front of the growth cone of *Aplysia* neurons (4). Analogues of cyclicAMP have also been shown to promote survival and neurite outgrowth in cultures of rat sympathetic and sensory neurons (5).

In a series of experiments, we have tested the effect of an extracellular gradient of cyclicAMP or other related compounds in orienting growth cone extension. The gradient was produced by repetitive ejection of picoliter volumes of test solutions, 100 μm from the growth cone and 45° from the direction of neurite extension, and the effect on growth cone orientation was examined by video microscopy. The results showed that gradients of dB-cyclicAMP or membrane-permeable phosphodiesterase inhibitor isobutyrylmethylxanthine (IBMX) produced significant turning response within 2 hr of application. Similar gradients of sucrose, (underivatized) cyclicAMP, or dB-cyclicGMP were ineffective. Figure 1a shows representative responses of the growth cone toward gradients of dB-cyclicAMP. The path of growth cone extension during the 2-hr period was drawn from the recorded video images for all growth cones that showed net extension longer than 8 μm, the minimum length for reliable determination of the neurite extension. The drawings were superimposed in the composite graphs shown in Fig. 1c–e for the effect of sucrose (control), dB-cyclicAMP, and IBMX. Further quantitative analysis on the orientation and growth of the neurite showed that the differences of the average angles of turning between the dB-cyclicAMP and that of sucrose, cyclicAMP, or dB-cyclicGMP were all statistically significant, whereas the differences between that of sucrose and that of cyclicAMP or dB-cyclicGMP were not significant. The net growth cone extension in various gradients is, however, relatively constant. Theoretical calculation of the gradient showed that, under repetitive pulse applications, the gradient produced is relatively stable at a distance of 100 μm from the source after about 10 sec, and the magnitude of gradient is approximately proportional to the frequency of the pulses. Under the conditions of the experiments shown in Fig. 1, the dB-cyclicAMP gradient that induced growth cone turning was about 0.1 μM/μm, or the difference of 1 μM extracellularly across a typical growth cone 10 μm in width. Because the concentration of dB-cyclicAMP at the growth cone reached a relatively stable level between 8 to 9 μM within 10 min after the onset of the gradient, the growth cone thus can respond to an approximate 10% difference in the concentration of external dB-cyclicAMP across the growth cone.

The turning behavior of the growth cone reported here is similar to the chemotactic response of leukocytes (6). In the latter case, it appears that binding of chemoattractant peptides to cell surface receptors increases polymerization of the cytoplasmic actin filaments, which are important components of filopodia and lamellipodia of the advancing edge of the cell. It remains to be determined whether a gradient of cytoplasmic cyclicAMP and the consequent activation of cyclicAMP–dependent enzymatic processes can promote actin polymerization on one side of growth cone cytoplasm, leading to net addition of new membrane material on that side. The observation that the gradient of dB-cyclicAMP affected the direction but not the rate of neurite extension suggests that the imposed cytoplasmic gradient of second messenger acts by redirecting the existing membrane precursor materials for growth, without mobilizing additional new ones.

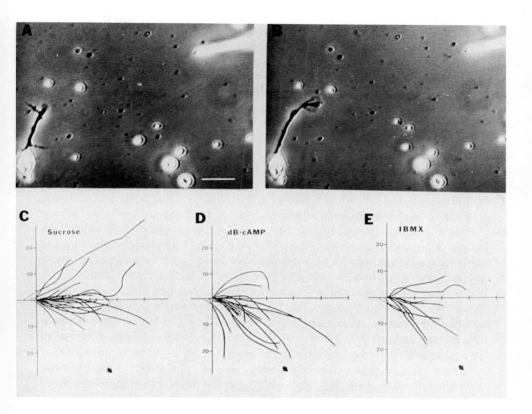

FIG. 1. Turning response of growing nerve processes of *Xenopus* spinal neurons in presence of chemical gradients. Representative phase-contrast micrographs of isolated neurons before (**A**) and 2 hr after (**B**) pulsatile application of dB-cyclicAMP from a micropipette, which was positioned at a distance of 100 μm from the center of the growth cone and an angle of 45° from the direction of neurite extension. Pulse frequency 0.5 Hz, pulse duration 4 msec, volume ejected per pulse 0.30 ± 0.02 pl. Concentration of dB-cyclicAMP in the pipette, 20 mM. Bar, 20 μm. **C–E:** Composite drawings of neurites under influence of chemical gradients. Graphs were made by superimposing individual drawings obtained by tracing video records of microscopic images of all neurites examined for a particular chemical gradient. Origin represents the position of the center of growth cone before application of the gradient. Original direction of the neurite extension, as defined by the last 50-μm segment of the neurite, was aligned with x-axis. Line drawings depict the path of the neurite after 2 hr of growth in the chemical gradient. *Arrows* point to radial direction of chemical gradients, which were produced by pulsatile application of sucrose (**A**), dB-cyclicAMP (**B**), and IBMX, respectively. Note that some neurites had retracted a short distance from the origin before subsequent extension (*dashed lines*). Scale, 10 μm.

TRANSMITTER SECRETION: MODULATION BY ELECTRICAL
ACTIVITY, CELL CONTACT, AND SECOND MESSENGERS

Neurite extension results from a net gain in material through exocytic and endocytic activities at the growth cone. At the presynaptic nerve terminal, impulse-dependent local influx of Ca^{2+} is responsible for triggering the exocytosis of synaptic vesicles, a process that leads to the incorporation of vesicular membrane components into the plasmalemma. Extension of mature nerve terminals does not occur during synaptic activity, presumably because of an effective endocytic process for membrane retrieval. Growth cones of cultured neurons are also capable of releasing neurotransmitter (7–9). In embryonic *Xenopus* spinal neurons (9), we found that growth cone secretion resembles in many ways the ACh secretion at mature nerve terminal: There is short delay of about 1 msec for excitation–secretion coupling, the secretion requires Ca^{2+} influx, and the growth cone exhibits posttetanic potentiation after a brief high-frequency firing of the neuron.

Figure 2 depicts an example of recording from a growth cone showing both contact-dependent and impulse-evoked ACh secretion. An excised patch of muscle membrane in outside-out configuration was used as a probe for extracellular ACh. The secretion was detected as bursting openings of ACh channels at the patch membrane. Spontaneous pulsatile ACh secretion was triggered by contact of the patch membrane with the growth cone (arrow 1). Evoked release was induced by suprathreshold stimulation of the neuron at the soma (arrow 3). The dependence of evoked secretion on Ca^{2+} influx is shown in Fig. 2b, where addition of 10 mm of Co^{2+} reversibly abolished the ACh secretion.

The spontaneous secretion at the growth cone, as induced by the muscle membrane contact, also shows much similarity with the quantal secretion reflected as miniature synaptic potentials at the presynaptic nerve terminal. In particular, we found the same sensitivity of the spontaneous ACh secretion to experimental manipulation of second-messenger systems. Bath application of 0.3 mm ATP, which acts through the binding to P_2-purinergic receptors and the activation of protein kinase C, greatly potentiates spontaneous ACh secretion from both the presynaptic nerve terminal and the growth cone (10). Similar potentiation is found for bath application of dB-cyclicAMP and forskolin. Modulation of either cyclicAMP or phosphoinositides metabolism has been shown to affect neurite growth in some systems (5,11). This suggests that neurite extension and transmitter secretion may be related phenomena at the growth cone, perhaps through their common involvement of exocytic processes. Experiments that aim to correlate neurite growth and transmitter secretion through combined high-resolution optical and electrophysiological recordings are currently in progress.

The capability of the growth cone to release ACh in response to nerve impulses bears important consequences in synaptogenesis. Functional synaptic transmission can be established between the growth cone and any cell bearing sufficient ACh receptors on its surface. Indeed, suprathreshold-evoked responses were observed in the muscle cell within the first minute after growth cone contact (12–14). This early

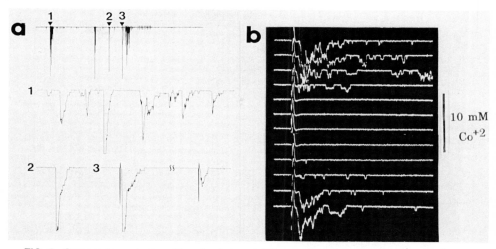

FIG. 2. Contact-dependent and impulse-induced ACh secretion from the growth cone. An excised patch of muscle membrane in outside-out fashion was prepared from a cultured *Xenopus* embryonic muscle cell and positioned near the growth cone of a co-cultured spinal neuron to detect presence of secreted ACh. Continuous trace depicts membrane current recorded at the excised patch. The patch was voltage-clamped at −60 mV. Spontaneous ACh release was triggered by deliberate contact of the patch membrane with the growth cone (at time marked by 1). Suprathreshold stimulation was applied at the soma of the neuron (at time marked by 3), using an extracellular patch electrode. Both contact-induced spontaneous ACh release and impulse-evoked release are observed as bursts of patch membrane currents with characteristic "staircase" pattern, reflecting activation of single ACh channels at the patch by a pulse of ACh nearby. Note that impulse-evoked ACh secretion from the neuron is signified by the preceding stimulus artifact (marked "s").

establishment of synaptic function, before any recognizable morphological differentiation characterizing the presynaptic ending, may be important for the maturation of the postsynaptic cell and of the synapse itself.

The above studies have shown that although spontaneous ACh secretion was rare before target cell contact, efficient ACh release can be readily induced by impulse activity. During *in vivo* development, many embryonic neurons are likely to have received dendritic or somatic inputs before growing axons have reached their target cells. Thus impulse-dependent transmitter secretion could occur during the process of target searching by the nerve processes. The findings that the growth cone possesses efficient cellular mechanisms for secretion of transmitter substances and other molecules (15) suggest the possibility that the growth cone is not merely a passive receiver of environmental cues but may also send out signaling molecules to the environment. Such two-way signaling between the growth cone and its environment may allow for more efficient target searching by the growth cone. Perhaps cell-type specific environmental cues are induced by the molecules secreted by the specific neuronal type.

REFERENCES

1. Letourneau PC. Nerve fiber growth and its regulation by extrinsic factors. In: Spitzer NC, ed. *Neuronal development*. New York: Plenum Press, 1982;1213–1254.
2. Bray D, Hollenbeck PJ. Growth cone motility and guidance. *Annu Rev Cell Biol* 1988;4:43–62.
3. Purves D, Lichtman J. *Principles of neural development*. Sinauer Associates, 1985.
4. Forscher P, Kaczmarek LK, Buchanan J, Smith SJ. Cyclic AMP induces changes in distribution and transport of organelles within growth cones of *Aplysia* bag cell neurons. *J Neurosci* 1987;7:3600–3611.
5. Rydel RE, Greene LA. cAMP analogs promote survival and neurite outgrowth in cultures of rat sympathetic and sensory neurons independently of nerve growth factor. *Proc Natl Acad Sci USA* 1988;85:1257–1261.
6. Devretoes P, Zigmond S. Chemotaxis in eukaryotic cells. *Annu Rev Cell Biol* 1988;4:649–686.
7. Hume RI, Role LW, Fischbach GD. Acetylcholine release from growth cones detected with patches of acetylcholine receptor-rich membranes. *Nature* 1983;305:632–634.
8. Young, SH, Poo M-m. Spontaneous release of transmitter from growth cones of embryonic neurons. *Nature* 1983;305:634–637.
9. Sun Y, Poo M-m. Evoked release of acetylcholine from the growing embryonic neuron. *Proc Natl Acad Sci USA* 1987;84:2540–2544.
10. Fu W, Poo M-m. ATP potentiates spontaneous ACh secretion at developing neuromuscular junction. *Neuron* 1991;6:837–843.
11. Traynor AE. The relationship between neurite extension and phospholipid metabolism in PC12 cells. *Dev Brain Res* 1984;14:205–210.
12. Xie Z, Poo M-m. Initial events in the formation of neuromuscular synapse. *Proc Natl Acad Sci USA* 1986;83:7069–7073.
13. Buchanan J, Sun Y, Poo M-m. Studies of nerve–muscle interactions in *Xenopus* cell culture: morphology of early functional contacts. *J Neurosci* 1989;9:1540–1554.
14. Evers J, Laser M, Sun Y, Xie Z, Poo M-m. Studies of nerve–muscle interactions in *Xenopus* cell culture: analysis of early synaptic currents. *J Neurosci* 1989;9:1523–1539.
15. Krystosek A, Seeds NW. Plasminogen activator release at the neuronal growth cone. *Science* 1981;213:1532–1534.

The Nerve Growth Cone, edited by P. C. Letourneau,
S. B. Kater, and E. R. Macagno, Raven Press, Ltd.,
New York © 1992.

20

Neural Recognition Molecules and Their Influence on Cellular Functions

Melitta Schachner

Department of Neurobiology, Swiss Federal Institute of Technology, Zürich, Switzerland, and University of Heidelberg, Heidelberg, West Germany

In the developing and adult nervous system, cell interactions have been elaborated to a high degree of precision. These interactions are, at least in part, governed by cell–cell and cell–substrate interactions, which mediate specific recognition between partners. The molecules involved in these interactions have been termed *adhesion molecules*, because in *in vitro* assay systems antibodies directed against these molecules were initially shown to interfere with the adhesion or "stickiness" among cells. Later on, the isolated molecules themselves were found to adhere directly to the cell surfaces of other cells or to the extracellular matrix (for reviews, see ref. 1). It was subsequently realized that these cell surface-exposed and substrate-bound glycoproteins not only make cells recognize each other but that the cells may display a broad repertoire of cellular responses that result in either adhesive, inhibitory, or repulsive cell behavior. Because recognition is the primary event that triggers either one or a mixture of these cellular responses, it is conceivable that cell behavior may depend on the blend of adhesion molecules exposed on one cell, the intracellular make-up of the cell type expressing or binding the adhesion molecules, and the developmental stage, environment, and life history of the cell. Such molecules should thus better be termed *recognition molecules*, because, depending on these circumstances, they are likely to trigger different cellular responses.

Cell recognition is the first decisive step in the morphogenesis of an extremely complex organ, the nervous system. Recognition events lie at the basis of a neural cell's decision whether to proliferate, how to migrate from its birthplace to its final destination, where to extend its axons or dendrites, with which other cells it should engage in synapse formation, whether to regenerate after damage in the adult nervous system, whether to maintain stable synapses, and whether to engage in sprouting of new neurites, resulting in novel synapses. For these complex events to occur, a simple static recognition process between cells is, however, not sufficient. Rather, a simple "lock-and-key" recognition process has to lead into a cascade of dynamic cellular responses that ultimately shape the cell's response toward its environment.

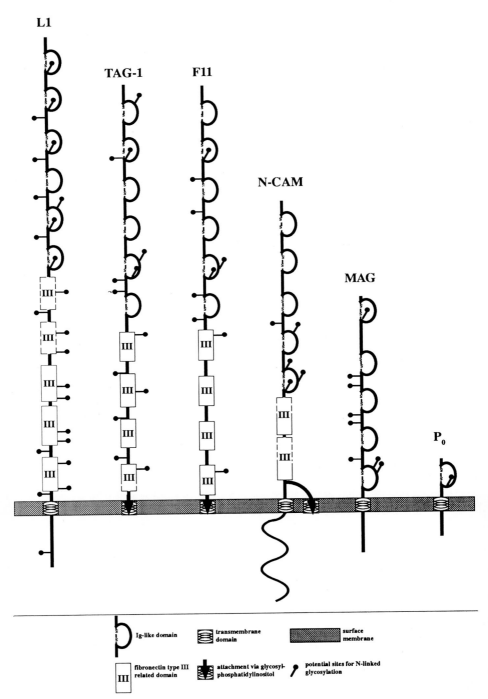

FIG. 1. Schematic presentation of the molecular structure of several neural recognition molecules of the immunoglobulin and fibronectin type III superfamilies.

The behavioral mechanisms by which a neural cell achieves the integration of recognition events on the one hand and cellular response on the other are yet unknown. The dissection of the probably multiple steps involved in the cellular responses after recognition are aggravated by the fact that a particular cell expresses more than one recognition molecule. Recognition molecules are likely to share common pathways of intracellular reactions but may also engage in distinct pathways that will be extremely difficult to distinguish from each other in the complex interplay of intracellular messenger systems. Transduction of the recognition process is likely to involve the cell's entire assembly of intracellular metabolic machinery, ranging from plasma membrane-associated regulatory proteins and cytoskeletal elements to the modification of gene expression. In this orchestrated interplay, the neuronal growth cone appears to be a strategically important integrator of cell surface cues, the final processing of which determines whether a neurite would engage in stable interactions with its partner cells and its environment, whether it performs transient interactions, or whether it is discouraged from engaging in any interactions and is finally inhibited or repelled. Thus, insights into individual transduction processes initiated by recognition molecules in various types of live cells will be crucial for our understanding of growth cone behavior in an extremely complex milieu.

The aim of this review is to describe several recognition molecules in their ability to transduce recognition events into cellular functions, most of which have been identified to be associated with distinct intracellular partners mediating the consequences of the triggering of recognition molecules at the cell surface. Several types of recognition molecules have been described that, on the basis of structural similarities, can be grouped into families within which the members are likely to perform related functions (Fig. 1).

FAMILIES OF RECOGNITION MOLECULES

The immunoglobulin superfamily derives its name from the structural features of immunoglobulin domains originally described in antibodies (2). These domains appear to confer self-binding, "homophilic" reactivity in which one member of the superfamily binds to itself and binding may be increased by cooperativity via a carbohydrate-dependent, "assisted homophilic" reactivity, with another member (3). Interactions with nonself, "heterophilic" partners have also been observed (4). Recognition molecules of the immunoglobulin superfamily are the neural recognition molecules N-CAM, L1, the myelin-associated glycoprotein MAG, TAG-1, the contactin/F3/F11-group, and the major peripheral nervous system glycoprotein P_o in vertebrates. Neuroglian and the fasciclins II and III in *Drosophila* are also members of the immunoglobulin superfamily (for review, see ref. 5). The fibronectin type III domain, originally described in the extracellular matrix recognition molecule fibronectin, is another structural feature common to some members of the immunoglobulin superfamily, such as N-CAM, L1, TAG-1, and the contactin group, and extracellular matrix glycoproteins, such as J1/tenascin/cytotactin, which also carries domains homologous to epidermal growth factor-like repeats.

The cadherin group of homophilic recognition molecules and the integrin family of cell surface ligands for extracellular matrix glycoproteins are structurally distinct from the immunoglobulin and fibronectin type III families and do not show any resemblance to each other or to other molecules of which the primary sequence is known (for review, see ref. 6). Another founding member of recognition molecules has arisen in the adhesion molecule on glia AMOG, which is structurally identical to the so-called β_2 subunit of Na^+/K^+-ATPase (7). AMOG and β_2 are structurally homologous but not identical to the β_1 subunit, which had been identified two decades ago along with the catalytic α subunit of the enzyme, but its function has so far remained elusive, except that without it the α subunit is not active. Other β-like subunits have recently been discovered, but their roles in cell recognition and interactions have not yet been studied.

Carbohydrate structures common to subsets of recognition molecules form the bases of other family traits and are themselves involved in recognition (8,9). It is tempting to speculate that these characterized carbohydrate structures and possibly many others contribute to the fine-tuning of the recognition process by their immense possibilities of combination in expression on the protein backbone of a single recognition molecule.

The involvement of some of these recognition molecules in signal transduction processes leading to distinct features in neural cell behavior will now be discussed.

NEURAL RECOGNITION MOLECULES L1 AND N-CAM INFLUENCE SECOND-MESSENGER SYSTEMS

The recognition molecules L1 and N-CAM are involved in adhesion between cells in the nervous system. N-CAM appears early during development and is involved in neuron–neuron, neuron–glia, and neuron–muscle interactions. L1 is more restricted in its expression and has been detected in the central nervous system on subpopulations of some postmitotic neurons. L1 and N-CAM do not act independently of each other in cell adhesion and aggregation, and carbohydrate structures appear to be involved in the functional association between the two molecules (3,10). The extracellular domain of N-CAM has been found in many alternatively spliced forms that appear to be regulated in a developmental and cell type–specific fashion (11,12). Although some binding properties of the extracellular domains of the two molecules have been characterized, the intracellular consequences of the involvement in cell interactions have remained largely obscure.

The question whether neural recognition molecules may trigger second messenger systems inside the cell lies at the basis of our understanding of transducing mechanisms. We have used a well-studied cell line with neural properties, the rat PC12 pheochromocytoma, as a model and have triggered the two neural recognition molecules by their respective antibodies, following the paradigm studies in hormone receptors, whereby specific antibodies directed against distinct epitopes on the hormone receptor could mimic some of the functions of the hormone itself

(13). Using this paradigm, antibodies to L1 and N-CAM were used as substitutes for the putative ligands of these molecules. After the application of antibodies to L1 and N-CAM to live monolayer cultures of PC12 cells, intracellular levels of D-myo-inositol 1,4-biphosphate (IP_2) and D-myo-inositol 1,4,5-triphosphate (IP_3) were reduced, whereas intracellular levels of cyclicAMP were unaffected. The antibodies also reduced intracellular pH and increased intracellular Ca^{2+} concentrations by opening Ca^{2+} channels, as could be shown by blocking these responses with the Ca^{2+} channel blockers verapamil and diltiazem. The triggering of these responses could also be induced by Fab fragments of the L1 and N-CAM antibodies, suggesting that cross-linking of molecules on the cell surface is not required for the signal transduction process to occur. Unrelated antibodies or monoclonal N-CAM antibodies reacting with the cell surface of PC12 cells did not change these cellular parameters. Because the antibody effects were blocked by pertussis toxin and the phorbol ester, TPA, the involvement of a G protein and protein kinase C in the signal transduction process was suggested. The extent of the intracellular responses was dependent on antibody concentration. They could be elicited by allowing adhesion of single PC12 cells to each other to occur, thus underscoring the physiological significance of the observed changes. The combined observations suggest that recognition molecules induce changes in second messenger systems that are specific and physiological. Although the functional consequences of these alterations in second messenger systems remain unknown, it is likely that they are important and ultimately affect cellular parameters that, among others, influence growth cone mobility, stabilization or destabilization of cell contacts, activity of ion channels in neurites and at the synapse, and cell death. Although such effects will have to be directly demonstrated, our study has given the first evidence that neural cell recognition provides a molecular trigger for cell transduction events.

ANTIBODIES TO N-CAM MODULATE K^+ CHANNELS IN CULTURED GLIAL PRECURSOR CELLS

Using the same experimental rationale, namely, triggering the neural recognition molecule N-CAM by its antibodies, a further link of N-CAM to regulation of ionic milieu could be discovered. Oligodendroglial precursor cells *in vitro* express the two isoforms of N-CAM with apparent molecular weights of 120 and 140 kDa (14). The investigation of these cells with respect to the ability of N-CAM to influence channel properties was prompted by the observation that these immature glial cells express several distinct ion channels (15). Thus, the specificity of the influence of N-CAM on various channels could be studied. Using the whole-cell patch-clamp technique, it could be shown that both the A-type and delayed rectifier K^+ currents are reduced in amplitude within a few minutes after application of either poly- or monoclonal antibodies against N-CAM (Fig. 2) (16). Tetrodotoxin-sensitive Na^+ channels were not influenced by application of the antibodies. Specificity of the effect was further shown by using other mono- and polyclonal antibodies reactive

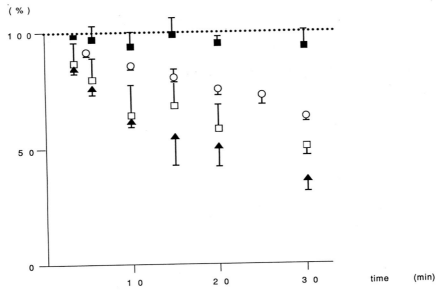

FIG. 2. Time course of the relative current amplitude of cultured oligodendroglial precursor cells in absence or presence of antibodies to N-CAM and liver membranes or in presence of the phorbol ester PMA. Peak currents obtained in response to a voltage step from -110 mV to 20 mV in absence and presence of antibodies were normalized and plotted as a function of application time. Points correspond to the mean values of five individual cells for antibodies to liver membranes, seven cells for polyclonal antibodies to N-CAM, three cells for monoclonal antibodies to N-CAM, and four cells for PMA. *Bars* show standard deviations. The *dotted line* (100%) corresponds to the control current measured as the mean current amplitude within 15 min before application. Antibodies to liver membranes (antiliver, *filled squares*) did not signifi-cantly alter the current amplitude within 30 min. In contrast, both polyclonal and monoclonal N-CAM antibodies (*open squares* and *open circles*, respectively) reduced the mean current amplitude in a time-dependent manner. An effect similar to that with polyclonal N-CAM anti-bodies was seen with PMA (*filled triangles*). (Modified from ref. 16.)

with the surface of glial precursor cells but not eliciting any responses in the membrane currents. Interestingly, the transition from an O4 antigen-positive oligo-dendroglial precursor cell to an O1 antigen-positive more mature oligodendrocyte in culture has been found to be associated with a down-regulation of those voltage-activated K^+ channels that are affected by N-CAM antibodies. Thus, contacts of N-CAM-expressing glial precursor cells with their partner ligand(s), such as neurons, may be responsible for the modulation of ion channels that are down-regulated during differentiation. It is interesting in this context that other glial cells, the Schwann cells of the peripheral nervous system and astrocytes of the central ner-vous system, could be inhibited in their proliferation by blocking voltage-activated K^+ channels (17). These combined observations invite the speculation that N-CAM-dependent adhesion of glial precursor cells with their partner cells may not only influence membrane properties in general but, in particular, proliferation of these glial precursor cells by modulating K^+ channels.

The mechanisms by which N-CAM antibodies affect K^+ currents remain to be clarified. An involvement of second messenger systems and kinases, possibly mediating phosphorylation of the K^+ channels, appears likely, particularly because the same currents are down-regulated by activation of protein kinase C. Down-regulation of K^+ currents in cultured ovine oligodendrocytes has also been observed after application of the protein kinase C activator phorbol ester (18). However, all attempts to detect a link between activation of protein kinase C and the N-CAM antibody-dependent regulation of K^+ channel activity in glial precursor cells have so far failed. It is also unknown whether the 120- or 140-kDa components or both of N-CAM are involved in the modification of K^+ channels.

PROTEIN KINASE ACTIVITIES ASSOCIATED WITH THE NEURAL CELL RECOGNITION MOLECULE L1

Another link between cell recognition molecules and posttranslational modifications has become apparent in studies on kinase activities tightly copurifying with the L1 molecule during stringent isolation procedures. Two distinct activities have been recognized in preparations of L1 from adult mouse brain (19). One of these phosphorylates casein but not L1, uses ATP as well as GTP and is strongly inhibited by heparin. These features suggest that the kinase could be similar or identical to casein kinase II. The other protein kinase specifically phosphorylates L1, uses ATP but not GTP, and is only weakly inhibited by heparin. This protein kinase phosphorylates L1 in its intracellular domain on serine residues. Because the primary sequence of L1 shows no homology with the short sequence motifs that are highly conserved between the catalytic domains of kinases and because the size of the intracellular part of L1 appears too short to contain the catalytic site, it appears that the kinase activities associated with L1 do not reside in the molecule itself but are due to enzymes that copurify with the molecule, withstanding the stringent washing procedures used during the immunopurification of L1. Recent evidence suggests that another protein kinase, a protein kinase C, is able to phosphorylate L1 (Sadoul and Schachner, *unpublished results*). Thus, L1 can be phosphorylated by two different kinases, which are protein kinase C, which does not copurify with L1, and a kinase that copurifies with it. These relationships between L1 and protein kinases suggest the possibility that L1 may influence the phosphorylation of other proteins and that it itself may be regulated in its functions by phosphorylation. These functions may implicate both the intra- and extracellular domains of the molecule. It is conceivable that intracellular phosphorylation modifies the recognition properties of the extracellular domain and that the transduction events themselves are influenced by the phosphorylation state of the L1. Thus, L1 appears to be subject to diverse regulatory signals that impinge on it, on the one hand, and, on the other, is itself able to influence protein phosphorylation, thereby interdigitating into the complex network of phosphorylation mechanisms.

THE ADHESION MOLECULE ON GLIA (AMOG) AND ITS INFLUENCE ON THE IONIC MILIEU

The link between triggering of cell surface molecules and secondary events gains a new dimension with the adhesion molecule on glia, AMOG, which is structurally and functionally associated with an ion pump, the Na^+/K^+-ATPase (7). AMOG is expressed by glial cells in the central nervous system and is involved in neuron–astrocyte but not astrocyte–astrocyte adhesion, as shown by antibody inhibition experiments (20). The direct role of AMOG in the recognition event is indicated by its ability to bind to cells after purification and incorporation into liposomes (Fig. 3) (21). AMOG is expressed during morphogenetically active periods, such as the migration of cerebellar granule neurons along Bergmann glial cells. Fab fragments of monoclonal antibodies strongly inhibit this migration. After completion of granule cell migration, AMOG continues to be expressed by astrocytes, predominantly in the cerebellum and less in other brain regions but always where the packing density of neuronal cell bodies appears to be high (22).

Sequence analysis of AMOG reveals a 40% amino acid identity with the ATPase β_1 subunit whose exact functional role has remained elusive. A 100-kDa component that tenaciously copurifies with AMOG by immunoaffinity chromatography is identical with the $\alpha2$ and possibly also $\alpha3$ isoforms of the ATPase catalytic subunit. A functional link between AMOG and Na^+/K^+-ATPase has been shown by the ability of monoclonal AMOG antibodies, when added to live cultured astrocytes, to increase the ouabain-inhibitable uptake of radioactive Rb^+, indicative of K^+ uptake and thus ion pump activity. AMOG-mediated adhesion occurs both at 4°C, where the pump is inactive, and in the presence of ouabain, an inhibitor of the catalytic activity of the enzyme, further underscoring that AMOG is indeed a recognition molecule. Whether the inhibition of granule cell migration on Bergmann glial cells exerted by monoclonal antibodies to AMOG results from triggering of ion pump activity in Bergmann glial cells or by modification of the recognition process itself is presently unknown. This dichotomy in the influence of antibodies on cellular functions will have to be taken into account more generally in the future, when the effects of antibodies on the behavior of live cells *in vitro* and *in situ* are interpreted.

FIG. 3. Double-immunofluorescence staining of monolayer cultures of early postnatal mouse cerebellum after 4 days *in vitro*, using polyclonal antibodies against L1 (**B**, using tetramethyl rhodamine-coupled second antibodies) and carboxyfluorescein-labeled AMOG-containing liposomes (**C**). When liposomes are preincubated with Fab fragments of monoclonal AMOG antibody, binding of AMOG-containing liposomes to cerebellar cells is blocked (**E**). AMOG-containing liposomes bind to cultured pheochromocytoma PC12 cells (**G**). AMOG-containing liposomes do not bind to cultures of embryonic mouse spinal cord maintained for 10 days *in vitro* (**I**). **A, D, F, H:** The phase-contrast micrographs corresponding to fluorescence images **B** and **C** and **E**, **G**, and **I**, respectively. Bar in **H**, 50 μm. (From ref. 20, with permission.)

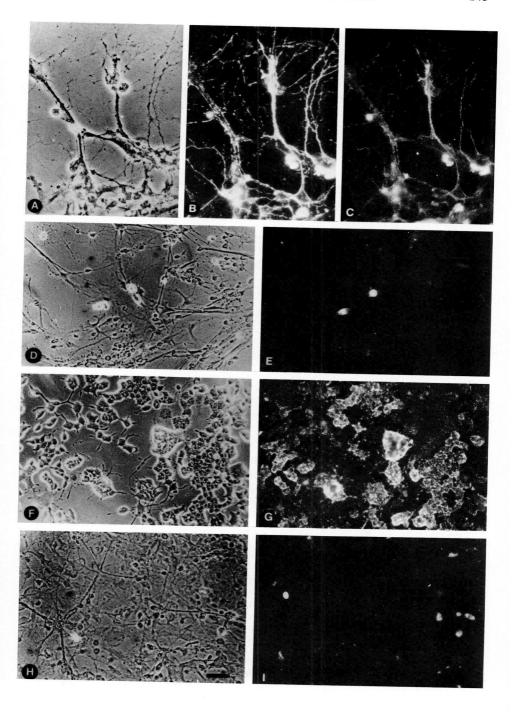

Several implications of the association between cell adhesion and ion pump activity are worth considering in the context of neuron–glia interactions during development and the support of neuronal activity by astrocytes in the adult. Binding of the putative AMOG receptor on neurons to AMOG on glial cells may modulate Na^+/K^+-ATPase activity directly or indirectly. The activities of both Na^+ and K^+ are known to determine the membrane potential, size of the extracellular space, and cell volume. Local changes in pump activity affecting only certain parts of a cell may thus influence cell shape in a polarized manner. The way by which AMOG may modulate these parameters could be by influencing ATPase activity. AMOG-mediated morphogenetic events, such as neuronal migration along the radial processes of Bergmann glial cells, may thus result from the dynamic interplay between recognition and changes in the intra- and extracellular ionic environment. In the adult, expression of AMOG at the neuron–glia interface may indicate that cell contacts between neurons and glia remain instrumental in regulating the ionic symbiosis between neurons and glia. Regulation of the ionic milieu inside and outside the cell may be particularly relevant in the modulation of neuronal excitability and synaptic efficacy.

N-CAM 180 AND ITS ROLE IN MEDIATING CELL CONTACTS

N-CAM occurs in the central nervous system in three major molecular components, which are generated by alternative splicing from one gene. Two of these, the 120- and 140-kDa components designated N-CAM 120 and N-CAM 140, have been mentioned to be expressed by oligodendrocyte precursor cells (see above). All three forms have been observed to carry identical extracellular domains, with each component able to express various alternatively spliced constructs, but are different in the size of their intracellular domains. N-CAM 180, the largest component of N-CAM, has the longest cytoplasmic domain, which has been suggested to be involved in the stabilization of cell contacts via its interaction with brain spectrin, which is a membrane glycoprotein–cytoskeleton linker protein (for reference, see ref. 23).

→

FIG. 4. Immunoelectron-microscopic localization of N-CAM 180 (**a, b,** and **d**) and N-CAM total (N-AM 180, 140, and 120) (**c**) in the cerebellum (**a**) and hippocampus (**b–d**) of 21-day-old mice by preembedding peroxidase staining procedures. **a:** Molecular layer of the cerebellum; **b:** hilus of the gyrus dentatus; (**c:** stratum moleculare of the gyrus dentatus; **d:** stratum radiatum of the CA3 region. Some postsynaptic densities are labeled by N-CAM 180 antibodies (*arrowheads,* **a, b,** and **d**), whereas others are not stained (*arrows,* **a, b,** and **d**). N-CAM 180 antibodies are never observed to stain pre- or postsynaptic membranes not associated with postsynaptic densities (**a, b,** and **d**). Polyclonal antibodies reacting with all three components of N-CAM (N-CAM total) stain all pre- and postsynaptic membranes (*arrowheads,* **c**) and less in postsynaptic densities (*arrows,* **c**). Ax, axon; d, dendrite; m, mitochondrion; t, Purkinje cell dendritic thorn. Bars: 0.3 μm (**a**), 1.0 μm (**b–d**). (From ref. 23, with permission.)

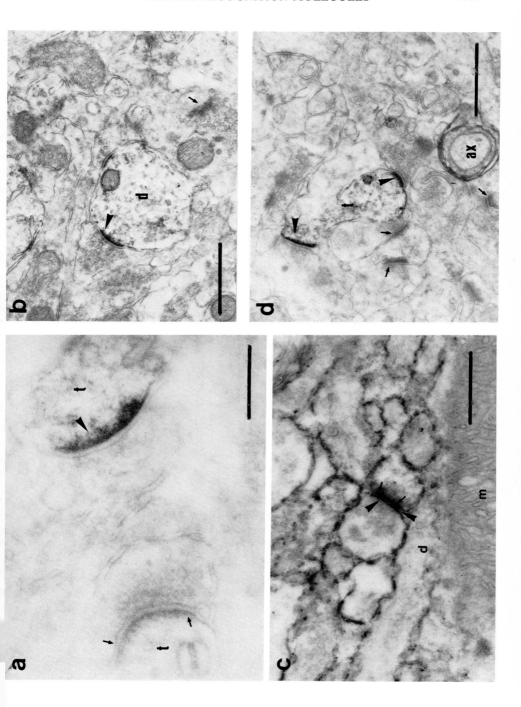

Important in the context of our interest in the functional consequences of the ability of N-CAM 180 to interact with the cytoskeleton is the finding that N-CAM 180 is accumulated at the postsynaptic membrane (23). The N-CAM 180–specific epitope, which is recognized by a monoclonal antibody, is concentrated in post-synaptic densities as observed by immunoelectron microscopy (Fig. 4). In contrast to the specific localization of N-CAM 180, antibodies to all three components of N-CAM react uniformly with pre- and postsynaptic surface membranes. Inter-estingly, some types of synapses show no detectable N-CAM 180 postsynaptically, such as the mossy fiber synapse in the hippocampus. Also, the climbing fiber–Purkinje cell synapse is only transiently N-CAM 180-positive, whereas in the adult, N-CAM 180 is no more detectable at these synaptic contacts. All other types of synapses investigated in hippocampus and cerebellum of adult mice show partial expression of N-CAM 180 (i.e., not all synapses of a particular type express N-CAM 180). These observations, together with our knowledge that Ca^{2+} influx into cells is enhanced by triggering N-CAM on the surface of PC12 cells, that Ca^{2+} is needed to stabilize the interaction of surface membrane glycoproteins with the cytoskeleton, and that Ca^{2+} influx into the postsynaptic compartment is enhanced by synaptic activity, suggest the possibility that N-CAM 180 may be involved in stabilizing the affinity of synaptic surface membranes with each other as a result of synaptic activity. This modulation may implicate several other molecular mecha-nisms discussed above in the context of N-CAM- and L1-mediated transduction signals.

GLIAL RECOGNITION MOLECULES DEMARCATING BOUNDARIES OR BARRIERS

How multifactorial such transduction events may be has become apparent from recognition molecules in the extracellular matrix, the J1 family of glycoproteins, which affect the interacting partner cell types in distinct manners. The J1 glycopro-teins are synthesized by the glial cells of the central and peripheral nervous system. The J1 family contains several members with different apparent molecular masses and functions (24). The members of the high-molecular-weight group, the predomi-nant components of which are J1/200 and J1/220, are immunochemically related to if not identical with tenascin and cytotactin in the chicken and hexabrachion in the human. They are expressed by astrocytes and Schwann cells and are involved in neuron–glia recognition (25,26). The members of the low-molecular-weight group, the predominant components of which are J1/160 and J1/180, are expressed by oligodendrocytes and myelin in the central nervous system and become detectable late during development (27). Although they are structurally related, they are dis-tinct from each other and from J1/tenascin.

The high-molecular-weight J1 components most likely mediate nerve–muscle interactions at the regenerating neuromuscular junction and are locally generated by proliferating fibroblast-like cells (28,29). Like L1, they are up-regulated after lesioning of peripheral but not central nerves in the adult mouse, so they may be involved in regenerative axonal regrowth (26).

In the central nervous system, the expression of J1/tenascin demarcates and appears to confine functional neuronal assemblies (30–32). This is indicated by its distribution in a brain region characterized by distinctive local groupings of neurons: the vibrissae-related barrel fields in the somatosensory cortex of the mouse.

The barrel fields are the cortical representatives of the whiskers on the mouse's snout. Each barrel, representing a single whisker, has a wall of cell bodies surrounding a core of neuropil and cell bodies. Setting up the boundaries of the barrels seems to be induced by the activity of the input neurons from the thalamus, which begin to innervate the somatosensory cortex early in postnatal life. Before these afferents arrive, J1/tenascin can be detected in the barrel field cortex but is less localized topographically than it is once the first thalamic axons arrive. It even seems as if the thalamic afferents hollow out the boundaries of their individual barrel fields from a more evenly distributed background of J1/tenascin expression (Fig. 5).

Once the afferent maps are established, J1/tenascin-positive boundaries are no longer detectable. This decrease in J1/tenascin expression may imply that neuronal activity can regulate J1/tenascin expression. Regulation of J1/tenascin during the initial phase of establishing the topographic map sets up the barrel field boundaries, which may constrain axons that arrive later into their prospective territories and shape the assembly of cell bodies and associated dendritic target fields of postsynaptic cells. It is not known whether this phase involves the up- or down-regulation of J1/tenascin expression by glial cells. Further increase in neuronal activity in the second phase shuts down J1/tenascin expression completely.

These observations are intriguing on the basis of our knowledge on the functional roles of J1/tenascin in neuronal attachment and neurite outgrowth in culture. J1/tenascin exhibits diverse functional effects, depending on its particular cellular and molecular environment in which it is presented. When provided *in vitro* as a substrate in combination with an adhesive substrate such as polyornithine, J1/tenascin inhibits cell attachment in situations in which neurons at high densities are confronted with the choice of a more adhesive substrate (33). Without the choice of a more adhesive substrate and at low cell densities, J1/tenascin does not interfere with adhesion of cell bodies and increases neurite extension compared with the adhesive substrate alone (34). This differential behavior of neurons is likely to result from the hierarchy of adhesive forces in situations, where there is or is not a choice between more or less adhesive cell surface and cell-to-substrate interactions. As soluble additive to the culture medium, J1/tenascin blocks neurite outgrowth on adhesive substrates. Such differential cell responses are likely to be mediated by different molecular domains and receptor qualities of the neurons that transduce the binding of J1/tenascin into differential cascades of intracellular events underlying the cell's decision whether to interact positively or negatively.

The low molecular group of the J1 family, J1/160 and J1/180, which is expressed by oligodendrocytes and myelin in the central nervous system but not in the periph-

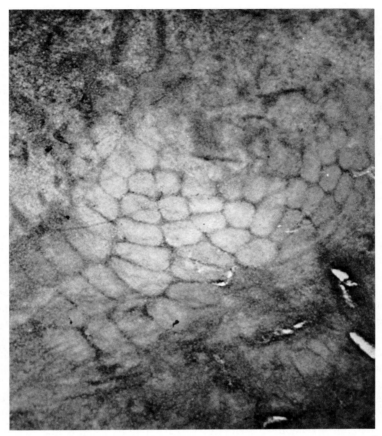

FIG. 5. Immunohistological localization of J1/tenascin in the somatosensory cortex of a 6-day-old mouse as visualized by the indirect immunoperoxidase labeling technique. (Courtesy of Dr. D. Steindler.)

eral nervous system of mice, seems to play a functional role in maintaining the cytoarchitecture at the node of Ranvier in the optic nerve (27,35).

J1-160/180 molecules are implicated in a recognition process between cells that merges into stabilization of cell contacts or adhesion for astrocytes and destabilization of cell interactions or repulsion for neurons. *In vitro,* the purified J1/160 and J1/180 molecules are nonpermissive substrates for the adhesion and spreading of astrocytes, fibroblasts, and small cerebellar neurons (27). Mixed with laminin, the J1-160/180 molecules are repulsive for neuronal cell bodies and growth cones (Fig. 6) but not for astrocytes or fibroblasts. In short-term adhesion assays between oligodendrocytes and neurons or between purified J1-160/180 and neurons, these molecules mediate transitory recognition between oligodendrocytes and neurons that re-

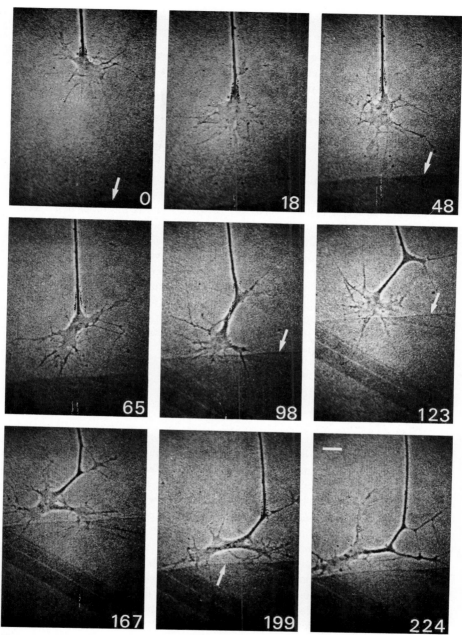

FIG. 6. Frames of a video time-lapse cinematographic investigation of a growth cone of a dorsal root ganglion neuron from 8-day-old chicken embryos advancing toward the boundary between the laminin substrate on which the growth cone extends toward the border of a J1-160 substrate marked with colloidal gold (at the bottom and indicated by *arrows*). Cultures were filmed between 12 and 24 hr after plating *in vitro*. *Numbers* indicate minutes of consecutive filming in real-time. Note that between 65 and 167 min, the growth cone, having met the border, advances more slowly, when compared with the previous hour (0–65). The growth cone then grows along the J1/160-laminin border (167–224). Bar, 10 μm. (Courtesy of Dr. J. Taylor.)

verses into inhibition of adhesion as the time of interaction between the cells increases (36). In the interaction of oligodendrocytes with astrocytes, however, J1-160/180 plays an adhesive role at all times tested.

Thus, recognition between interacting partners may lead not only to cell adhesion, as a result of stabilization of cell contacts over longer times, but it may also provoke inhibition of adhesion, which results in cell repulsion. The term *repulsion* signifies that there is active inhibition of adhesion, which results from an initial step of recognition and leads to de-adhesion. Important in the definition of *repulsion* is the requirement for the anti- or de-adhesive molecule to exert its repulsive action in mixture with an adhesive molecule. We, therefore, propose to use the term *repulsion* for this particular cellular behavior. However, unless the molecular mechanisms are understood that underlie cell repulsion, the definition of a precise terminology remains a futile exercise.

It is likely that the two opposite effects on cell behavior elicited by the J1 molecules result from differential intracellular responses to a cell surface trigger. Variety in responses may derive from different cell surface receptors and/or different consequences in intracellular signaling networks. Thus, recognition events mediated at the cell surface are decisive but not unequivocal determinants of a cell's behavior, because the cell integrates the triggering signals into a constantly changing dynamic interplay of its intracellular affairs.

OUTLOOK

With the realization that recognition molecules act as signal transducers between extracellular cues and the intracellular network of modulators of cellular functions, the understanding of the mechanisms by which recognition molecules may influence cell behavior has reached a new era. It is foreseeable that recognition molecules will be uncovered to be among the many players with opportunities to contribute individually in the concert of the immensely complex repertoire of molecular responses that a cell is capable of. This repertoire has been found to range from influences on the intra- and extracellular ionic milieu, second messenger systems, protein phosphorylation, and cytoskeleton and is likely to encompass the genomic level. The diverse and individual effects of the growing families of recognition molecules on the formation and modification of interactions between the various cell types mediated by intracellular events are likely to be important attributes to the multifaceted patterns of nervous system function in development and, in the adult organism, maintenance, plasticity, and regeneration. To unravel the functional interdigitations of different neural recognition molecules either individually or in combination will turn out to be more intricate than the understanding of cellular functions in more simple organs but will profit from the generally increasing knowledge of the molecular functioning of cells in general.

ACKNOWLEDGMENTS

I am grateful to my colleagues who have contributed to the work presented in this review and to Deutsche Forschungsgemeinschaft, Bundesministerium für Forschung und Technologie, Hermann und Lilly Schilling-Stiftung, Gemeinnützige Hertie-Stiftung, Schweizerischer Nationalfonds, Ciba-Geigy Basel, and Kommission zur Förderung der Wissenschaftlichen Forschung for support. Some portions of this review have been modified from a chapter in *Neurobiology of Glia*, R. Mirsky and K. Jessen (eds.), Seminars in the Neurosciences, Saunders Scientific Publications, 1990.

REFERENCES

1. Edelman GM, Cunningham BA, Thiery JP. *Morphoregulatory molecules*. New York: John Wiley and Sons, 1990.
2. Williams AF. A year in the life of the immunoglobulin superfamily. *Immunol Today* 1987;8:298–303.
3. Kadmon G, Kowitz A, Altevogt P, Schachner M. The neural cell adhesion molecule *N*-CAM enhances L1-dependent cell–cell interactions. *J Cell Biol* 1990;110:193–208.
4. Werz W, Schachner M. Adhesion of neural cells to extracellular matrix constituents. Involvement of glycosaminoglycans and cell adhesion molecules. *Dev Brain Res* 1988;43:225–234.
5. Lander AD. Understanding the molecules of neural cell contacts: emerging patterns of structure and function. *Trends Neurosci* 1989;12:189–195.
6. Takeichi M. Cadherins: a molecular family important in selective cell–cell adhesion. *Annu Rev Biochem* 1990;59:237–252.
7. Gloor S, Antonicek H, Sweadner KJ, et al. The adhesion molecule on glia (AMOG) is a homologue of the β subunit of the Na,K-ATPase. *J Cell Biol* 1990;110:165–174.
8. Künemund V, Jungalwala FB, Fischer G, Chou DKH, Keilhauer G, Schachner M. The L2/HNK-1 carbohydrate of neural cell adhesion molecules is involved in cell interactions. *J Cell Biol* 1988; 106:213–223.
9. Fahrig T, Schmitz B, Weber D, Kücherer-Ehret A, Faissner A, Schachner M. Two monoclonal antibodies recognizing carbohydrate epitopes on neural adhesion molecules interfere with cell interactions. *Eur J Neurosci* 1990;2:153–161.
10. Kadmon G, Kowitz A, Altevogt P, Schachner M. Functional cooperation between the neural adhesion molecules L1 and *N*-CAM is carbohydrate-dependent. *J Cell Biol* 1990;110:209–218.
11. Barthels D, Santoni MJ, Wille W, et al. Isolation and nucleotide sequence of mouse *N*-CAM cDNA that codes for a M_r 79,000 polypeptide without a membrane-spanning region. *EMBO J* 1987;6:907–914.
12. Cunningham BA, Hemperly JJ, Murray BA, Prediger EA, Brackenbury R, Edelman GM. Neural cell adhesion molecule: structure, immunoglobulin-like domains, cell surface modulation, and alternative splicing. *Science* 1987;263:799–805.
13. Schuch U, Lohse MJ, Schachner M. Neural cell adhesion molecules influence second messenger systems. *Neuron* 1989;3:13–20.
14. Trotter J, Bitter-Suermann D, Schachner M. Differentiation-regulated loss of the polysialylated embryonic form and expression of the different polypeptides of the neural cell adhesion molecule by cultured oligodendrocytes and myelin. *J Neurosci Res* 1989;22:369–383.
15. Sontheimer H, Trotter J, Schachner M, Kettenmann H. Channel expression correlates with differentiation stage during the development of oligodendrocytes from their precursor cells in culture. *Neuron* 1989;2:1135–1145.
16. Sontheimer H, Kettenmann H, Schachner M, Trotter J. The neural cell adhesion molecule *N*-CAM modulates K^+ channels in cultured glial precursor cells. *Eur J Neurosci* 1991;3:230–236.

17. Chiu SY, Wilson GF. The role of potassium channels in Schwann cell proliferation in Wallerian degeneration of explant rabbit sciatic nerves. *J Physiol* 1989;408:199–222.
18. Soliven B, Szuchet S, Arnason BGW, Nelson DJ. Forskolin and phorbol ester decrease the same K^+ conductance in cultured oligodendrocytes. *J Membr Biol* 1988;105:177–186.
19. Sadoul R, Kirchhoff F, Schachner M. A protein kinase activity is associated with and specifically phosphorylates the neural cell adhesion molecule L1. *J Neurochem* 1989;53:1471–1478.
20. Antonicek H, Persohn E, Schachner M. Biochemical and functional characterization of a novel neuron-glia adhesion molecule that is involved in neuronal migration. *J Cell Biol* 1987;104:1587–1595.
21. Antonicek H, Schachner M. The adhesion molecule on glia (AMOG) incorporated into lipid vesicles binds to subpopulations of neurons. *J Neurosci* 1988;8:2961–2966.
22. Pagliusi SR, Schachner M, Seeburg PH, Shivers BD. The adhesion molecule on glia (AMOG) is widely expressed by astrocytes in developing and adult mouse brain. *Eur J Neurosci* 1990;2:471–480.
23. Persohn E, Pollerberg GE, Schachner M. Immunoelectron-microscopic localization of the 180 kD component of the neural cell adhesion molecule *N*-CAM in postsynaptic membranes. *J Comp Neurol* 1989;288:92–100.
24. Kruse J, Keilhauer G, Faissner A, Timpl R, Schachner M. The J1 glycoprotein—a novel nervous system cell adhesion molecule of the L2/HNK-1 family. *Nature* 1985;316:146–148.
25. Faissner A, Kruse J, Chiquet-Ehrismann R, Mackie E. The high-molecular weight J1 glycoproteins are immunochemically related to tenascin. *Differentiation* 1988;37:104–114.
26. Martini R, Schachner M, Faissner A. Enhanced expression of the extracellular matrix molecule J1/tenascin in the regenerating adult mouse sciatic nerve. *J Neurocytol* 1990;19:601–616.
27. Pesheva P, Spiess E, Schachner M. J1-160 and J1-180 are oligodendrocyte-secreted nonpermissive substrates for cell adhesion. *J Cell Biol* 1989;109:1765–1778.
28. Sanes JR, Schachner M, Covault J. Distribution of several adhesive macromolecules in embryonic, adult, and denervated adult skeletal muscles. *J Cell Biol* 1986;102:420–431.
29. Gatchalian CL, Schachner M, Sanes JR. Fibroblasts that proliferate near denervated synaptic sites in skeletal muscle synthesize the adhesive molecules J1/tenascin, *N*-CAM, fibronectin, and a heparin sulfate proteoglycan. *J Cell Biol* 1989;108:1873–1890.
30. Steindler DA, Cooper NGF, Faissner A, Schachner M. Boundaries defined by adhesion molecules during development of the cerebral cortex: the J1/tenascin glycoprotein in the mouse somatosensory cortical barrel field. *Dev Biol* 1989;131:243–260.
31. Steindler DA, Faissner A, Schachner M. Brain "cordones": transient boundaries of glia and adhesion molecules that define developing functional units. *Comments Dev Neurobiol* 1989;1:29–60.
33. Faissner A, Kruse J, Kühn K, Schachner M. Binding of the J1 adhesion molecules to extracellular matrix constituents. *J Neurochem* 1990;54:1004–1015.
34. Lochter A, Lloyd V, Kaplony A, Prochiantz A, Schachner M, Faissner A. J1/tenascin in substrate-bound and soluble form displays contrary effects on neurite outgrowth. *J Cell Biol* (*in press*).
35. ffrench-Constant C, Miller RH, Kruse J, Schachner M, Raff MC. Molecular specialization of astrocyte processes at nodes of Ranvier in rat optic nerve. *J Cell Biol* 1986;102:844–852.
36. Morganti MC, Taylor J, Pesheva P, Schachner M. Oligodendrocyte-derived J1-160/180 extracellular matrix glycoproteins are adhesive or repulsive depending on the partner cell type and time of interaction. *Exp Neurol* 1990;109:98–110.

The Growth Cone in Intact Developing Systems

The Nerve Growth Cone, edited by P. C. Letourneau,
S. B. Kater, and E. R. Macagno, Raven Press, Ltd.,
New York © 1992.

21

Introduction

Carol Ann Mason

*Department of Pathology and Anatomy and Cell Biology, Center for Neurobiology and
Behavior, Columbia University College of Physicians and Surgeons,
New York, New York 10032*

For those of us who study the developing nervous system in its native state, this is a timely celebration. After the many decades since Ramón y Cajal's work (1), it has only been in the last decade that we have been able to "see" selected populations of growth cones. By the 1980s, descriptions of the natural history of developing insect neurons, spectacularly outlined by intracellular dye injection, set the standard for observing the behaviors of individual growth cones in their natural setting. This work established the "labeled pathways" hypothesis and brought to light the importance of pioneer and guidepost neurons in pathfinding.

Progress was much slower in defining pathways and growth cone interactions in higher nervous systems, because of the difficulty of visualizing the shapes of individual neurons in the CNS during developmental periods. The interactions of growth cones with their target *cells* were particularly inaccessible, because of the difficulty of tracing the fine projections of axons and growth cones and of seeing the target cells selectively within the target region. A major turning point came in 1988, when the application of lipophilic carbocyanine dyes to fixed tissue revealed the paths and forms of growth cones in vertebrate brains.

This section on embryogenesis focuses on the growth cone in the context of the intact nervous system and addresses the role of the growth cone in the formation and navigation of paths and in the assembly of synaptic connections. The analysis of pathfinding in mammalian embryos has approached the level of analysis of pathfinding in insect and lower vertebrate embryos, focusing on single neurons of identified populations. In each of the systems discussed in these papers, new hypotheses and models have been posed on growth cone interactions in paths and targets. The development of new experimental preparations, as well as improvements in video imaging and microscopic techniques, has made it possible to chronicle growth cone behavior in real-time in relatively intact tissue. Together, the *in vitro* and real-time approaches verify information extracted from static observations of the intact nervous system and offer additional assays for molecules important for growth cone functioning.

Four themes emerge from the new work: (a) the strategies and rules for growth in pathways and to and within targets; (b) the meaning of alterations in growth cone form in different locales in paths and targets; (c) cues for general growth or inhibition of growth and for specific changes in trajectory; and (d) the molecular changes that occur in and on the axon and growth cone as it extends in paths and contacts targets.

STRATEGIES OF AXON PATHFINDING AND TARGET RELATIONS: NATURAL HISTORY AND RULES

In *pathways*, two new scenarios have been unfolded, and detailed behavior of growth cones in more well-known paths elucidated. The chapter by Easter and colleagues describes exploration of the uncharted earliest paths in the CNS of vertebrates. A simple scaffold consisting of five tracts and four commissures provides the highway system for the subsequent growth of other axonal systems, such as the later-developing retinal axon system. An exciting finding, novel to the vertebrate CNS, is the characterization of identified neurons that pioneer one of these tracts. Easter's analysis raises an interesting issue, recently demonstrated in a number of other systems: The first growth cones relate to pial basal lamina or neuroepithelial cells, and subsequently follower axons relate primarily to other axons.

Another system that has yielded a novel model for unraveling mechanisms of guidance is the optic chiasm. The long-standing problem of how fibers from each eye distribute themselves to each side of the brain at the optic chiasm has been attacked with DiI tracing in mouse embryos (chapter by Mason and Godement). The remarkable feature of the decussation or sorting out process is that fibers destined for the ipsilateral side of the brain do not grow straightaway into the ipsilateral optic tract but rather begin to cross, then make a hairpin turn back toward the ipsilateral side. The discrete locus of this turn suggests that an inhibitory cue for the uncrossed fibers is associated with the chiasm midline.

The chapter by Bentley and O'Connor presents, in the well-described grasshopper limb preparation, the detailed steps in growth cone behavior in elongation and turning, during steering and contact with guidepost cells. Some of these strategies, such as filopodial expansion, resemble those used by retinal axon growth cones in the chiasm during turning (chapter by Mason and Godement).

Advances in dye labeling, coupled with experimental ablations, immunocytochemistry, and tissue culture, have shed light on growth cone interactions in *target* regions and with specific target cells. In the leech, the simplicity and size of identified neurons allows manipulation of neurons that project within the CNS and to peripheral targets. Macagno and colleagues (chapter by Wolszon and Macagno) demonstrated that the target regulates the extent to which the initial excessive growth is remodeled. In addition, in the central projections of segmentally repeated neurons and in the peripheral arbors of the same neurons, growth cones participate in cell–cell communication with resultant "space-sharing" mechanisms. This communication by growth cones is contact-mediated and may involve intercellular junctions.

In rodent brain, the orchestration of afferent ingrowth and contact with target cells is more closely timed than previously thought with older tracing techniques (chapter by Kalil and Norris and chapter by Mason and Godement). Rather than arriving "early," to wait in subcellular zones before advancing toward target cells, callosal afferents to the hamster cortex, and climbing fiber afferents to the mouse cerebellum, enter the target tissue immediately after arriving in its vicinity.

Dye labeling in combination with electron microscopy has also allowed analysis of the relationships of ingrowing axons and their growing tips within target regions. Callosal afferents enter the cortex orthogonal to their direction of growth in the corpus callosum, entwined along radial glial fibers, which also serve as scaffolds for migrating target cells. This arrangement may afford a mechanism for connecting callosal axons with appropriate columnar targets in the contralateral cortex. In contrast to previously held views, both callosal and corticospinal axons enter targets and initially arborize quite precisely, rather than display exuberant growth followed by elimination of excess branches (chapter by Kalil and Norris).

Once afferent growth cones enter target regions, the larger, more elaborate forms of growth cone in decision regions and in straight paths collapse or condense into tapered buds (chapters by Kalil and Norris and by Mason and Godement). This dramatic transformation suggests that the growth cone machinery shuts down after contact with targets and "shifts gears" to build a synaptic contact, a rather protracted process in the mammalian CNS. The role of target cells in regulating afferent extension, in effect, arresting growth, has been demonstrated in mouse cerebellum, a region from which purified target cells can be obtained in high yield (chapter by Mason and Godement). The growth-promoting, arresting, or even inhibitory properties of different targets cells within a given brain region has also been implicated by the regeneration and transplant studies described in the chapters by Sotelo et al. and Bray.

THE SIGNIFICANCE OF CHANGES IN GROWTH CONE FORM IN PATHS AND TARGETS

Ramón y Cajal was the first to note in Golgi-impregnated material that growth cones in a single region, the spinal cord, displayed different forms, depending on the locale in which they were found (1). Although he did not relate the variety of forms with cellular interactions, he presented the different designs as examples of the remarkable sensitivity of the growth cone as it responds to different cues in the immediate environment.

As growth cones were more readily visualized with new methodologies, the meaning of the various forms became an issue. Observations in fixed tissue revealed that growth cones positioned at different points along a given neural pathway had characteristically different shapes. Growth cones have simple morphologies and straight trajectories in common or straight paths. In regions where axons that have followed a common path diverge, commonly referred to as "decision regions," growth cones display complex alterations in trajectory and morphology. Within targets, small reduced endings correspond to contact with target cells (chapters by Bentley and O'Connor, Easter et al., Nordlander, Mason and Godement, and Kalil and Norris). A striking example of this principle is presented in the optic chiasm, where the most complex and wide-ranging growth cones are in the process of turning, apparently avoiding an inhibitory cue near the midline (chapter by Mason and Godement). This dramatic exhibition of different forms and behavior in different locales has been held as evidence, as Cajal thought, that growth cones respond to specific cues in their microenvironment, to extend, to explore or turn, or to cease growing.

Several of the studies presented here challenge the view that growth cones at the same position have uniform shapes. First, the real-time studies reveal that within a single locale individual growth cones undergo astonishingly rapid and diverse shape changes during changes in trajectory, as well as during straight extension (chapters by Mason and Godement and by Bentley and O'Connor). Thus, the uniform growth cone shapes observed in static preparations may represent only the average or predominant form at any one time and place. The shapes that have been catalogued so far should be considered as indicators of interactions at that moment. Because the shape ultimately reflects cellular and molecular interactions, the argument can be made that shape is primarily interaction-specific. A single type of interaction can occur among growth cones in one locale, such as fasciculation in a tract, whereas more varied interactions, with a wider range of growth cone forms, take place in decision regions. Second, with antibodies to cell-specific neurotransmitters, the chapter by Nordlander demonstrates intrinsic differences in the form of growth cones of neurons of different populations, when growing in the same position in closely apposed tracts. Third, the chapters by Kalil and Norris and by Nordlander demonstrate that in the corpus callosum, and diagonal tract of sensory ganglion cell axons, growth cone complexity can occur even in straight paths.

CUES THAT REGULATE NEURITE ELONGATION
IN PATHS AND TARGETS

A key issue in many of the chapters is to discern the cues used by growth cones to grow, cease growing, or change direction in paths and targets. A number of studies give new insight on the molecules, the kinds of cells and tissues serving as cues and in which these molecules reside, and to what extent they operate by contact or long-range diffusion.

Bentley and colleagues (chapter by Bentley and O'Connor) systematically deleted various tissues in the grasshopper limb to find that mesodermal cells and basal lamina are dispensable for guidance. Important guidance cues were found to be the epithelial segment boundary cells, offering surfaces of low affinity and therefore less attractive to the growth cone. Distal to these boundary cells is a circumferential band of cells of high affinity, where growth cones selectively adhere and turn. In concert, these cellular regions reorient the growth cone toward guidepost cells. The notion that axonal growth cones are guided by a series of environmental components, including guidepost neurons, segmental boundaries, and processes of other neurons, is stressed.

The chapter by Eisen and Pike probes whether individual pairs of identified motoneurons in the zebrafish are necessary for outgrowth of their partners. After laser-ablating the secondary motoneurons, the primary pioneering motor neurons can quite easily make their way in specific paths. When the primary motoneurons are ablated, surprisingly the secondary motoneurons at first are arrested in their growth, then recover to develop after a lag time. The ease of manipulation of these identified single neurons allows another sort of experiment, that of plucking them out of their home territory at very early stages and transplanting them to other sites, to determine when they acquire their "identity."

Work on the chick motoneuron system in the innervation of the limb has defined two types of cues (chapters by Landmesser and by Tosney). Previous work showed that after spinal cord rotations or ablations or motoneuron pools, motoneurons can still find their way to specific targets. If motoneurons are displaced great distances from their home site, however, they will enter foreign plexus and muscle, as though the cues were not recognized. Landmesser advanced the notion that there are both specific guidance cues, read as the "local language," and more general cues, a universal or "global" language, providing permissive highways that motoneurons could follow regardless of ethnic identity.

Tosney and colleagues have shown that general cues consist of paths and barriers. Paths are tissues such as anterior sclerotome, which express permissive molecules. Barriers express markers of early cartilage differentiation, large matrix molecules that are inhibitory to axon growth. Other inhibitory components are identified in the zebrafish, where myotomal boundaries express fibronectin, whereas permissive areas express a laminin-like molecule (chapter by Eisen and Pike). Thus, identification of potentially inhibitory molecules strengthens the notion that inhibition as well as growth promotion are crucial to guidance (see also chapters by Baier and Bonhoeffer and by Raper, et al).

A much talked-about locus for cues is the midline of the neuraxis. Specialized glial cells in the midline of the insect central nervous system facilitate crossing of certain growth cones, which fail to do so if these cells are ablated or defective in mutants (chapter by Goodman et al.). In the optic chiasm, a radial glial structure has been defined with the proper register and temporal appearance for the inhibitory cue for uncrossed retinal axons (chapter by Mason and Godement).

A strong case for a tropic cue is made by Tosney. Epaxial motor neurons orient toward dermamyotome muscle precursors. If these precursors are deleted, the epaxial motoneurons do not grow out. In addition, this is distance-dependent, suggesting that a diffusible cue emanates from the muscle precursor. This is an example of a specific cue, essential only for the development of epaxial innervations, and one that provides information regarding direction of travel. In contrast, general cues determine where axons can and cannot advance.

Tosney has emphasized that there must be multiple cues for axon guidance, some used in concert in a given situation. In addition to multiple cues, not all cues are positive or elicit outgrowth. How do we distinguish among multiple mechanisms that the varied cues in an axon's path imply? Tosney argues that multiple assays must be used, each of which, on its own, gives a restricted view of a given mechanism, but when considered together, would present a more complete understanding of the possible mechanisms. Although the permutations and combinations of multiple cues and mechanisms at present seems daunting, for each set of neurons there is likely to be a sequential hierarchy of cues important for proper guidance.

MOLECULAR CHANGES ON GROWING AXONS

In the insect CNS, pioneer neurites set down a scaffold, and later-extending growth cones follow specific pathways, selectively fasciculating along certain axons. The work of Goodman and colleagues resulted in the proposal that neighboring paths are differentially labeled by surface recognition molecules, allowing growth cones to distinguish between them. Monoclonal antibody techniques allowed the molecules to be isolated and characterized as surface glycoproteins. Some of these molecules are members of the immunoglobulin superfamily, which includes adhesion molecules expressed by vertebrate neurons.

Now that the genes encoding the neuronal recognition or surface molecules have begun to be identified and characterized, particularly in *Drosophila*, Goodman and colleagues have probed mutations with genetic and molecular techniques (chapter by Goodman et al.). Simply tampering with or knocking out one gene for one gene product does little to affect process outgrowth. However, double mutations, for instance of fasciclin 1 and abl, a protoncogene homologue that encodes a cytoplasmic tyrosine kinase, can substantially alter the trajectory of the RP1 neuron, which does not cross the midline as in the normal embryo.

Landmesser and colleagues present molecular changes that occur spatially and temporally in a distinct pattern on growing axons in the chick limb. The phosphorylated epitope 5E10 is expressed in motoneurons in the distal portion of the axon as it enters the plexus, or decision region, where axons enter different nerve branches. Landmesser speculates that response to a specific guidance cue, via phosphorylation of such a molecule, may result in reorganization of the cytoskeleton to change growth.

Much of the effort to unveil molecules underlying "specificity" of neuronal identity and therefore formation of connections, via monoclonal technology, has been disappointing. The 5A5 monoclonal is not a cell-specific marker but recognizes the highly sialated form of NCAM. Surprisingly, this marker also distinguishes motoneuron axons projecting to different regions (chapter by Landmesser). Because Landmesser's work has also shown that tampering with the levels of polysialic acid with endosialidase can alter the pattern of intramuscular nerve branching in the same motoneuron, this molecule and its posttranslational modification comprise an interesting candidate for regulating morphogenesis and for providing differences between neurons, perhaps one basis for "specificity," without altering or requiring extensive genetic expression of multiple molecules.

THE FUTURE

We are now entering an exciting period of understanding how the various forms of growth cones mirror cellular and molecular interactions, and the identity of the soluble and bound cues that underlie these interactions. New dye-labeling technology will continue to expand our view of growth cone interactions in the intact nervous system, especially in real-time. The improved definition of the events of pathfinding and target interactions will serve as a basis for demonstrating the molecular correlates of different phases of development. Genetics will be a powerful tool for the systems that have had a head-start on clarifying pathfinding and principles of guidance, such as *Drosophila*. It should soon be possible to correlate the varied forms and transitions of growth cone in different locales, with functions of specific molecules. By this approach, the "sign language" of varied growth cone shapes can be "decoded" into cellular and molecular terms. We are well on the way to better define guidance cues, their generality, multiplicity, and how they are housed. One challenge will be to test for the effects of diffusible factors of the sort discussed in Part 2, within the confines of the intact nervous system.

An aim for those working in the intact embryo will be to link the analyses in the first part of the book, to probe the surface of the growth cone, and to look "inside" to examine its workings. We need to unravel how functionally relevant molecules are perceived and how this information affects second-messenger systems, which in turn alter the cytoskeleton to result in extension, changes in trajectory, or development of a synaptic ending. Such multimodal approaches in turn should elucidate the requirements for successful pathfinding and synaptogenesis, during normal development and regeneration.

REFERENCE

1. Ramón y Cajal S. *Histologie du Système Nerveux de l'Homme et des Vertébrés*, vol 1. Paris: Maloine, 1911:598.

The Nerve Growth Cone, edited by P. C. Letourneau,
S. B. Kater, and E. R. Macagno, Raven Press, Ltd.,
New York © 1992.

22

Guidance and Steering of Peripheral Pioneer Growth Cones in Grasshopper Embryos

David Bentley and Timothy P. O'Connor

*Department of Molecular and Cell Biology, University of California,
Berkeley, California 94720*

PERIPHERAL NERVES OF GRASSHOPPER LIMBS

Early in the development of the grasshopper embryo, a pair of afferent neurons arises from the epithelium at the distal tip of each limb bud. The neurons, termed the *tibial* (Ti1) *pioneers*, extend axons along a stereotyped route through the limb to the central nervous system (CNS) (Fig. 1). These cells have proven to be a useful model for analysis of several aspects of directed nerve outgrowth, including the role of pioneer neurons in establishing nerve routes, the nature of guidance information for growth cone migration, and the mechanisms of growth cone steering in response to such information. In this article, we briefly review current understanding of these issues in this system.

Grasshopper limbs are operated by a complex musculature and contain an extensive array of proprioceptors and surface mechano- and chemoreceptors. Motor and sensory neuron axons course through a stereotyped pattern of major nerve trunks and subsidiary nerve branches (1). The nerve trunks are free-floating in the limb interior (being anchored at the CNS and at their connections to effectors or sensory structures), are ensheathed and subdivided by an extensive extracellular and glial investiture, and are generally of mixed motor and sensory composition (2). They may contain from 10 to 100 motor neurons and thousands of afferent axons. How does this stereotyped pattern of nerves arise?

Grasshoppers are hemi-metabolous insects, having a period of embryonic development within an egg resulting in a hatchee resembling a diminutive adult, a postembryonic period of several nymphal stages, and finally a molt to the adult form. During embryogenesis, most or all the thoracic motor neurons that will innervate the limb are generated (3). It seems likely that all proprioceptive sensory neurons that leave the epithelium and come to lie in the limb interior also arise during embryogenesis (4). Although epithelial sensory neurons that innervate cuticular structures are generated throughout postembryonic development, the first set of

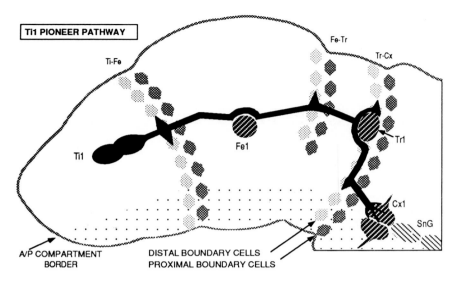

FIG. 1. Schematic representation of the Ti1 pioneer neuron pathway in a 34% stage limb bud. The pioneer cell bodies lie within the tibia. Growth cones migrate proximally across the tibia/femur (Ti-Fe) boundary, contact guidepost cell Fe1, cross the femur/trochanter (Fe-Tr) boundary, encounter the Tr1 guidepost cell, turn ventrally along the trochanter/coxa boundary (Tr-Cx), and extend to the pair of Cx1 guidepost cells that lie at the ventral anterior–posterior compartment boundary. Between the Cx1 cells and the CNS (to *right*) lie several adepithelial cells that may be segmental nerve root glial cells (SnG). At each limb segment boundary is an interface between a distal band of epithelial cells, which has high affinity for the growth cones, and a proximal band of cells, which has lower affinity. The proximally located Tr-Cx boundary differentiates before the more distally located segment boundaries. The Ti-Fe and Fe-Tr segment boundaries are not fully differentiated at the time of Ti1 pioneer growth cone migration.

these neurons also is produced during embryogenesis (5). At the end of embryogenesis, the characteristic peripheral nerve pattern, containing both motor and sensory neurons, is in place. Thus the formation of this pattern is an embryonic event.

The first neurons to undergo axonogenesis in the limb are the sibling afferent Ti1 pioneer neurons (6), which arise from a single mother cell situated in the limb tip epithelium at about 30% of embryogenesis (7). Concomitant with the generation of these neurons, two additional neurons, the Cx1 cells, emerge individually from anterior and posterior limb epithelium, migrate ventrally, and extend axons to the CNS (8). During the ensuing 20% of embryogenesis, single neurons, pairs, or in two cases, small clusters of neurons, arise at specific locations throughout the elongating limb bud and also extend axons along specific routes through the limb (9). Where they encounter each other, these axons fasciculate, so that all the pioneer axons become collected into a few bundles more proximally in the limb. This initial scaffold of axons from the pioneer neurons in different limb regions establishes the pattern of afferent nerve trunks along which large numbers of later arising sensory neurons fasciculate. Thus, the routes of these trunks are the result of the paths through the limb taken by the initial set of pioneer growth cones.

Motor growth cones emerge from the CNS soon after the arrival of the first afferent growth cones (10). In some cases, motor axons extend along afferent pathways, but they also frequently establish their own routes, either initially or by diverging from the afferent nerves, particularly at the location of muscle pioneer cells (10,11).

At 30% of embryonic development, when afferent pioneer axonogenesis begins, the limb comprises an ectodermal epithelium and an interior of mesodermal cells (Fig. 2). The mesodermal cells are rearranging from an initially layered configuration to a looser mesenchyme, which presages the formation of muscles and other limb structures. These two layers are separated by a thick basal lamina (12). The pioneer growth cones migrate along the basal surface of the epithelium, on the epithelial side of the basal lamina (13). Thus the epithelium is the substrate on which the pioneer scaffold is constructed. Soon after the period of peripheral axonogenesis, the axons become invested with glial cells of undetermined origin (14).

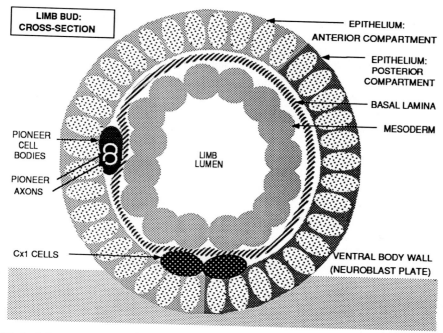

FIG. 2. Schematic representation of a limb bud, showing the external layer of ectodermal epithelium, the basal lamina, and an internal layer of mesoderm. Pioneer cell bodies emerge from the epithelium and lie between the epithelium and the basal lamina, where pioneer growth cone migration occurs. Anterior and posterior Cx1 guidepost cells emerge from the anterior and posterior epithelial compartments (8,48), respectively, and migrate to the ventral midline of the limb bud.

The pioneer axons enwrapped by these glial cells subsequently lose their attachment to the epithelium and become displaced into the interior of the limb. This displacement appears to require movement of the nerve through the basal lamina.

In summary, the grasshopper limb has a stereotyped pattern of peripheral nerves, which arises during embryogenesis. The routes of these nerves are determined by the sites of origin of a small set of early arising pioneer neurons and by the migration paths of the axonal growth cones of these afferent cells as well as efferent growth cones emerging from the CNS. Once in place these pioneer axons provide a substrate for the migration of later arising axons and, by accrual of such axons, are transformed into nerve trunks.

DEVELOPMENTAL ROLE OF PIONEER NEURONS

Are pioneer neurons simply the first neurons to undergo axonogenesis, or do they play a specific role in generation of the PNS? In particular, would the development of the PNS be different in their absence? Experimental deletion of specific neurons indicates that some pioneers do play an essential role in development and that this results from the place and time of their birth rather than distinctive phenotypic features.

In crickets, afferent axons in the cerci, posterior sensory appendages, are collected into two major nerves. Early laser ablation of the pioneer neurons that found these nerves results in the development of many small axon bundles rather than the normal pair of nerves (15).

In grasshopper limbs, two afferent neurons, Fe1 and Tr1 (Fig. 1), normally arise along the pioneer pathway after passage of the pioneer growth cones and extend fasciculating axons along this pathway. If the Ti1 neurons are photoablated at the onset of axonogenesis, Fe1 and Tr1 still extend axons along the path that would have been taken by the Ti1 axons (16). These results indicate that the Ti1 growth cones do not have unique pathfinding capability and that the growth cones of other afferent neurons are able to follow the same guidance cues as the Ti1 pioneers if they encounter them. In general, growth cones from different afferent neurons appear to make the same steering decisions when encountering guidance features in the limb.

However, place and time of birth do confer unique pathfinding opportunities on pioneer growth cones. Differentiation of the Ti1 pioneer neurons can be prevented by timed heat-shock of the whole egg. Embryogenesis can then be allowed to proceed to later developmental stages, and the effects of the absence of the pioneers on late-arising neurons located in distal limb regions assessed. Under these circumstances, one of the major limb nerves fails to develop (17). The axons of afferent neurons distal to the Ti1 neurons and growing toward the CNS are blocked at a limb segment boundary. Similarly, if the Cx1 neurons (Figs. 1 and 3) are selectively ablated by UV microbeam, the Ti1 growth cones are unable to cross the proximally located trochanter/coxa boundary normally (18). Once differentiated, limb segment

has been observed both in limbs where Fe1 has been relatively slow to differentiate (31) and where differentiation of Fe1 has been prevented by timed heat-shock. In the absence of Fe1, the pioneer growth cones are more branched than usual and may be migrating more slowly, but still migrate proximally. Both proximal migration and also the ventral turn at the trochanter/coxa boundary occur when differentiation of Tr1 has been prevented by heat-shock. By contrast, the presence of the Cx1 cell pair does appear necessary for normal pathway formation. If the Cx1 cells are ablated with a UV microbeam before arrival of the pioneer growth cones, the growth cones fail to leave the trochanter/coxa boundary and to grow proximally to the CNS at the normal time and location (18).

Nerve Root Glial Cells

Extending from the Cx1 cells to the site where the pioneer growth cones and the Cx1 growth cones enter the CNS is a chain of three or four adepithelial cells. These cells occasionally label with anti-HRP serum antibodies (22,41). Detailed observation of the relationship of the pioneer growth cones to these cells suggests that the growth cones do not migrate between the cells and the epithelium, but rather on the luminal aspect of the cells. The morphology of growth cones in this region is uniquely narrow and focused. These cells may be grasshopper homologues of the nerve root glial cells described in *Drosophila* (42).

GROWTH CONE STEERING

Oriented neurite elongation in response to guidance cues comprises growth cone steering. *In vitro*, two general modes of axon elongation have been observed (43). Generally, filopodia or microspikes are extended from the leading edge of a growth cone, possibly driven by actin polymerization. Flat lamellae or veils then extend between the filopodia, and these veils secondarily expand with the intrusion of organelles and cytoplasmic material. Finally, at the base of the growth cone this expanded region is converted into a more mature neurite with an interior core of bundled microtubules. In rapidly advancing growth cones, veils may co-extend with the microtubule bundles so that such bundles appear as ribs within the veil, rather than as filopodia. Veil extension without well-defined microtubule bundles also can occur.

An alternative mode of growth cone advance, reported *in vitro* in two cases, comprises the conversion of a single filopodium into the neurite (44). In these cases, a single filopodium extending across a region of relatively low affinity contacts either a higher-affinity substrate or the surface of a glial cell. The filopodium then increases in diameter to become the neurite.

Elongation *In Situ*

In the grasshopper limb fillet preparation, pioneer neurons can be viewed in Nomarski optics and labeled with the fluorescent lipophilic dyes Dil or DiO (36). The dye diffuses rapidly throughout the plasma membrane so that individual filopodia are readily observed (Fig. 4). Using computer-shuttered halogen or mercury illumination, SIT or CCD image intensifiers, and computer image enhancement, time-lapse videos of growth cone migration and interactions with guidance cues can be obtained. Of particular interest are the growth cone behaviors of pioneer neurons at steering decision points.

On the *in situ* substrate, the two modes of axon elongation seen *in vitro* both occur (Fig. 5). When the pioneer growth cones are first emerging from the cell bodies and are extending across intrasegmental epithelium within the femur, they advance by *veil extension* (36). In this region, a relatively small number of filopodia are extended within a roughly 45-degree quadrant in advance of the growth cone. Veils then extend between subsets of these filopodia, and no single filopodium is followed for more than a few micrometers. Similar growth cone migration by veil extension is also seen when growth cones are migrating ventrally along the high-affinity cell band at the trochanter/coxa boundary. Thus migration by veil extension appears to occur where growth cones are advancing over relatively homogeneous

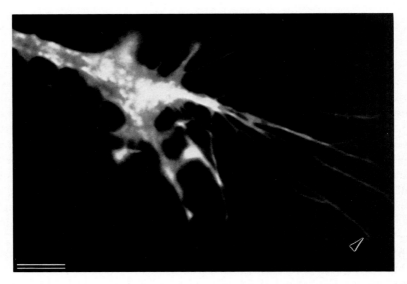

FIG. 4. Single live Ti1 pioneer growth cone, labeled with DiO, migrating on intrasegmental epithelium in the proximal region of the femur in a 32.5% stage limb bud. The position, number, and length of individual filopodia extending in advance of the growth cone are readily resolved (*arrowhead*). Proximal, to right: dorsal, up. Scale, 5 μm.

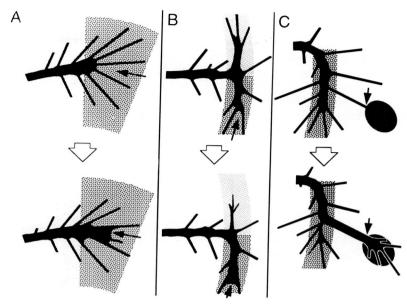

FIG. 5. Schematic diagram of the types of steering events seen in pioneer growth cones migrating on the *in situ* substrate. **A:** In regions that appear to have a relatively homogeneous substrate (which may feature a shallow gradient of affinity), growth cones migrate by the extension of lamellar veils between filopodia. Preferential extension of veils between more proximally oriented filopodia mediates a series of shallow angle turns that maintain axial growth. **B:** At limb segment boundaries, where growth cones encounter an orthogonal interface between a high-affinity and a low-affinity substrate, proximal migration ceases, and the growth cones remain on the higher-affinity substrate by extending robust branches in both directions on that substrate. Subsequently, the dorsal branch is withdrawn and further growth occurs in the ventral direction. Thus this steering decision is mediated by a process of selective branch retraction. **C:** When a growth cone migrating on a favorable substrate establishes a single filopodial contact (*arrow*) with a high-affinity guidepost cell, that filopodium expands in diameter and becomes the sole path of the elongating neurite.

substrates. In this situation, differences in substrate affinity between the tips of different filopodia and between filopodia and the base of growth cone should be relatively small.

By contrast, where a filopodium contacts the surface of a guidepost cell, the growth cone can advance directly along that filopodium by *filopodial expansion* (36). Where the filopodium contacts the cell surface, it often begins to expand into a palmate configuration from which secondary filopodia are subsequently extruded. The shaft of the filopodium does not expand smoothly and usually has several intervening sites of local expansion. Eventually, the expanding filopodium reaches the diameter of the axon so that the growth cone has advanced along the length of the filopodium in a single saltation. This mode of advance, as also seen *in vitro* (44), appears to occur where a marked difference in substrate affinity exists between the substrate at the tip of the filopodium and the substrate at the growth cone and at other filopodia.

Steering *In Situ*

During growth cone migration on the fillet substrate, three kinds of steering events have been observed (Fig. 5) (36). Where growth cones are advancing over a relatively homogeneous substrate in the intrasegmental region of the femur, a generally proximal course along the limb axis is maintained by preferential extension of veils between more proximally extended filopodia. This type of steering can be viewed as a series of small-angle steering events mediated by selective veil extension.

At the trochanter/coxa limb segment boundary, the growth cones encounter an orthogonal interface between a higher-affinity and a lower-affinity substrate. In this situation, branches fail to become established on the lower-affinity substrate, and substantial branches are formed in both the dorsal and ventral directions on the higher-affinity substrate. Subsequently, the dorsal branch, which frequently forms first and can extend at least 20 μm, is withdrawn and the ventral branch becomes the axon. Thus, this steering event occurs by selective branch withdrawal. A similar response, where growth cones encounter an interface between substrates, occurs *in vitro* (43) and has been termed *micropruning*.

The third type of steering event observed *in situ* is mediated by filopodial expansion. Where a growth cone is migrating in one direction and a single off-axis filopodium contacts a guidepost cell, the entire growth cone can reorient along the filopodium. The most consistent example of this phenomenon is seen where growth cones are migrating ventrally along the trochanter/coxa boundary. Although these cells are a highly adhesive substrate, a single contact with the Cx1 cells results in reorientation of the growth cones. This phenomenon indicates that events occurring at the tip of a filopodium can initiate the transmission of signals along that filopodium, which results in the highly selective accrual of material from the growth cone into the base of the filopodium. The presence of such signals also is suggested by the ability of filopodia that find themselves on favorable substrates to elongate selectively, even in new directions (36). A key question in growth cone steering is the nature of such signals.

NEW DIRECTIONS

Microtubule Disposition

The morphological configuration of a neuron is maintained by the disposition of its microtubules. In migrating growth cones, the regions in which microtubules become stabilized will establish the configuration of branches or axons and determine the course of migration. Consequently, the mechanisms that control the disposition of microtubules in the growth cone will determine growth cone steering decisions. Possible models for the process of regional disposition of microtubules in the growth cone include random microtubule extension into the periphery followed by selective stabilization, directional displacement of randomly extended microtubules, and initial directionally selective extension of microtubules (45).

In the grasshopper pioneer preparation, it is possible to monitor changes in microtubule disposition during growth cone steering events (46). Rhodaminated bovine tubulin can be injected into the neuron cell bodies in the fillet preparation. The tubulin is transported to the growth cone where it rapidly becomes incorporated into microtubules. Using a cooled CCD camera, which has a 1300×1024 pixel chip, image resolution is adequate to resolve microtubules. Injected, time-lapse imaged growth cones make their normal stereotyped steering decisions on this *in situ* preparation. In growth cones containing labeled tubulin, unitary linear structures that appear to be single microtubules are observed. Preliminary observations indicate that microtubules intrude into only a subset of filopodia extended from the leading edge of the growth cone and that after these initial insertions, a characteristic sequence of microtubule accrual and spacing occurs. Substantiation of these observations and experimental manipulation of the system during microtubule monitoring should yield illuminating information on the process of microtubule control during steering events.

Intracellular Signaling

The ability of single filopodial contacts to reorient the growth cone indicates that effective signals can be transmitted along single filopodia. Such signals might be mechanical, as effected by changes in tension or transport of intracellular material, but they could also involve a variety of intracellular second-messenger systems. Cytosolic calcium ion concentration, for example, is a critical controller of growth cone motility, an effect that appears to be mediated at least in part by control of actin microfilament polymerization (47). Possible roles for such signals may be evaluated by monitoring intracellular signals during growth cone steering events.

A beginning of such monitoring has been made by examining cytosolic calcium ion concentration in pioneer growth cones at different single stages of their migration, using intracellularly injected fura-2 (40). The initial results indicate that calcium ion concentrations are relatively low in preaxonogenesis neurons and become elevated in migrating growth cones; that in such growth cones they are in the greater than 100-nM range seen in a variety of neurons *in vitro*; that there is often a shallow concentration gradient that is most elevated at the growth cone; and that calcium ion concentration in the pioneer neurons is lowered by diffusion into coupled guidepost cells. It is now desirable to determine, with time-lapse imaging, whether spatial or temporal differences in calcium concentration in leading filopodia are associated with filopodial expansion or selective veil extension and whether such differences may mediate growth cone steering decisions.

ACKNOWLEDGMENTS

Support was provided by NIH NS09074 and the March of Dimes Birth Defects Foundation (D.B.), and a Canadian MRC Postdoctoral Fellowship (T. O'C).

REFERENCES

1. Campbell JI. The anatomy of the nervous system of the mesothorax of *Locusta migratoria migratoriodes* R. and F. *Proc Zool Soc Lond* 1961;137:403–432.
2. Zill SN, Underwood MA, Rowley JC, Moran DT. A somatotopic organization of groups of afferents in insect peripheral nerves. *Brain Res* 1980;198:253–270.
3. Shepard D, Bate CM. Spatial and temporal patterns of neurogenesis in the embryo of the locust (*Schistocerca gregaria*). *Development* 1990;108:83–96.
4. Kutsch W. Formation of the receptor system in the hind limb of the locust embryo. *Roux's Arch Dev Biol* 1989;198:39–47.
5. Shankland M, Bentley D. Sensory receptor differentiation and axonal pathfinding in the cercus of the grasshopper embryo. *Dev Biol* 1983;97:468–482.
6. Bate CM. Pioneer neurons in an insect embryo. *Nature* 1976;260:54–56.
7. Keshishian H. The origin and morphogenesis of pioneer neurons in the grasshopper metathoracic leg. *Dev Biol* 1980;80:388–397.
8. Bentley D, Toroian-Raymond A. Pre-axonogenesis migration of afferent pioneer cells in the grasshopper embryo. *J Exp Zool* 1989;251:217–223.
9. Ho RK, Goodman CS. Peripheral pathways are pioneered by an array of central and peripheral neurones in grasshopper embryos. *Nature* 1982;297:404–406.
9a.Keshishian H, Bentley D. Embryogenesis of peripheral nerve pathways in grasshopper legs. 1. The initial nerve pathway to the CNS. *Dev Biol* 1983;96:89–102.
9b.Keshishian H, Bentley D. Embryogenesis of peripheral nerve pathways in grasshopper legs. 2. The major nerve routes. *Dev Biol* 1983;96:103–115.
10. Ball EE, Ho RK, Goodman CS. Development of neuromuscular specificity in the grasshopper embryo: guidance of motoneuron growth cones by muscle pioneers. *J Neurosci* 1985;5:1808–1819.
11. Whitington PM. The early development of motor axon pathways in the locust embryo: the establishment of the segmental nerves in the thoracic ganglia. *Development* 1989;105:715–722.
12. Anderson H, Tucker R. Spatial and temporal variation in the structure of the basal lamina in embryonic grasshopper limbs during pioneer neurone outgrowth. *Development* 1989;106:185–194.
13. Anderson H, Tucker RP. Pioneer neurones use basal lamina as a substratum for outgrowth in the embryonic grasshopper limb. *Development* 1988;104:601–608.
14. Toroian-Raymond A, Bentley D. Embryonic development of an insect antennal nerve (*Abstr*). *Soc Neurosci Abstr* 1981;6:374.
15. Edwards JS, Chen S, Berns MW. Cercal sensory development following laser microlesions of embryonic apical cells in *Acheta domesticus*. *J Neurosci* 1981;1:250–258.
16. Keshishian H, Bentley D. Embryogenesis of peripheral nerve pathways in grasshopper legs. 3. Development without pioneers. *Dev Biol* 1983;96:116–124.
17. Klose M, Bentley D. Transient pioneer neurons are essential for formation of an embryonic peripheral nerve. *Science* 1989;245:982–984.
18. Bentley D, Caudy M. Pioneer axons lose directed growth after selective killing of guidepost cells. *Nature* 1983;304:62–65.
19. Caudy M, Bentley D. Pioneer growth cone behavior at a differentiating limb segment boundary in the grasshopper embryo. *Dev Biol* 1987;119:454–465.
20. Kutsch W, Bentley D. Programmed death of peripheral pioneer neurons in the grasshopper embryo. *Dev Biol* 1987;123:517–525.
21. Lefcort F, Bentley D. Organization of cytoskeletal elements and organelles preceding growth cone emergence from an identified neuron *in situ*. *J Cell Biol* 1989;108:1737–1749.
22. Caudy M, Bentley D. Pioneer growth cone steering along a series of neuronal and non-neuronal cues of different affinities. *J Neurosci* 1986;6:1781–1795.

23. Lefcort F, Bentley D. Pathfinding by pioneer neurons in isolated, opened and mesoderm-free limb buds of embryonic grasshoppers. *Dev Biol* 1987;119:466–480.

24. Ball EE, deCouet HG, Horn PL, Quinn JMA. Haemocytes secrete basement membrane components in embryonic locusts. *Development* 1987;99:255–259.

25. Montell SJ, Goodman CS. *Drosophila* laminin: sequence of B2 subunit and expression of all three subunits during embryogenesis. *J Cell Biol* 1989;109:2441–2453.

26. Condic ML, Bentley D. Removal of the basal lamina *in vivo* reveals growth cone–basal lamina adhesive interactions and axonal tension in grasshopper embryos. *J Neurosci* 1989;9:2678–2686.

27. Levinson G, Bradley TJ. Removal of insect basal laminae using elastase. *Tissue Cell* 1984;16:367–375.

28. Koefoed BM. The ability of an epithelium to survive removal of the basal lamina by enzymes. *Tissue Cell* 1987;19:65–70.

29. Condic ML, Bentley D. Pioneer neuron pathfinding from normal and ectopic locations *in vivo* after removal of the basal lamina. *Neuron* 1989;3:427–439.

30. Locke M. The cuticular pattern in an insect: the behaviour of grafts in segmented appendages. *J Insect Physiol* 1966;12:397–402.

30a.Bohn H. Regeneration of proximal tissues from a more distal amputation level in the insect leg (*Blaberus cranifer*, Blatteria). *Dev Biol* 1976;53:285–293.

31. Caudy M, Bentley D. Pioneer growth cone morphologies reveal proximal increases in substrate affinity within leg segments of grasshopper embryos. *J Neurosci* 1986;6:364–379.

32. McKenna MP, Raper JA. Growth cone behavior on gradients of substratum bound laminin. *Dev Biol* 1988;130:232–236.

33. Caudy M, Bentley D. Epithelial cell specialization at a limb segment boundary in the grasshopper embryo. *Dev Biol* 1986;118:399–402.

34. Letourneau PC. Possible roles for cell-to-substratum adhesion in neuronal morphogenesis. *Dev Biol* 1975;44:77–91.

35. Condic ML, Bentley D. Pioneer growth cone adhesion *in vivo* to boundary cells and neurons after enzymatic removal of basal lamina in grasshopper embryos. *J Neurosci* 1989;9:2687–2696.

36. O'Connor TP, Duerr JS, Bentley D. Pioneer growth cone steering decisions mediated by single filopodial contacts *in situ. J Neurosci* 1990;10:3935–3946.

37. O'Connor TP, Gorodezky L, Toroian-Raymond A, Bentley D. Circumferential guidance cues for pioneer growth cone migration in grasshopper embryonic limb buds (*Abstr*). *Soc Neurosci Abstr* 1990;16:626.

38. Condic ML, Lefcort F, Bentley D. Selective recognition between embryonic afferent neurons of grasshopper appendages *in vitro. Dev Biol* 1989;135:221–230.

39. Taghert PH, Bastiani MJ, Ho RK, Goodman CS. Guidance of pioneer growth cones: filopodial contacts and coupling revealed with an antibody to lucifer yellow. *Dev Biol* 1982;94:391–399.

40. Guthrie PB, Kater SB, Bentley D. Guidepost cells act as calcium sinks for pioneer growth cones *in vivo* (*Abstr*). *Soc Neurosci Abstr* 1989;15:1261.

41. Jan LY, Jan YN. Antibodies to horseradish peroxidase as specific neuronal markers in *Drosophila* and grasshopper embryos. *Proc Natl Acad Sci USA* 1982;79:2700–2704.

41a.Snow PM, Patel NH, Harrelson AL, Goodman CS. Neural-specific carbohydrate moiety shared by many glycoproteins in *Drosophila* and grasshopper embryos. *J Neurosci* 1987;7:4137–4144.

42. Bieber AJ, Snow PM, Hortsch M, Patel N, Jacobs JR, Traquina ZR, Schilling J, Goodman CS. *Drosophila* neuroglian: a member of the immunoglobin superfamily with extensive homology to the vertebrate adhesion molecule L1. *Cell* 1989;59:447–460.

43. Aletta JM, Greene LA. Growth cone configuration and advance: a time-lapse study using video-enhanced differential interference contrast microscopy. *J Neurosci* 1988;8:1425–1435.

43a.Burmeister DW, Goldberg DJ. Micropruning: the mechanism of turning of *Aplysia* growth cones at substrate borders *in vitro. J Neurosci* 1988;8:3151–3159.

43b.Goldberg DJ, Burmeister DW. Looking into growth cones. *Trends Neurosci* 1989;12:503–506.

44. Letourneau PC. Cell-to-substratum adhesion and guidance of axonal elongation. *Dev Biol* 1975;44:92–101.

44a.Hammarback JA, Letourneau PC. Neurite extension across regions of low cell–substrate adhesivity: implications for the guidepost hypothesis of axonal pathfinding. *Dev Biol* 1986;117:655–662.

45. Mitchison T, Kirschner M. Cytoskeletal dynamics and nerve growth. *Neuron* 1988;1:761–772.

46. Sabry J, O'Connor T, Evans L, Toroian-Raymond A, Kirschner M, Bentley D. Microtubule behavior during guidance of pioneer neuron growth cones *in situ. J Cell Biol* (*in press*).

47. Forscher P, Smith SJ. Actions of cytochalasins on the organization of actin filaments and microtubules in a neuronal growth cone. *J Cell Biol* 1988;107:1505–1516.
47a.Lankford KL, Letourneau PC. Evidence that calcium may control neurite outgrowth by regulating the stability of actin filaments. *J Cell Biol* 1989;109:1229–1243.
47b.Mattson MP, Kater SB. Calcium regulation of neurite elongation and growth cone motility. *J Neurosci* 1987;8:4034–4043.
48. Patel NH, Martin-Blanco E, Coleman KG, et al. Expression of *engrailed* proteins in arthropods, annelids, and chordates. *Cell* 1989;58:955–968.

The Nerve Growth Cone, edited by P. C. Letourneau,
S. B. Kater, and E. R. Macagno, Raven Press, Ltd.,
New York © 1992.

23

Molecular Genetics of Neural Cell Adhesion Molecules in *Drosophila*

*Corey S. Goodman, *Gabriele Grenningloh, and
*†Allan J. Bieber

*Howard Hughes Medical Institute, Department of Molecular and Cell Biology,
University of California Berkeley, Berkeley, California 94720, and
†Department of Biological Sciences, Purdue University, West Lafayette, Indiana 47907

In the developing insect central nervous system (CNS), once the scaffold of axon pathways has been established by pioneering growth cones, most later growth cones display a remarkable ability to choose among and extend along specific axon pathways, a process called *selective fasciculation*. Based on a series of descriptive and experimental studies on the mechanisms of selective fasciculation in the grasshopper (1–5), Raper, Bastiani, and Goodman proposed that neighboring axon pathways must be differentially labeled by surface recognition molecules, which allow growth cones to distinguish among them, a notion they called the *labeled pathways hypothesis*. Subsequent cellular analysis from our lab in both the grasshopper (6–8) and a simple vertebrate (the fish spinal cord; see ref. 9) further supported this hypothesis. At about the same time, other studies from our lab, in collaboration with Michael Bate in Cambridge, England, showed that what had been learned from the large grasshopper embryo with its highly accessible identified neurons could be directly applied to the much smaller fruitfly, *Drosophila*, with its powerful genetics (10), thus opening the door to a combined cellular, classical genetic, and molecular genetic analysis of this problem (e.g., ref. 11).

Several years ago, in an attempt to identify molecules that impart this type of specificity on the developing nervous system, our lab began a series of monoclonal antibody screens to identify surface glycoproteins that are differentially expressed during development on subsets of axon pathways in the insect embryo (12–14). The long-term goal of this work is to identify and characterize the genes encoding these neuronal recognition molecules in *Drosophila*, to identify mutations in these genes, and to use these mutations as the starting point for a detailed genetic analysis of neuronal recognition.

We initially identified and subsequently cloned the genes encoding four different surface glycoproteins that are dynamically expressed on different overlapping subsets of growth cones, axon fascicles, and glia during embryonic development (12–14). Fasciclin I and fasciclin II were initially characterized and cloned in grasshopper (15–17) and subsequently the homologous genes were identified in *Drosophila* (16,18; G. Grenningloh and E. Rehm, *unpublished results*). Fasciclin III and neuroglian, however, were initially characterized and cloned in *Drosophila* (13,14,19), and subsequently the neuroglian homologue was identified in grasshopper (18; G. Grenningloh and E. Rehm, *unpublished results*).

One striking result from these molecular genetic studies was the finding that three of the four proteins (fasciclin II, neuroglian, and fasciclin III) are members of the immunoglobulin (Ig) superfamily. Fasciclin II and neuroglian are highly related to a series of vertebrate neural cell adhesion molecules including such molecules as NCAM (20,21), MAG (22,23), L1 (24), contactin/F11 (25,26), and TAG-1 (27). Within this group, fasciclin II is related to and shares a common evolutionary ancestor with NCAM (17), whereas neuroglian is related to and shares a common ancestor with L1 (14). The third of these proteins, fasciclin III, was initially described as possessing a novel structure (19). However, subsequent analysis indicated that fasciclin III is, in fact, composed of three Ig domains that are much more divergent than those found in fasciclin II or neuroglian (18). The other protein uncovered by our initial immunological screen, fasciclin I, has a novel sequence and structure that is unrelated thus far to any previously described proteins (16). *In vitro* aggregation assays show that all four of these proteins can function as homophilic cell adhesion molecules capable of mediating cell aggregation and cell sorting (18,19,28; A. Bieber and G. Grenningloh, *unpublished results*).

In this paper, we review what we have learned about the structure and function of these four molecules in *Drosophila*, focusing in particular on the three proteins that are members of the Ig superfamily: fasciclin II, neuroglian, and fasciclin III. We also consider the prospects for using genetic approaches in *Drosophila* to study the function of neural cell adhesion molecules during growth cone guidance.

EXPRESSION OF FASCICLIN GLYCOPROTEINS

Within each neuromere of the developing insect CNS there develops a scaffold of axon pathways, including a pair of bilaterally symmetric longitudinal axon tracts, a pair of commissural tracts (anterior and posterior) connecting the two sides, and a pair of nerve roots exiting the CNS on each side (the segmental and intersegmental nerve roots). Each of the major tracts is subdivided into an array of distinct axon bundles, or fascicles. In the insect CNS, the first growth cones extend largely toward and along the surfaces of special glial cells (and some neurons) and, in so doing, establish the initial axon pathways (29–33).

As development proceeds, however, the growth cones of the bulk of later-born neurons find themselves in an environment increasingly dominated by other axons. Most of these later growth cones do not contact the glia but rather only contact the growth cones and axons of other neurons. As the scaffold of axon pathways grows larger and more complex within the CNS, these later growth cones show remarkable selectivity in their ability to recognize and extend along specific axonal surfaces, a process called *selective fasciculation* (1,2). Experimental studies on the mechanisms of selective fasciculation in insects (3–8) led to the prediction (the labeled pathways hypothesis) that neighboring axon pathways are differentially labeled by surface recognition molecules, which allow growth cones to distinguish among them. This model led to the search for glycoproteins expressed on subsets of fasciculating embryonic axons.

Candidates for axonal recognition molecules were identified by generating monoclonal antibodies that recognize surface antigens expressed on subsets of axon fascicles in insect embryos. These antibodies were used to characterize and purify and generate further antibodies against four different membrane-associated glycoproteins, fasciclin I and fasciclin II in grasshopper (12) and fasciclin III and neuroglian in *Drosophila* (13,14). Antibodies against the fasciclin I and fasciclin II homologues in *Drosophila* were subsequently generated (fasciclin I: 16,34; fasciclin II: 18; G. Grenningloh and E. Rehm, *unpublished results*).

The expression of these four axonal glycoproteins is consistent with their potential involvement in neuronal recognition and growth cone guidance (Fig. 1); all four proteins are dynamically expressed on subsets of growth cones and fasciculating axons and, in some cases, on the glia they extend along during the period of axon outgrowth. The pattern of expression of each protein changes during development, and in some cases, the expression of a particular protein on an individual neuron is transient during a particular stage of axon outgrowth. Each of the proteins is also expressed outside of the developing nervous system in particular patches or stripes of cells (12–14,35; G. Grenningloh and E. Rehm, *unpublished results*; L. McAllister and K. Zinn, *unpublished results*).

The four axonal glycoproteins are expressed on different but overlapping subsets of axon fascicles, neuroglian being the most widely distributed of the four and fasciclin I, fasciclin II, and fasciclin III being expressed on more restricted subsets of axon fascicles (Fig. 1A). For example, one form of *Drosophila* neuroglian (the long form; see ref. 35) is expressed at high levels on all the axons in the intersegmental nerve root, whereas the other form of neuroglian (the short form) is expressed on the glia of this nerve root along which the axons extend. All the axons in the intersegmental nerve root also express fasciclin I, whereas only a subset of these axons express fasciclin III, and this subset stays tightly bundled within the larger nerve (J. Jacobs, *unpublished results*). In contrast, some axon pathways express only one of these four proteins, and others express none at all (Fig. 1A), leading to the suggestion that there are likely to be additional fasciclin-like proteins still awaiting future discovery.

Some features of the expression of these proteins have been remarkably conserved across many hundreds of millions of years of insect evolution. For example, fasciclin I is expressed on the surface of the aCC but not the pCC neuron in both grasshopper and *Drosophila* (12,16), and fasciclin II is expressed at high levels on the axons of the MP1/dMP2 fascicle in both grasshopper (17) and *Drosophila* (G.

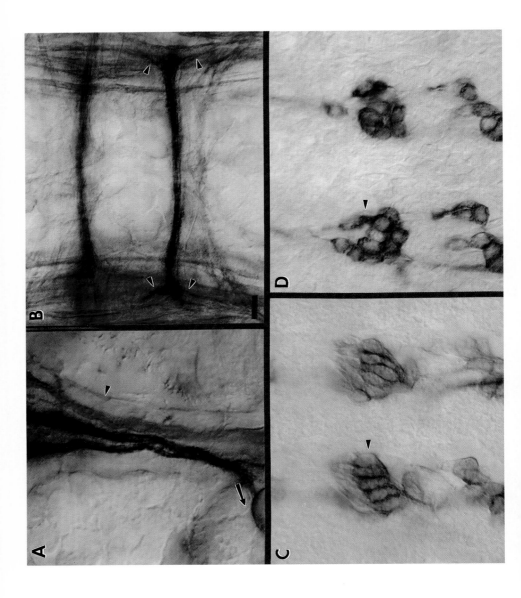

Grenningloh and E. Rehm, *unpublished results*). However, some features have changed over evolution; perhaps most striking is the evolutionary change in the forms and expression of neuroglian between grasshopper and *Drosophila* (G. Grenningloh and E. Rehm, *unpublished results*; 35), described in a later section of this chapter.

Most neurons in the insect CNS are interneurons, and many of these interneurons have long projection axons that cross the midline in one of the commissures and then extend rostrally or caudally in one of the longitudinal pathways. The growth cones of these neurons typically show no affinity for the homologous longitudinal pathway on their own (ipsilateral) side, but then dramatically change as they turn and follow the same pathway on the other (contralateral) side after crossing the midline. The simplest hypothesis to explain this change in growth cone behavior

---

FIG. 1. Expression of fasciclin I and fasciclin II in grasshopper and expression and function of neuroglian in *Drosophila*. **A,B:** Dynamic and regional expression of the fasciclin I (*black label*) and fasciclin II (*brown label*) axonal glycoproteins in the grasshopper embryo as revealed by two rounds of anti-HRP immunocytochemistry using monoclonal antibodies and nickel enhancement for the black color. **A:** View of the longitudinal connective on the left side between two segments in a 35% grasshopper embryo, showing the first three longitudinal axon fascicles. The *arrowhead* marks the inside-most vMP2 fascicle, which does not express either fasciclin I or fasciclin II; the middle, brown-stained fascicle is the MP1/dMP2 fascicle, which expresses fasciclin II; and the outside, black-stained fascicle is the U fascicle, which expresses fasciclin I. Note that two different bundles of black-stained axons come together to form the U fascicle and also that many of these axons turn laterally (*arrow*) to extend out the intersegmental nerve root. **B:** A single neuromere of a 40% grasshopper embryo showing the expression of fasciclin I (*black label*) on one large fascicle in the anterior commissure and one large fascicle in the posterior commissure. Many of the longitudinal bundles express fasciclin II (*brown label*). The *arrowheads* mark the choice point regions on each side where axons change from commissural pathways to longitudinal pathways and where some of these axons change from fasciclin I to fasciclin II. **C,D:** The lateral cluster of sensory neurons in the A2 and A3 segments of a (**C**) wild-type and (**D**) *neuroglian* mutant *Drosophila* embryo as stained with the (**C**) BP104 MAb and (**D**) 22C10 Mab, respectively, showing that the null mutation in the *neuroglian* gene leads to disruption of sensory neurons. **C:** Neuroglian is normally expressed at high levels at point of membrane apposition between sensory neurons in the *Drosophila* embryo PNS, as shown here by HRP immunocytochemistry with an antineuroglian monoclonal antibody (BP104; see ref. 35). This photo shows the normal pattern of lateral sensory neurons (including in particular the five chordotonal neurons (*arrows*)) in a wild-type embryo. **D:** A null lethal mutation in the *neuroglian* gene, *l(1)RA35,* leads to disruption of sensory neurons. At a gross level, the overall structure of the CNS and PNS, and in particular the peripheral nerve roots and CNS axon pathways, develops in a relatively normal way in *nrg* mutant embryos. However, although neurons do not become "unglued," there is a consistent although more subtle phenotype in *nrg* mutant embryos: The orientation and extent of contact among the normally neuroglian-positive sensory neurons in the PNS is abnormal. As shown here, the five lateral chordotonal neurons in each abdominal hemisegment normally line up in a tight row, with each cell body having extensive membrane apposition with the neurons on either side of it; the chordotonal neurons are normally flattened against one another and lie in the same focal plane. In contrast, in *nrg* mutant embryos, the five chordotonal neurons are more randomly organized in a looser group with less membrane apposition, resulting in a disorganization in the alignment of their dendrites. Similar types of phenotypes are seen with other clusters of sensory neurons as well. Scale bar: **A,** 10 μm; **B,** 20 μm; **C,D,** 6 μm.

after crossing the midline is to postulate that the expression of axonal recognition molecules is both dynamic and regional, dynamic in that the molecules controlling the selective affinity for a particular longitudinal pathway are not expressed until after the growth cone crosses the midline, and regional in that the molecules controlling the selective affinity for a particular commissural pathway are likely not to be expressed after the growth cone crosses the midline and turns onto a longitudinal pathway. This dynamic and regional expression of axonal glycoproteins was one of the predictions of a more detailed discussion of the labeled pathways hypothesis (see Fig. 11 in ref. 36).

In the initial characterization of fasciclin I, fasciclin II, and fasciclin III (12,13), one of the key observations was that these three proteins are regionally expressed in just this predicted fashion: For example, some interneurons express fasciclin I on their commissural processes and then express fasciclin II on their longitudinal axon segments after crossing the midline (Fig. 1B). The discovery of the regional expression of axonal glycoproteins is not isolated to insects; similar changes have been seen in the vertebrate spinal cord, as projection interneurons express TAG-1 on their commissural processes and then express L1 on their longitudinal processes after crossing the midline (37). The mechanisms that regulate this "switch" in the temporal and spatial expression of axonal glycoproteins is presently unknown.

FASCICLIN II, FASCICLIN III, AND NEUROGLIAN ARE MEMBERS OF THE IMMUNOGLOBULIN SUPERFAMILY

Monoclonal antibody affinity columns were used to purify microgram quantities of fasciclin I, fasciclin II, fasciclin III, and neuroglian proteins from kilogram quantities of lysates of grasshopper (fas I and fas II) and *Drosophila* (fas III and nrg) embryos (12–15). This purified protein was used to generate serum antibodies against all four proteins (for cDNA expression cloning) and for protein microsequencing. N-terminal sequence was obtained for fasciclin I and neuroglian, and chemically generated fragments were microsequenced for fasciclin II and neuroglian (14,15). Oligonucleotide probes based on protein microsequence data were used to isolate cDNA clones for fasciclin I and fasciclin II from a grasshopper embryo cDNA library (15). The serum antibody probes were used to screen a cDNA expression library to isolate cDNA clones for fasciclin III and neuroglian in *Drosophila* (13,14). The cloning of the genes encoding three of the proteins was confirmed by comparing the deduced amino acid sequence from the cDNA clones with the protein microsequence data; the cloning of the gene encoding the fourth protein (fasciclin III) was confirmed by genetic deficiency analysis.

Full length cDNA clones encoding fasciclin I and fasciclin II were initially isolated in grasshopper (15–17). The cDNAs for the *Drosophila* homologues of both were subsequently isolated, fasciclin I using low-stringency hybridization (16) and fasciclin II using the polymerase chain reaction (PCR) method (18; G. Grenningloh and E. Rehm, *unpublished results*). Fasciclin III and neuroglian, however, were initially characterized and cloned in *Drosophila* (13,14,19). PCR was also used to clone a cDNA for the neuroglian homologue in grasshopper (18; G. Grenningloh and E. Rehm, *unpublished results*).

Analysis of fasciclin I cDNAs from both grasshopper and *Drosophila* reveals a deduced structure consisting of four tandem 150-amino-acid domains with evolutionarily conserved ~40-amino-acid repeats at the ends of domains 2, 3, and 4 (16); these tandem domains are novel in sequence and structure and appear unrelated to

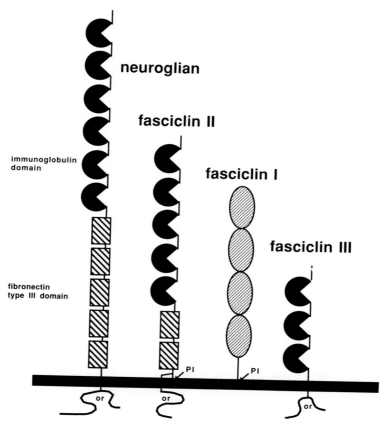

FIG. 2. Schematic domain structure of the neuroglian, fasciclin II, fasciclin I, and fasciclin III axonal glycoproteins. Three of the four axon glycoproteins are members of the immunoglobulin superfamily. Two of these proteins, neuroglian and fasciclin II, have multiple Ig domains followed by multiple fibronectin type III domains; the third, fasciclin III, has more divergent Ig domains (see text). Fasciclin I has a novel structure made up of four tandem domains (16) and is anchored to the membrane via a phosphatidylinositol (PI) lipid membrane anchor (34). Neuroglian (35) and fasciclin III (P. Snow and Z. Traquina, *unpublished results*) have alternative cytoplasmic domains; fasciclin II also comes in different forms including one with a putative PI membrane anchor (G. Grenningloh and E. Rehm, *unpublished results*) and as a transmembrane protein with a cytoplasmic domain (17).

anything else in the data bank (16). Biochemical analysis of the fasciclin I glycoprotein indicates that it is tightly associated with the lipid bilayer by a phosphatidylinositol (Pl) lipid moiety (34).

In contrast to the novel structure of fasciclin I, cDNA sequence analysis reveals that the other three proteins (fasciclin II, neuroglian, and fasciclin III) are members of the Ig superfamily (Fig. 2). What defines proteins as members of the Ig superfamily is a common domain structure (of ~100 amino acids), typically (but not always) with two cysteines in each domain (separated by ~50 amino acids), with many other conserved amino acids (particularly around the cysteine residues) and with a conserved deduced three-dimensional structure, called the *immunoglobulin fold* (e.g., refs. 38,39). Ig domains typically fold to form a globular structure containing two β sheets, each consisting of three to four antiparallel β strands of 5 to 10 amino acids each. Intrachain disulfide bonding between the conserved cysteine residues stabilizes the structure. A common characteristic of Ig-related molecules is that most of them function in some form of adhesion or recognition at the cell surface. Three types of Ig domains have been proposed: V, C1, and C2 type domains (39).

Most of the Ig domains of the neural cell adhesion molecules (including NCAM, L1, MAG, F11/contactin, TAG-1, fasciclin II, neuroglian, and fasciclin III) are of the C2 type (38). In addition to these tandem Ig domains, most of these neural cell adhesion molecules (all listed above except MAG and fasciclin III) have another type of tandem conserved repeat near to their transmembrane domains; these repeats are called *fibronectin* (Fn) *type III domains* (Fig. 2) based on their homology to a repeat motif first found in the extracellular matrix adhesion molecule fibronectin (40). Fasciclin II has five Ig C2-type domains followed by two Fn domains; neuroglian has six Ig C2-type domains followed by five Fn domains (14,17). As described in a later section, fasciclin III has three divergent Ig domains and no Fn domains (18).

FASCICLIN II IS RELATED TO NCAM

In 1988 came the discovery of the first two members of the Ig superfamily outside of the chordates: amalgam in *Drosophila* (41) and fasciclin II in grasshopper (17). When fasciclin II was first cloned in grasshopper, its extracellular portion, consisting of five Ig C2-type domains followed by two Fn domains, was shown to have the

→

FIG. 3. Summary of comparisons of *Drosophila* and grasshopper fasciclin II and mouse NCAM and of *Drosophila* and grasshopper neuroglian and mouse L1. *Numbers* shown are percent amino acid identity in each domain compared between the two species immediately above and below the number (Ig domains are measured here as including 20 amino acids outside the two characteristic cysteine residues; fibronectin type III domains are measured as including 20 amino acids outside the characteristic tryptophan and tyrosine residues). Because these molecules have alternative cytoplasmic domains and in some cases alternative membrane linkages, all that is shown here are the extracellular regions of each protein.

membrane attachment (Fig. 2). In none of the three cases can we detect alternative splicing in the extracellular domain. [Fasciclin I does appear to have alternative splicing in its extracellular domain (L. McAllister, K. Zinn, E. Rehm, and C. Goodman, *unpublished results*), a topic outside the scope of this review.] Most vertebrate genes encoding Ig superfamily molecules have introns between each Ig domain, with some such as NCAM having additional introns in the middle of each Ig domain. In contrast, fasciclin II (G. Grenningloh and E. Rehm, *unpublished results*) and neuroglian (A. Bieber, M. Hortsch, and Z. Traquina, *unpublished results*) do not have introns between their Ig domains and, for that matter, have very few introns in the region coding their extracellular domains. [Amalgam, another Ig superfamily molecule in *Drosophila*, also has no introns between its Ig domains (41).]

The initial grasshopper fasciclin II cDNA that was sequenced encodes a protein with a transmembrane domain of 25 amino acids and a ctyoplasmic domain of 108 amino acids (17). A more detailed characterization of the fasciclin II gene in *Drosophila* has revealed several different mRNAs on Northern blots, the most abundant of which in the embryo encodes a deduced protein that, according to cDNA sequence analysis, does not have a transmembrane domain but rather appears to have a Pl lipid membrane anchor (G. Grenningloh and E. Rehm, *unpublished results*). Thus it is likely that fasciclin II comes in at least two different forms, one of which is Pl-linked, and the other of which has a transmembrane domain. The existence of multiple forms of a neural cell adhesion molecule and in particular different forms of membrane attachment is reminiscent of NCAM (20,45–51), the molecule with which fasciclin II shares a common ancestor.

The *neuroglian* gene in *Drosophila* generates at least two different protein products by tissue-specific alternative splicing (35). The two protein forms differ in their cytoplasmic domains; thus far, there is no evidence for a Pl-linked form of neuroglian, just as there is no evidence for a Pl-linked form of vertebrate L1, its closest relative. Although identical in their extracellular domains, after the transmembrane domain, the two neuroglian protein forms share only the first 68 amino acids of their cytoplasmic domains. The short, more abundant form of the protein continues for another 17 amino acids. However, in contrast to the short form, the long form of the protein extends for another 62 amino acids. The entire cytoplasmic domain of the long form of the neuroglian protein form encompasses 148 amino acid residues compared with 85 amino acids in the cytoplasmic domain of the short form. The long form is restricted to the surface of neurons in the CNS and neurons and some support cells in the PNS; in contrast, the short form is expressed on a wide range of other cells and tissues. Thus, whereas the mouse *L1* gene appears to encode only one protein, which functions largely as a neural cell adhesion molecule, its closest *Drosophila* relative, the *neuroglian* gene, encodes at least two protein forms, which may play two different roles, one as a neural cell adhesion molecule and the other as a more general cell adhesion molecule involved in tissue and imaginal disc morphogenesis.

Some striking differences appear to have evolved in the alternative splicing of the *neuroglian* gene during the 300 million years of evolution that separate the more advanced insect, *Drosophila*, from the more primitive one, grasshopper. Whereas the *Drosophila neuroglian* gene generates two different forms of the protein with different cytoplasmic domains (which are easily detectable on Western blots), the grasshopper gene appears to generate only one protein form as detected on Western blots (G. Grenningloh and E. Rehm, *unpublished results*). This single form in grasshopper is expressed throughout many tissues of the embryo, much as is the short form of the *Drosophila* protein. Thus, although *Drosophila* does have a nervous system–specific, alternatively spliced form of neuroglian, the more primitive grasshopper apparently does not. This conclusion is supported by the observation that the two alternatively spliced cytoplasmic domains in *Drosophila* may have recently evolved by an exon duplication. The short-form specific exon encodes for another 17 amino acids, eleven of which are conserved in the protein sequence encoded by the long-form specific exon (35).

Just as with fasciclin II and neuroglian, so too *Drosophila* fasciclin III is alternatively spliced to generate at least two different protein forms with different cytoplasmic domains, each of which has a different spatial and temporal pattern of expression (P. Snow, T. Elkins, and Z. Traquina, *unpublished results*).

ALL FOUR PROTEINS CAN FUNCTION AS HOMOPHILIC CELL ADHESION MOLECULES

Fasciclin II is related to NCAM, a homophilic neural cell adhesion molecule, and neuroglian is related to L1, another homophilic neural cell adhesion molecule. Fasciclin III is also a member of the Ig superfamily. Fasciclin I has a novel structure. Do any of these four *Drosophila* axonal glycoproteins function as neural cell adhesion molecules, as some of their structures predict? To answer this question, we have used DNA transfection methods to test if these proteins can confer cell aggregation *in vitro* in the nonadhesive *Drosophila* S2 cells, an experimental paradigm modeled after the studies on vertebrate cadherins begun by Takeichi and colleagues (52). The first aggregation experiments using transfected *Drosophila* cDNAs and the *Drosophila* S2 cell line showed that fasciclin III can function as a homophilic cell adhesion molecule (19). In subsequent studies, we have shown that fasciclin I (28), neuroglian (18), and fasciclin II (18) can each function as a homophilic cell adhesion molecule *in vitro*. We have also shown that when the fasciclin I–transfected S2 cells are heterogeneously mixed with the fasciclin III-transfected S2 cells (28), the fasciclin I–transfected S2 cells with the neuroglian-transfected S2 cells (A. Bieber, *unpublished results*), or the fasciclin III–transfected cells with the neuroglian-transfected S2 cells (A. Bieber, *unpublished results*), they undergo cell-type-specific sorting into homogeneous aggregates. These *in vitro* results lead to the suggestion that these neural cell adhesion molecules (the three Ig superfamily proteins, fasciclin II, neuroglian, and fasciclin III, and the novel protein, fasciclin I) might play a similar role in cell sorting during development *in vivo*, particularly during axonal guidance in which they are expressed on specific growth cones and the axon pathways they follow.

MUTATIONS HAVE BEEN IDENTIFIED IN ALL FOUR GENES

The *Drosophila* genes encoding all four neural cell adhesion molecules have been mapped to the polytene chromosomes and are located as follows: Neuroglian and fasciclin II are on the X chromosome, neuroglian at band 7F and fasciclin II at band 4B; fasciclin III is on the left arm of the second chromosome at band 36E, and fasciclin I is on the right arm of the third chromosome at 89D. We have identified and/or generated mutations in all four neural cell adhesion molecules, including a viable, null mutation in the *fasciclin I* gene (which leads to uncoordinated motor behavior; 53); a lethal, null mutation in the *neuroglian* gene (14); a lethal, null mutation in the *fasciclin II* gene (G. Grenningloh, *unpublished results*); and a viable, null mutation in the *fasciclin III* gene (M. Elkins et al., *unpublished results*). It is interesting to note that null mutations in two of the four neural cell adhesion molecules are viable. To our knowledge, the mutations in the *fasciclin II, fasciclin III*, and *neuroglian* genes are first known null mutations in Ig superfamily cell adhesion molecules. Of the mutations in the three Ig superfamily neural cell adhesion molecules, the one that has been analyzed in greatest detail thus far is in *neuroglian*.

A lethal mutation *l(1)RA35* (ref. 54), leads to mutant embryos that completely lack neuroglian expression; this is a null mutation in the *neuroglian* (*nrg*) gene. We have used a variety of nervous system markers for our initial analysis of the phenotype of *nrg* mutant embryos. The most striking observation is that, at a gross level, the overall structure of the CNS and PNS, and in particular the peripheral nerve roots and CNS axon pathways, develops in a relatively normal way. Clearly, normally neuroglian-positive axon pathways do not become "unglued" when this *Drosophila* L1 homologue is genetically deleted, suggesting some functional overlap in overall axonal and glial adhesion systems.

However, although neurons do not become "unglued," there is a consistent although more subtle phenotype in *nrg* mutant embryos: The orientation and extent of contact among the normally neuroglian-positive sensory neurons in the PNS is abnormal (Fig. 1C,D). For example, the five lateral chordotonal neurons in each abdominal hemisegment normally line up in a tight row with each cell body having extensive membrane apposition with the neurons on either side of it; the chordotonal neurons are normally flattened against one another and lie in the same focal plane. In contrast, in *nrg* mutant embryos, the five chordotonal neurons are more randomly organized in a looser group with less membrane apposition, resulting in a disorganization in the alignment of their dendrites. Similar types of phenotypes are seen with other clusters of sensory neurons as well.

FUTURE PROSPECTS

Studies in vertebrates, in which antibodies were used to perturb neurite outgrowth and axon fasciculation *in vitro*, suggest that the systems that mediate neural cell adhesion are redundant in that perturbation of more than one system is required before major functional disruptions occur (55–59). Presumably, in the developing organism, these systems are not simply redundant but rather each of the overlapping systems has a subtly different function. If such overlap of adhesion systems is indeed at play in *Drosophila* as it appears to be in vertebrates, multiple mutations that simultaneously remove more than one cell adhesion system may be necessary to produce gross disruptions of nervous system development. In this light, it is perhaps not so surprising that the *nrg* mutant does not lead to a grossly abnormal CNS in which axon pathways and peripheral nerve roots become "unglued" and highly disorganized. Rather, the *nrg* mutant does lead to a more subtle phenotype in the disruption of the precise patterning of sensory neurons, which makes us wonder if there might also be subtle abnormalities in the guidance and patterning of axons in the CNS that are not as easy to detect.

It will be of interest in the future to look for more subtle phenotypes in the behavior of individual growth cones, axons, and arborizations in flies carrying null mutations in either the *nrg, fas I, fas II*, or *fas III* genes. In the case of *fas I* (53), the null mutation leads to a behavioral defect (uncoordinated motor behavior) that suggests changes in CNS wiring. Just what changes are associated with this behavioral defect awaits future study, as does a more detailed analysis of the growth of individual neurons in the *fas II, fas III,* and *nrg* mutants. For example, in *fas II* mutant Drosophila embryos, the CNS displays no gross phenotype, but the MP1 fascicle fails to develop (G. Grenningloh and E. Rehm, *unpublished results*). The MP1, dMP2, and vMP2 growth cones fail to recognize one another or other axons that normally join the MP1 pathway. During their normal period of axon outgrowth, these growth cones stall and do not join any other neighboring pathway.

Another genetic approach to this problem is to look for more gross phenotypes in embryos carrying mutations in more than one gene, for example, in two or more neural cell adhesion molecules, or in a neural cell adhesion molecule and a signal transduction molecule. To this end, we previously studied the development of the axon commissures and the extension of individual growth cones in embryos doubly mutant for *fas I*, which on its own does not lead to a gross defect in CNS morphogenesis, and in the *Drosophila abelson* (*abl*) protooncogene homologue (which encodes a cytoplasmic tyrosine kinase that is expressed during embryogenesis primarily in developing CNS axons; 60), which on its own also does not lead to gross defects in CNS morphogenesis (53). However, embryos doubly mutant for *fas I* and *abl* display major defects in CNS axon pathways, particularly in the commissural tracts where the expression of these two proteins normally overlaps. The double

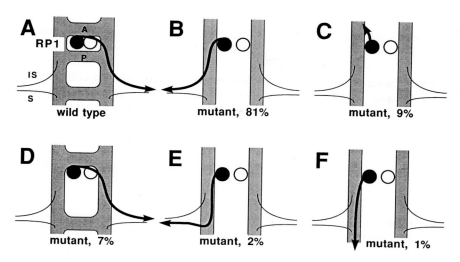

FIG. 5. The range of pathfinding defects by the RP1 growth cone in embryos doubly mutant for the *fasciclin I* and *abelson* genes. **A:** The RP1 axon in wild-type embryos. The RP1 growth cone extends across the midline as it pioneers one of the first axon fascicles in the anterior commissure. After crossing the anterior edge of the contralateral RP1 cell body, it then turns posteriorly and then laterally to exit the CNS in the contralateral intersegmental nerve root. **B–F:** The RP1 axons in abl^2 fas I^{TE} double mutant embryos (*fasciclin I* encodes a neural cell adhesion molecule, and *abl* encodes a cytoplasmic tyrosine kinase; see ref. 53). **B:** In 81% of hemisegments examined ($n = 100$), the RP1 axon did not extend across the midline, but rather extended out the intersegmental nerve on its own side. **C:** In 9% of the hemisegments, the RP1 axon stalled in an abnormal location a short distance from the cell body. **D:** In 7% of the hemisegments, the RP1 axon behaved similar to wild type. **E:** In 2% of the hemisegments, the RP1 axon failed to cross the midline and instead turned posteriorly and then laterally out the segmental nerve (the wrong pathway) in the next posterior segment. **F:** In 1% of the hemisegments, the RP1 failed to cross the midline and instead turned posterior and extended beyond the next posterior segment. IS, intersegmental nerve; S, segmental nerve; A, anterior commissure; P, posterior commissure; gray area, major axon tracts.

mutant shows a clear defect in growth cone guidance; for example, the RP1 growth cone (normally *fas I*-positive) does not follow its normal path across the commissure (Fig. 5). These results suggest the role of two functionally parallel pathways for commissural axon guidance, with one of them including a tyrosine kinase (*abl*) and the other a neural cell adhesion molecule (*fasciclin I*). We interpret these results to suggest that mutations in either pathway alone do not lead to a major disruption in growth cone guidance, whereas mutations in two different pathways do disrupt the guidance of commissural growth cones.

The power of genetics is likely to be a valuable tool in studies on the molecular mechanisms underlying growth cone guidance. The ability to identify mutations in the genes encoding neural cell adhesion molecules, to put these mutations in combination with other mutations, and to conduct second site enhancer or suppressor screens (on the background of an existing mutation) to look for interacting genes and parallel pathways should lead to a deeper understanding of the molecules and molecular pathways involved in the guidance of neuronal growth cones. Given the common ancestry and similar structure and function of arthropod and chordate neural cell adhesion molecules (e.g., fasciclin II and NCAM; neuroglian and L1), there is ample reason to believe that the molecular mechanisms of growth cone guidance will be equally well-conserved between arthropods and chordates.

ACKNOWLEDGMENTS

Many people who have been in the Goodman lab made contributions to the work described in this review, and thus we thank Michael Bastiani, the late Tom Elkins, Allan Harrelson, Michael Hortsch, J. Roger Jacobs, Linda McAllister, Nipam Patel, E. Jay Rehm, Peter Snow, Jim Schilling, Zaida Traquina, and Kai Zinn. We thank Andrew Smith and Alan Williams for sharing with us their unpublished analysis of the structure of fasciclin III and Nipam Patel for allowing us to use his photographs in panels A–C of Fig. 1. This work was supported by postdoctoral fellowships from the Deutsche Forschungsgemeinschaft to G.G. and NIH to A.B. and by grant HD 21294 to C.S.G., who is an investigator with the Howard Hughes Medical Institute.

REFERENCES

1. Raper JA, Bastiani MJ, Goodman CS. Pathfinding by neuronal growth cones in grasshopper embryos: I. Divergent choices made by the growth cones of sibling neurons. *J Neurosci* 1983;3:20–30.
2. Raper JA, Bastiani MJ, Goodman CS. Pathfinding by neuronal growth cones in grasshopper embryos: II. Selective fasciculation onto specific axonal pathways. *J Neurosci* 1983;3:31–41.
3. Raper JA, Bastiani MJ, Goodman CS. Guidance of neuronal growth cones: selective fasciculation in the grasshopper embryo. *Cold Spring Harbor Symp Quant Biol* 1983;48:587–598.
4. Bastiani MJ, Raper JA, Goodman CS. Pathfinding by neuronal growth cones in grasshopper embryos. III. Selective affinity of the G growth cone for the P cells within the A/P fascicle. *J Neurosci* 1984;4:2311–2328.
5. Raper JA, Bastiani MJ, Goodman CS. Pathfinding by neuronal growth cones in grasshopper embryos. IV. The effects of ablating the A and P axons upon the behavior of the G growth cone. *J Neurosci* 1984;4:2329–2345.
6. Bastiani MJ, du Lac S, Goodman CS. Guidance of neuronal growth cones in the grasshopper embryo. I. Recognition of a specific axonal pathway by the pCC neuron. *J Neurosci* 1986;6:3518–3531.
7. du Lac S, Bastiani MJ, Goodman CS. Guidance of neuronal growth cones in the grasshopper embryo. II. Recognition of a specific axonal pathway by the aCC neuron. *J Neurosci* 1986;6:3532–3541.
8. Doe CQ, Bastiani MJ, Goodman CS. Guidance of neuronal growth cones in the grasshopper embryo. IV. Temporal delay experiments. *J Neurosci* 1986;6:3552–3563.

THE SEARCH FOR THE TARGET

Much work has been done in the past decade examining the behavior of growth cones in the context of the development of neuronal branching patterns and connectivity in the embryonic leech. One conclusion that may be drawn from the results of this work is that initial axon extension by leech neurons displays features that differ according to cell type as well as species. For example, motor neurons appear to grow exuberantly in many directions and then retract processes that do not reach the target, whereas sensory neurons grow more parsimoniously and directly toward the appropriate peripheral fields. In considering these results, we discuss the possible interactions and responses of growth cones in their search for peripheral targets.

Motor Neuron Strategies

In the hirudinid leech *Hirudo medicinalis*, certain motor neurons extend many axons initially and then eliminate those that do not find the peripheral target. Perhaps the best example of such a neuron is the RPE, found as a bilateral pair in SG6. The RPEs innervate the penile sheath and cause the male organ to evert, presumably during copulation (7). In adult *Hirudo*, each RPE has two axons that project out of the ganglion contralaterally and reach the target; one exits laterally through the anterior root of SG6, and the other exits SG6 anteriorly and travels along the connective to SG5, where it also exits through the anterior root (Fig. 2A). During embryogenesis, however, RPEs extend axons profusely, in many directions, including away from the target (Fig. 2B) (10). Every available path, whether within the CNS or in the periphery, appears acceptable to the RPE growth cones, and no evidence of a tropic signal from the target can be discerned. A few days after some growth cones contact the target, all others become thin, lose their filopodia, and are eventually eliminated. By comparison, those growth cones that do establish contact with the target begin to branch profusely, forming secondary and tertiary processes with much simpler growing tips than those of the parent axons (see chapters by Mason and Godement and by Kalil and Norris).

If the male genitalia are ablated on the 10th day of embryogenesis (E10— embryogenesis of *Hirudo* takes about 30 days at 23°C), the extra processes are instead retained and grow exuberantly (Fig. 2C), as though they were endlessly searching for the missing organ (10). This finding suggests that, in the normal animal, the cell initially is in a "general search" mode, until some of its processes find the correct target. At this time, the neuron responds globally, in that axons contacting the target are stabilized while all others are signaled to retract.

If the male organ is transplanted to another segment at E10, the RPE neuron can often find it, even using axons that would not normally be retained in the adult (Fig. 2D). In fact, sometimes RPE processes take extremely aberrant paths to reach and make functional synapses with the ectopic organ (10). Although it has not been

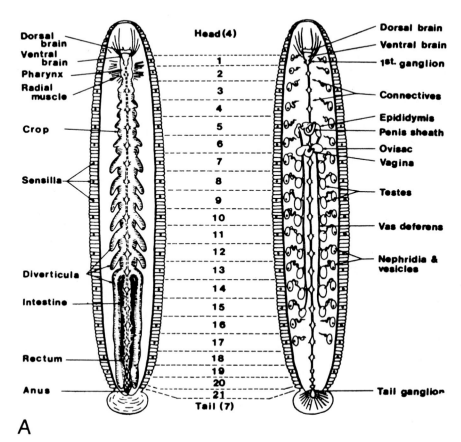

A

FIG. 1. Diagrams of a leech and a segmental ganglion. In both panels, anterior is up and the dorsal aspect is toward the viewer. **A:** Schematic drawings of an opened leech, showing the internal organs and the ventral nerve cord. The diagram on the *left* shows the digestive system and CNS, and the one on the *right* indicates the nephridia, sex organs, and CNS. (From ref. 4, with permission.) **B:** Diagram of a segmental ganglion in an embryo, showing a representative motor neuron with several axons bearing growth cones at their tips. The axons extend into the anterior and posterior connectives (*longitudinal projection*) and out to the periphery through the nerve roots (*lateral projections*). As noted, the growth cones on the connectives are presumed to recognize guidance cues and neural targets, and those in the periphery presumably recognize guidance cues and nonneural targets (cf. Fig. 3A).

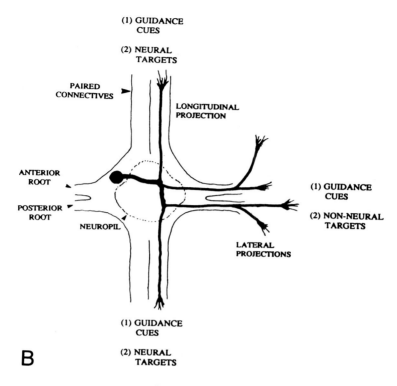

FIG. 1. *Continued*

tested definitively in either the normal or the experimentally modified cases, the neuron does not seem to form synapses with any other tissue during its search. Growth cones of this neuron are therefore able to navigate new paths, identify unambiguously their displaced target, and then signal the rest of the cell to abandon the search and eliminate other projections.

The Rz cells in SG5 and SG6 respond to growth cone contact with the genitalia in a similar global fashion: They withdraw their projections in the connectives while maintaining the lateral ones through the nerve roots (11,12). Indeed, cutting the roots of these ganglia early in development can lead to the retention of the normally retracted longitudinal projections, which then innervate the target through an adjacent ganglion (W. Gao and E. Macagno, *unpublished data*). Furthermore, the interaction of their growth cones with the genitalia modifies the fate of Rz5 and Rz6 in several ways (e.g., with respect to their synaptic inputs) (13). In contrast, the Rz cells in other segments normally retain their longitudinal projections in the adult, which implies that whatever the targets in those segments are, they do not communicate a signal leading to process withdrawal. Thus, the response of the cell depends

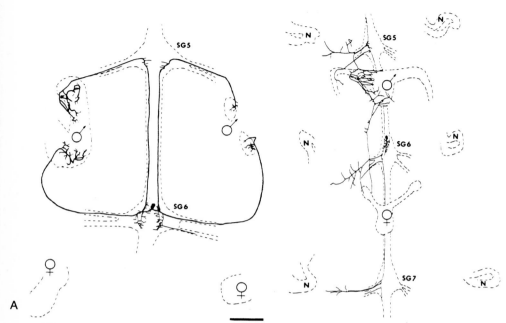

FIG. 2. Camera lucida drawings of rostral penile evertor (RPE) motor neurons in whole mounts, from normal and operated animals. The neurons were filled with horseradish peroxidase. The segmental ganglia (SG) are numbered according to body segment; male and female genitalia are labeled with symbols. Anterior is up and dorsal is toward the viewer. Nephridia (N) are outlined with *dashed lines*. In **A, C,** and **D** the genitalia were divided into two pieces during dissection and moved away from the midline to aid visualization of the CNS. Bar, 200 μm. **A:** RPEs from a 50-day-old juvenile. The two extraganglionic projections that persist in adult animals can be seen to innervate the male genitalia exclusively. The cell on the left retains a much thinner projection in the right posterior nerve root, but it does not reach the male genitalia. Many of the secondary branches in the neuropil and the terminals at the target have not been drawn. **B:** Right RPE from a 15-day-old animal. Many extraganglionic projections that are eliminated later can be seen at this stage exiting from SG5 to SG7 in all the available contralateral pathways. Although the peripheral ramifications are most profuse on the male genitalia, several other tissues also receive branches of the cell.

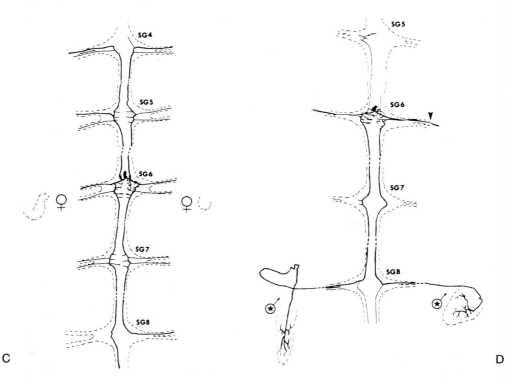

C

D

C: RPEs in a 50-day-old animal that had the male genitalia removed at 10 days of development. Both cells have longitudinal projections that reach SG4 and SG8 and have branches that exit the CNS from each ganglion. To compress the length of the nerve cord the interganglionic connectives have been shortened. **D:** Drawing of RPEs in a 60-day-old animal with the transplanted male genitalia located just posterior to SG8. The host's male genitalia were ablated at the time (E10) when the transplant was made. Both cells have thick axons in the posterior connectives of SG6 that travel to and exit from SG8 and branch extensively at the ectopic target. Note that these are projections that are normally eliminated. Other remaining projections have significantly smaller diameters and do not innervate the male genitalia. *Arrowhead* indicates the origin (in the anterior root of SG6) of one of the axons that travel in the posterior connective. (Modified from ref. 10, with permission.)

not only on establishing contact with the target, but also on the nature of the target itself.

In *Hirudo*, motor neurons such as the HAs (14), APs (15), and AEs (15,16) also retract extra processes after contacting their targets and thus also operate with an initial target-search mode whereby many growth cones are generated that can extend into all permissible paths. For example, until about E15, the APs extend four major axons: Two go out the contralateral nerve roots and grow into the body wall to their peripheral targets, and two extend into the anterior and posterior longitudinal connectives, toward but without reaching the adjacent ganglia (Fig. 3A). However, sometime around E14-E15, the longitudinal processes begin to retract and eventually disappear (15), so that only the contralateral root projections remain in the adult (Fig. 3B).

The results of an experimental manipulation suggest that the peripheral target is

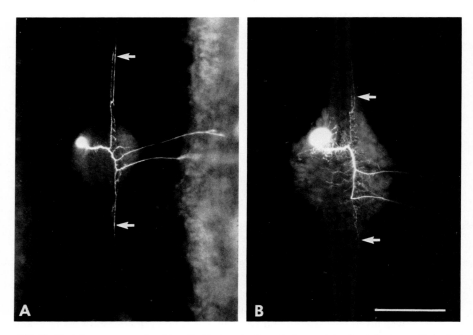

FIG. 3. Certain neurons extend longitudinal projections in the early embryo that are eliminated later. Photomicrographs of embryonic anterior pagoda (AP) motor neurons in midbody segmental ganglia shown in whole mounts. The cells are filled with Lucifer yellow by iontophoresis. Anterior is up, dorsal is toward the viewer. *Bar*, 100 μm. **A:** AP neuron from an E10 embryo. Longitudinal projections are present at this stage (*arrows*), along with the lateral ones exiting through the nerve roots contralateral to the soma. Note that the projections in the connectives do not reach the adjacent ganglia. **B:** AP neuron from an E25 embryo. Longitudinal projections have almost entirely disappeared by this time, although some fine processes can still be seen entering the connectives (*arrows*). A much more profuse secondary arborization in the ganglionic neuropil is apparent. (Modified from ref. 15, with permission.)

probably also involved in process retraction for the AP neuron. When the contra-lateral nerve roots were cut, thereby removing the lateral pathways to the periphery, the longitudinal projections were not retracted. They instead grew into the next ganglia and exited to the periphery there, thus innervating the target by abnormal paths (17). In contrast to the RPEs or Rz cells, however, process retraction by the APs (and AEs and HAs as well) depends not only on interactions with the target but, in addition, on interactions between growth cones of segmental homologues, a sub-ject that will be discussed in the next section.

Unlike those in *Hirudo*, motor neurons in *Haementaria ghilianii*, a species be-longing to a different leech family, do not send an excessive number of growth cones in many directions. The AE (18) and L (19) motor neurons in this species extend axons only laterally toward their peripheral target muscles. Apparently, they are capable of growing longitudinal projections, for when the L motor neuron is prevented from exiting the ganglion contralaterally, it exits ipsilaterally and along the anterior and posterior connectives (19). We are left with the conclusion that during normal development, the motor neurons in these two families of leeches use two different growth strategies: selective, directed growth in glossiphoniids and excessive, multidirectional growth in the hirudinids.

Central Mechanosensory Neurons

The genesis of extraganglionic projections is somewhat different for these neu-rons than for motor neurons, and furthermore, there does not seem to be a species difference as noted above. During development, central mechanosensory neurons extend only those peripheral projections that they will have in the adult, with only one exception. Kuwada and Kramer (18,20,21) examined the development of the pressure (P) and touch (T) sensory neurons in the glossiphoniid leech *Haementaria ghilianii*. They found that growth cones are large and have many filopodia extend-ing from the early primary peripheral axons exiting laterally from the ganglion, but that the later, secondary growth cones are thin, with few or no filopodia (18). Moreover, in most cases, the primary axons grow to the area of skin (dorsal, lateral, or ventral) that they eventually innervate before they begin to arborize significantly; no excessive branching with subsequent pruning was observed. Similar directed growth was subsequently reported for T cells in *Hirudo* (22) (see Fig. 4). Only one exception was noted by Kuwada and Kramer (18,21): The P neuron that innervates the dorsal body wall, which is also one of the earliest cells to grow out of the CNS to the periphery, initially extends several elaborate peripheral growth cones. One of these then grows rapidly and directly to its target area while all others are elimi-nated. Kuwada (21) suggested that this cell, as a pioneer neuron, might require multiple growth cones to ensure filopodial contact with appropriate peripheral guid-ance cues, a reasonable possibility that warrants further experimental testing.

In sum, the growth cones of motor neurons and mechanosensory neurons in *Hirudo* appear to differ from each other in one important aspect: The former trans-

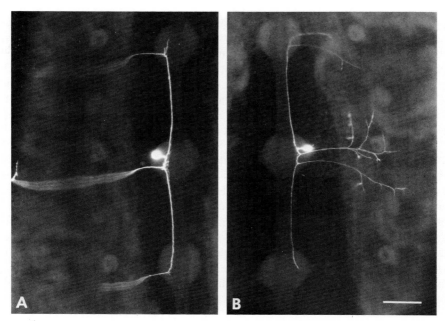

FIG. 4. Photomicrographs of two touch (T) mechanosensory neurons filled with Lucifer yellow in 10-day embryos in whole mounts. **A:** T cell innervating dorsal skin (T_D); **B:** T cell innervating ventral skin (T_V). The dorsal aspect of the animals is toward the viewer; anterior is up. Three segmental ganglia can be seen in these low-power micrographs, as well as peripheral tissues on the sides innervated by the T cells. Each cell sends lateral projections directly to the periphery from the middle ganglion and longitudinal projections to the two adjacent ganglia. Peripheral projections can be seen to exit from three of these four ganglia. Anterior projections grow slightly ahead of those traveling to the posterior ganglion, as can be seen by comparing the extent of peripheral branching in the adjacent ganglia; projections from the posterior ganglion in **B** would be found in slightly older embryos. In **A,** the peripheral projections of the T_D cell can be seen to travel unbranched to the left edge of the micrograph, which is where the dorsal midline is located. In **B,** the T_V cell can be seen to branch profusely in the ventral region adjacent to the nerve cord. Bar, 100 μm. (Modified from ref. 22, with permission.)

mit a message when they contact the target that causes global changes in the cell, leading to excess process retraction, whereas the latter do not provide such a signal. The advantages of either of these strategies are presently unknown. However, the two types of neurons have one characteristic in common: Both will continue to search for their target until told to stop. This raises the question of what tells them to stop and why. Although one answer to this question might be that the target tells them to stop to make a synapse, this is not the whole story. As we shall discuss below, another stop signal comes from other axons, either those of homologous cells or those of another branch of the same cell. These stop signals play a role in how territory is divided between competing axons.

leted early in development (15). Moreover, leeches grow thoughout their lives, and so does the area of the body wall that is innervated by these neurons. We may presume that neuronal arbors increase in extent accordingly. The answer to this question may lie in the *manner* in which target area is shared by the homologues, which is unknown for the motor neurons we are considering in this review.

Although the peripheral fields of homologues overlap extensively in the antero-posterior direction, little or no overlap is seen across the ventral or dorsal midlines of the animal. Whether this is because growth cones extending circumferentially are different from those extending longitudinally in the periphery or because the left–right boundaries pose special obstacles to growth is not known. An earlier report bearing in part on this question (29) showed that when a T-cell innervating dorsal skin was killed by pronase injection in an adult, the contralateral homologue could expand its field across the dorsal midline. One interpretation of this result is that the two dorsal T cells inhibit each other's growth across the midline, but other explanations are possible. This experiment has not been done in early embryo-genesis, when an examination of the behavior of growth cones would be feasible.

The fact that the RPE neurons do partition their target does suggest, however, that there is an interaction between these homologues at the midline. Early in embryogenesis, the RPEs extend processes in many directions, as described in the previous section. The two axons that find the target and are therefore maintained into adulthood enter the contralateral periphery by projecting out the anterior nerve roots of SG5 and SG6 (Fig. 2A). By E15, a key feature of the adult morphology is already being established: The branches from one RPE stay on only one side of the organ and do not invade the territory of the other RPE (Fig. 2B). The mechanism underlying this phenomenon is unknown. It is possible that the two halves of the organ are labeled with different markers and that the growth cones of each RPE have an affinity for only one of them. This mechanism is unlikely, however, given that when one RPE is deleted at E10, the other expands over the entire surface of the organ by E15 (30). Alternative explanations are that there is a trophic substance on the target in limited supply that prevents the occupation of space by two different neurons or that the growth cones of the RPEs inhibit each other directly. At this point, we cannot distinguish between the two mechanisms, but evidence from other leech neurons would favor the latter.

Self-Inhibition of Growth

The pattern of peripheral innervation of the mechanosensory cells, which have axons projecting from several adjacent ganglia, shows a remarkable feature: The subfields innervated by each axon show little or no overlap among fields (26,31), in sharp contrast to the extensive overlap found among fields innervated by homologues. In their study of the formation of the receptive fields of mechanosensory cells in *Haementaria*, Kramer and Kuwada (20) found that the developing peripheral branches of a cell rarely crossed nor did they appear to come into contact with one another, although their filopodia did seem to contact each other as well as other branches. It is likely, therefore, that some form of contact inhibition of growth cones also takes place between branches of the same cell.

That the observed patterns are a result of interactions among processes of the same cell is also supported by experiments in which the order of growth of the projections was modified (32). When the outgrowth of one of the peripheral axons of an embryonic P cell was prevented or delayed by crushing one nerve root, the target territory of the absent or delayed branch was innervated by another axon of the same neuron, shifting the boundaries between isoneuronal target fields (32). Therefore, it would appear that the presence of a sibling neurite may be sufficient to exclude others from expanding into the occupied space.

The mechanism responsible for this "self-avoidance" (32) is not known. Whether the mechanism involves junctions such as those present in the case of growth inhibition by homologues discussed above has not been examined, and it is possible that the filopodia form electrical junctions when they contact each other. Kramer and Stent (32) proposed a mechanism for self-recognition and self-avoidance based on the spontaneous, idiosyncratic electrical activity of each cell. The temporal coherence of the spontaneous activity pattern throughout the cell's arborization could ensure that a growing axonal process recognizes other processes as being self or nonself. Electrical or chemical junctions could then be the conveyors of these electrical signals between branches.

FUTURE DIRECTIONS

Although much of the work discussed in this book is concerned with understanding the behavior of growth cones in the simplified and carefully controlled circumstances of isolation in culture, some of the chapters, this one included, present attempts to understand how growth cones behave *in situ*, where they are faced with a complex array of terrains and with multiple critical decisions and possible responses. One of the important goals of investigating growth cones in the developing animal is to obtain a clear idea of what tasks growth cones must perform as they travel toward and reach their targets, what interactions they undergo, and what responses by the parent cell they mediate.

Having identified and described some of these interactions and responses in the leech, the next stage will be to work out the cellular and molecular mechanisms involved. In terms of the general theme of this review, we must explain how local and global responses are mediated. For example, the localized response at a stopped growth cone could be produced by affecting the assembly of the cytoskeleton or its connection to membrane receptors. The electrical connections that we have found to exist between interganglionic processes could allow small molecules that affect the dynamics of growth to pass between the cells. Calcium ions, normally found in a higher concentration in the growth cone than in the axon stalk, might become redistributed once the two processes are coupled and thus change the dynamics of growth (see chapter by Davis et al.). In contrast, the more global response to contacting the peripheral target might be the result of a signal that biases axonal transport in favor of the axons that find the target relative to those that do not, as has been shown for *Aplysia* neurons in culture (33,34).

Identifying the molecules involved and explaining how they have their effects are tremendous but fascinating challenges for the future.

ACKNOWLEDGMENTS

We thank Nicholas Necles help with the photography. The work from our laboratory described here was supported in part by NIH grant NS-20336 and by NSF grant BNS 8819970.

REFERENCES

1. Cowan WM, Fawcett JW, O'Leary DM, Stanfield BB. Regressive events in neurogenesis. *Science* 1984;225:1258–1265.
2. Purves D, Lichtman JW. *Principles of neuronal development.* Sunderland, MA: Sinauer, 1985.
3. Macagno ER. Number and distribution of neurons in leech segmental ganglia. *J Comp Neurol* 1980;190:283–302.
4. Muller KJ, Nicholls JG, Stent GS, eds. *Neurobiology of the leech.* New York: Cold Spring Harbor Laboratory, 1981.
5. Kramer AP, Weisblat DA. Developmental neural kinship groups in the leech. *J Neurosci* 1985; 5:388–407.
6. Stewart RR, Gao W-Q, Macagno ER. Segmental differentiation in the leech nervous system: proposed segmental differentiation in the leech nervous system: proposed segmental homologs of the heart accessory neurons. *J Comp Neur (in press).*
7. Zipser B. Identifiable neurons controlling penile eversion in the leech. *J Neurophysiol* 1979;42:455–464.
8. Lent CM. Retzius cells within the nervous systems of leeches. *Prog Neurobiol* 1977;8:81–117.
9. Glover JC, Mason A. Morphogenesis of an identified leech neuron: segmental specification of axonal outgrowth. *Dev Biol* 1986;115:256–260.
10. Baptista CA, Macagno ER. Modulation of the pattern of axonal projections of the leech motor neuron by ablation or transplantation of its target. *Neuron* 1988;1:949–962.
11. Loer CM, Jellies J, Kristan WB. Segment-specific morphogenesis of leech *Retzius* neurons requires particular peripheral targets. *J Neurosci* 1987;7:2630–2638.
12. Jellies J, Loer CM, Kristan WB. Morphological changes in leech *Retzius* neurons after target contact during embryogenesis. *J Neurosci* 1987;7:2618–2629.
13. Loer CM, Kristan WB. Central synaptic inputs to identified leech neurons determined by peripheral targets. *Science* 1989;244:64–66.
14. Gao W-Q, Macagno ER. Extension and retraction of axonal projections by some developing neurons in the leech depends upon the existence of neighboring homologues. I. The HA cells. *J Neurobiol* 1987;18:43–59.
15. Gao W-Q, Macagno ER. Extension and retraction of axonal projections by some developing neurons in the leech depends upon the existence of neighboring homologues. II. The AP and AE neurons. *J Neurobiol* 1987;18:295–313.
16. Wallace BG. Selective loss of neurites during differentiation of cells in the leech central nervous system. *J Comp Neurol* 1984;228:149–153.
17. Gao W-Q, Macagno ER. Axon extension and retraction by leech neurons: severing early projections to peripheral targets prevents normal retraction of other projections. *Neuron* 1988;1:269–277.
18. Kuwada JY, Kramer AP. Embryonic development of the leech nervous system: primary axon outgrowth of identified neurons. *J Neurosci* 1983;10:2098–2111.

19. Kuwada JY. Normal and abnormal development of an identified leech motor neuron. *J Embryol Exp Morphol* 1984;79:125–137.
20. Kramer AP, Kuwada JY. Formation of the receptive fields of leech mechanosensory neurons during embryonic development. *J Neurosci* 1983;3:2474–2486.
21. Kuwada JY. Pioneering and pathfinding by an identified neuron in the embryonic leech. *J Embryol Exp Morphol* 1985;86:155–167.
22. DeRiemer SA, Macagno ER. Quantitative studies of the growth of neuronal arbors. In: Carew T, Kelley D, eds. *Perspectives in neural systems and behavior*. New York: Alan R. Liss, 1989;11–31.
23. Gillon JW, Wallace BG. Segmental variation in the arborization of identified neurons in the leech central nervous system. *J Comp Neurol* 1984;228:142–148.
24. Stuart A. Physiological and morphological properties of motoneurones in the central nervous system of the leech. *J Physiol* 1970;209:627–646.
25. Gao W-Q. Axonal extension and retraction by developing neurons in the leech central nervous system. Ph.D. Dissertation, Columbia University, 1989.
26. Yau K-Y. Physiological properties and receptive fields of mechanosensory neurones in the head ganglion of the leech: comparison with homologous cells in segmental ganglia. *J Physiol* 1976; 263:489–512.
27. Johansen J, Hockfield S, McKay RDG. Axonal projections of mechanosensory neurons in the connectives and peripheral nerves of the leech, *Haemopis marmorata*. *J Comp Neurol* 1984;226:255–262.
28. McGlade-McCulloh E, Muller KJ. Developing axons continue to grow at their tip after synapsing with their appropriate target. *Neuron* 1989;2:1063–1068.
29. Blackshaw SE, Nicholls JG, Parnas I. Expanded receptive fields of cutaneous mechanoreceptor cells after single neurone deletion in leech central nervous system. *J Physiol* 1982;326:261–268.
30. Macagno ER, Gao W-Q, Baptista CA, Passani MB. Competition or inhibition? Developmental strategies in the establishment of peripheral projections by leech neurons. *J Neurobiol* 1990;21:107–119.
31. Nicholls JG, Baylor DA. Specific modalities and receptive fields of sensory neurons in the C.N.S. of the leech. *J Neurophysiol* 1968;31:740–756.
32. Kramer AP, Stent GS. Developmental arborization of sensory neurons in the leech *Haementeria ghilianii*. II. Experimentally induced variations in the branching pattern. *J Neurosci* 1985;5:768–775.
33. Schacher S. Differential synapse formation and neurite outgrowth at two branches of the metacerebral cell of *Aplysia* in dissociated cell culture. *J Neurosci* 1985;5:2028–2034.
34. Goldberg DJ, Schacher S. Differential growth of the branches of a regenerating bifurcate axon is associated with differential axonal transport of organelles. *Dev Biol* 1987;124:35–40.

The Nerve Growth Cone, edited by P. C. Letourneau,
S. B. Kater, and E. R. Macagno, Raven Press, Ltd.,
New York © 1992.

25

Pathfinding by the Growth Cones of Primary and Secondary Motoneurons in the Embryonic Zebrafish

Judith S. Eisen and Susan H. Pike

Institute of Neuroscience, University of Oregon, Eugene, Oregon 97403

One of the central challenges of developmental neurobiology is to learn how the growth cones of developing neurons find and form synapses with appropriate targets. Work from a variety of systems has demonstrated that *en route* to their targets growth cones actively navigate and interact with a variety of environmental features that influence the pathways they select (1–3). The first axonal tracts are established by pioneer neurons whose growth cones navigate through axon-free territories. Pioneer growth cones often appear to be guided by nonneuronal cells (4–7) or undifferentiated neurons (8–10) whose absence can prevent or alter the formation of specific axonal pathways (6,11–13). The growth cones of later-developing neurons navigate through territories in which many axonal tracts may already be present, and they may require specific axonal tracts for accurate pathway navigation (14,15). Interactions between navigating growth cones and the environmental features that guide them to their targets appear to depend on appropriate temporal and spatial expression patterns of specific molecules, e.g., extracellular matrix (ECM) components (16,17), cell–surface glycoproteins (18,19), and diffusible factors (20–22).

The study of growth cone guidance has been facilitated by systems in which it is possible to manipulate the environment and watch how growth cones respond. *In vitro* systems have been particularly useful in this regard. However, except in cases in which individually identified neurons can be cultured (23,24), this technique is limited to observing cells taken from a larger population. Culture studies also require taking a cell out of its normal environment, and thus the study of growth cone guidance is limited to artificial environments. *In vivo* systems in which individual cells can be visualized permit the study of growth cone guidance in a natural environment. Embryonic zebrafish are well-suited to studies of growth cone guidance because they are optically clear and develop rapidly, and early in development they have relatively few differentiated neurons, many of which can be individually identified and followed during their entire development *in situ* in the live embryo (see chapter by Easter et al.). In addition, the embryonic environment is accessible to a variety of manipulations, including genetic mutations. We have taken advantage of these features of the embryonic zebrafish to study pathfinding by the growth cones of two populations of neurons, primary motoneurons and secondary motoneurons, that project to the same targets but at different times. Growth cones of the primary motoneurons pioneer nerve pathways that are later followed by the growth cones of the secondary motoneurons. Thus, the growth cones of the primary motoneurons navigate through an axon-free environment, whereas the growth cones of the secondary motoneurons appear to navigate along preexisting axonal tracts. These observations suggest that the two cell populations might use different mechanisms during axonal pathfinding. In this chapter we describe work that examines whether, in the absence of the primary motoneurons, growth cones of the later developing secondary motoneurons can pioneer nerve pathways.

Development of Primary Motoneurons

Primary motoneurons in adult zebrafish are individually identified. Every muscle segment of the adult zebrafish is innervated by three primary motoneurons whose somata are arranged in bilaterally paired clusters (25). Each primary motoneuron within a cluster can be uniquely identified by its soma position and the region of muscle it innervates (Fig. 1A). CaP, the *ca*udal *p*rimary, has the most caudally located soma and innervates muscle fibers in the ventral third of the ipsilateral muscle segment. RoP, the *ro*stral *p*rimary has the most rostrally located soma and innervates muscle fibers in the middle third of the ipsilateral muscle segment. The soma of MiP, the *mi*ddle *p*rimary, is between the CaP and RoP somata, and MiP innervates muscle fibers in the dorsal third of the ipsilateral muscle segment.

The specificity of each primary motoneuron for its target muscle might arise in a variety of different ways. During development, the growth cone of each primary motoneuron might extend directly to the region of muscle appropriate for its adult function. Alternatively, the growth cone might initially extend into both appropriate and inappropriate muscle regions and later retract inappropriate branches. To learn how the primary motoneurons developed their individual innervation patterns, we labeled motoneuronal progenitors and then followed the development of the progeny in living embryos (26,27). We found that the growth cones of the identified primary motoneurons extended directly to the regions of muscle appropriate for their adult functions without making obvious mistakes (Fig. 1B). Moreover, the primary motoneurons that innervate each muscle segment initiate axonal outgrowth in a stereotyped temporal sequence in which CaP is first, MiP is second, and RoP is third. The growth cones of all three primary motoneurons extend along a common pathway until they reach a choice point at the nascent horizontal septum separating the dorsal and ventral muscle of the segment. After pausing at the choice point, the growth cone of each primary motoneuron selects a cell-specific pathway along which to extend. As a result of cell-specific pathfinding, each growth cone arrives at the region of the muscle segment containing appropriate muscle fiber targets.

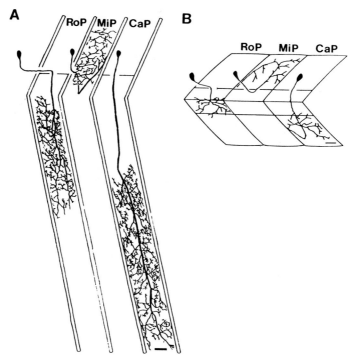

FIG. 1. Primary motoneurons are individually identified. **A:** Drawing of three segments of an adult zebrafish illustrating the soma positions and arbors of each of the primary motoneurons. *Diagonal lines* represent segment boundaries and the *horizontal line* represents the ventral edge of the spinal cord. RoP is to the left, MiP is in the middle, and CaP is to the right. Arbors were traced from individual primary motoneurons labeled by intracellular injection of HRP. Soma positions indicated were not reconstructed from the same cells. (Redrawn from ref. 25, with permission.) **B:** Drawing of three segments of a 72-h zebrafish embryo illustrating the soma positions and arbors of each of the primary motoneurons. RoP is to the left, MiP is in the middle, and CaP is to the right. These cells were labeled during the first day of development by application of Di-I, and their subsequent development was monitored using low-light-level video microscopy. Scale bars: A, 300 μm; B, 20 μm. (Redrawn from ref. 40, with permission.)

Interestingly, we found that in about half of the segments of the embryo there is a fourth primary motoneuron (28); because this cell is variably present, we have named it VaP for *variable primary* (Fig. 2). The VaP soma is adjacent to the CaP soma, and early in development the two cells cannot be distinguished. However, the VaP growth cone fails to extend beyond the horizontal septum choice point. Instead, most VaPs die without projecting an axon. A few VaPs (about 15%) survive and arborize in the region between the MiP and RoP arbors. Although these cells persist into larval development, they have not yet been observed in adults.

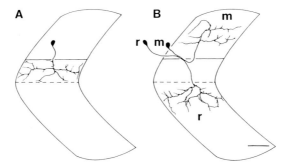

FIG. 2. VaP arborizes in a cell-specific muscle territory. **A:** Drawing of a Di-I-labeled VaP in an 89-h embryo. This cell arborized in a region of the myotome in which no other primary motoneurons had projections. **B:** Drawing of Di-I-labeled MiP (m) and RoP (r) in an 87-hr embryo. Arborizations of these cells complement but do not overlap the VaP arbor shown in **A**. Scale bar: 10 μm. (From ref. 28, by permission.)

Development of Secondary Motoneurons

Much less is currently known about the secondary motoneurons than about the primary motoneurons. The secondary motoneurons can be distinguished by their later birthdays, smaller sizes, and larger numbers from the earlier developing primary motoneurons. In addition, there are genetic differences between primary and secondary motoneurons (29), and the two types of neurons subserve different func-

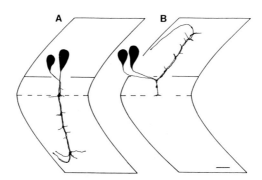

FIG. 3. Morphologies of early developing secondary motoneurons are similar to the morphologies of primary motoneurons. Cells shown here were drawn from experiments in which individual primary and secondary motoneurons were labeled by intracellular injection of fluorescent dyes. **A:** CaP motoneuron (*right*) and an early secondary motoneuron (*left*) with similar axonal morphology. Axons of these two cells appear to fasciculate. **B:** MiP motoneuron (*right*) and an early secondary motoneuron (*left*) with similar axonal morphology. This MiP had already withdrawn its ventral process (see ref. 26), whereas the secondary motoneuron still had a ventral process. Scale bar:10 μm.

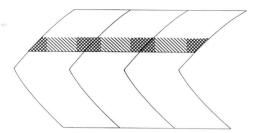

FIG. 4. Motoneuronal somata are regionally organized. Drawing of three segments of an embryonic zebrafish. Regions of the spinal cord with a single set of slanting lines contain motoneuronal somata that project axons into the ventral myotome. Regions of the spinal cord with crossed sets of slanting lines contain motoneuronal somata that project axons into the dorsal myotome.

tions during swimming behavior (30). Currently, we think that there may be two types of secondary motoneurons, a small population that arises within a few hours after the primary motoneurons, and a larger population that arises later; cells may be added to the second population over an extended period of time. Cells of the early secondary population may have distinctive morphologies that are similar to those of the primary motoneurons; preliminary results suggest there may be one to two secondary motoneurons whose morphology is similar to each primary motoneuron (Fig. 3).

Despite the differences between primary and secondary motoneurons, their somata appear to be organized similarly. We studied the positions of primary and secondary motoneuronal somata by retrogradely labeling them with Di-I applied to their axons from the periphery. We find that motoneurons that innervate ventral muscle have somata located in the spinal cord between the boundaries of the overlying myotomes. In contrast, motoneurons that innervate dorsal muscle appear to have somata only in the spinal cord underlying the myotomal boundaries (Fig. 4). Retrograde labeling of motoneurons in larval zebrafish with horseradish peroxidase revealed a similar organization (31).

PRESENT

Mechanisms of Pathfinding by Primary Motoneurons

With our colleagues, we have investigated a number of different components of the environment that might contribute to proper pathfinding by the growth cones of the primary motoneurons. Here we describe some of the roles played by extracellular matrix glycoproteins, target muscle cells, and the primary motoneurons themselves in growth cone pathway selection.

Extracellular Matrix Glycoproteins

Frost and Westerfield (32) determined the relationship between the distribution of two ECM glycoproteins, laminin and fibronectin, and the regions through which the primary motoneuronal growth cones navigate. They found that the regions traversed by the growth cones had laminin-like immunoreactivity, whereas the regions avoided by the growth cones, such as the myotomal boundaries, had fibronectin-like immunoreactivity. In addition, *in vitro*, putative primary motoneurons extended neurites on a laminin-rich substratum but not on a fibronectin-rich substratum. These observations suggest that the distribution of a fibronectin-like molecule may contribute to the segmental patterning of the motor axons by determining where they cannot grow. Interestingly, by the time the axons of the secondary motoneurons are extending in the region of the myotomal boundaries, the fibronectin-like immunoreactivity has disappeared. Because the growth cones of at least some secondary motoneurons can cross the myotomal boundaries (25), the disappearance of the fibronectin-like molecule at this time is consistent with the idea that it plays a role in axonal patterning by preventing the growth cones of the primary motoneurons from crossing the myotomal boundaries.

Target Muscles

Interactions between motoneurons and the muscles they innervate are likely to be important for the formation of normal axonal pathways (33–35). In embryonic zebrafish homozygous for the *spt-1* mutation (36), axonal outgrowth by the primary motoneurons is abnormal, resulting in primary motoneurons with aberrant morphologies. These abnormalities could be the result of a direct effect of the mutation on the primary motoneurons, or they could be due to alterations in the environment through which the growth cones of the primary motoneurons navigate. To test this idea, we created genetic mosaics by transplanting primary motoneurons between mutant and wild-type embryos (37). These experiments showed that the morphologies of the primary motoneurons depend on the phenotype of the host, not on the phenotype of the donor. Thus, primary motoneurons transplanted from mutant donors to wild-type hosts had wild-type morphologies, whereas primary motoneurons transplanted from wild-type donors to mutant hosts had mutant morphologies. These results suggest that the mutation affects the morphologies of the primary motoneurons indirectly, perhaps through an influence of the environment. The major environmental defect in *spt-1* embryos is deficiency and disorganization of the axial muscles caused by improper migration of their progenitors during gastrulation (36). Ho and Kane (38) showed that the disruption is due to a direct action of the mutation on the muscle precursors. Taken together, these experiments suggest that the target muscle normally affects the development of the primary motoneurons, but they do not reveal whether it plays a permissive or instructive role.

Interactions Among Motoneurons

Because the growth cones of the primary motoneurons reach their targets by directed pathfinding, it is tempting to speculate that these cells may have individual

their final destinations, growth cones extend to a series of intermediate targets. This idea is reminiscent of the extension of growth cones in the grasshopper limb (45; chapter by Bentley and O'Connor); these growth cones appear to be guided by a series of environmental components including guidepost cells, segmental boundaries, and the processes of other neurons. In the embryonic zebrafish, pathfinding by the primary and secondary motoneurons also appears to involve several steps that may include intermediate targets. Because the growth cones of both primary and secondary motoneurons can pioneer the common pathway, the cues along this pathway may be of a "general" nature (46; see chapter by Tosney et al.). In contrast, the cues along the cell-specific pathways may be recognized by only the growth cones of particular motoneurons. The axons of at least the primary motoneurons, but possibly also the secondary motoneurons, may provide guidance cues for specific growth cones. In the future, we would like to identify the molecules involved in guiding the growth cones of the primary and secondary motoneurons along the different pathway regions.

ACKNOWLEDGMENTS

We thank Ellie Brandenburg, Ed Sullivan, Sumita Ray, and Harrison Howard for technical assistance; Monte Westerfield and Charles Kimmel for criticism of the manuscript; and Pat Edwards for typing. This work was supported by NS23915, BNS8553146, HD07348, the Procter and Gamble Company, the American Heart Association, a Searle Scholar Award to JSE, and a Patricia Roberts Harris Fellowship to SHP.

REFERENCES

1. Lance-Jones C, Landmesser L. Pathway selection by chick lumbosacral motoneurons during normal development. *Proc R Soc Lond B* 1981;214:1–18.
2. Goodman CS, Raper JA, Ho RK, Chang S. Pathfinding by neuronal growth cones in grasshopper embryos. In: Subtelny S, Green PB, eds. *Developmental order: Its origin and regulation.* New York: Alan R. Liss, 1982;275–316.
3. Westerfield M, Eisen JS. Common mechanisms of growth cone guidance during axonal pathfinding. In: Easter SS, Barald KF, Carlson, BM, eds. *From message to mind: directions in developmental neurobiology.* Sunderland, MA: Sinauer, 1988;110–120.
4. Singer M, Nordlander RH, Egar M. Axonal guidance during embryogenesis and regeneration in the spinal cord of the newt: the blueprint hypothesis of neuronal pathway patterning. *J Comp Neurol* 1979;185:1–22.
5. Ho RK, Ball EE, Goodman CS. Muscle pioneers: large mesodermal cells that erect a scaffold for developing muscles and motoneurons in grasshopper embryos. *Nature* 1983;301:66–69.
6. Bastiani MJ, Goodman CS. Guidance of neuronal growth cones in the grasshopper embryos. III. Recognition of specific glial pathways. *J Neurosci* 1986;6:3542–3551.
7. Kuwada JY. Cell recognition by neuronal growth cones in a simple vertebrate embryo. *Science* 1986;233:740–746.
8. Bate CM. Pioneer neurons in an insect embryo. *Nature (Lond)* 1976;260:54–56.
9. Bentley D, Caudy M. Pioneer axons lose directed growth after selective killing of guidepost cells. *Nature (Lond)* 1983;304:62–65.

10. Bentley D, Caudy M. Navigational substrates for peripheral pioneer growth cones: limb-axis polarity cues, limb-segment boundaries, and guidepost neurons. *Cold Spring Harbor Symp Quant Biol* 1983;48:573–585.
11. Silver J, Lorenz SE, Wahlsten D, Coughlin J. Axonal guidance during development of the great cerebral commissures: descriptive and experimental studies, *in vivo*, on the role of preformed glial pathways. *J Comp Neurol* 1982;210:10–29.
12. Jellies J, Kristan WB, Jr. Embryonic assembly of a complex muscle is directed by a single identified cell in the medicinal leech. *J Neurosci* 1988;8:3317–3326.
13. Ball EE, Ho RK, Goodman CS. Development of neuromuscular specificity in the grasshopper embryo: guidance of motoneuron growth cones by muscle pioneers. *J Neurosci* 1985;5:1808–1819.
14. Raper JA, Bastiani MJ, Goodman CS. Pathfinding by neuronal growth cones in grasshopper embryos. IV. The effects of ablating the A and P axons upon the behavior of the G growth cone. *J Neurosci* 1984;4:2329–2345.
15. Landmesser L, Honig MG. Altered sensory projections in the chick hind limb following the early removal of motoneurons. *Dev Biol* 1986;118:511–531.
16. Tomaselli KJ, Reichardt LF, Bixby JL. Distinct molecular interactions mediate neuronal process outgrowth on non-neuronal cell surfaces and extracellular matrices. *J Dev Biol* 1986;103:2659–2672.
17. Sanes J. Roles of extracellular matrix in neural development. *Annu Rev Physiol* 1984;45:581–600.
18. Bastiani MJ, Harrelson AL, Snow PM, Goodman CS. Expression of fasciclin I and II glycoproteins on subsets of axon pathways during neuronal development in the grasshopper. *Cell* 1987;48:745–755.
19. Dodd J, Morton SB, Karagogeos D, et al. Spatial regulation of axonal glycoprotein expression on subsets of embryonic spinal neurons. *Neuron* 1988;1:105–116.
20. Letourneau PC. Chemotactic response of nerve fiber elongation to nerve growth factor. *Dev Biol* 1978;66:183–196.
21. Lumsden AGS, Davies AM. Chemotropic effect of specific target epithelium in the developing mammalian nervous system. *Nature* 1986;323:538–539.
22. Tessier-Lavigne M, Placzek M, Lumsden AGS, et al. Chemotropic guidance of developing axons in the mammalian central nervous system. *Nature* 1988;336:775–778.
23. Haydon PG, McCobb DP, Kater SB. Serotonin selectively inhibits growth cone motility and synaptogenesis of specific identified neurons. *Science* 1984;226:561–564.
24. Schacher S, Rayport SG, Ambron RT. Giant *Aplysia* neuron R2 reliably forms strong chemical connections *in vitro*. *J Neurosci* 1985;5:2851–2856.
25. Westerfield M, McMurray J, Eisen JS. Identified motoneurons and their innervation of axial muscles in the zebrafish. *J Neurosci* 1986;6:2267–2277.
26. Eisen JS, Myers PZ, Westerfield M. Pathway selection by growth cones of identified motoneurons in live zebrafish embryos. *Nature* 1986;320:269–271.
27. Myers PZ, Eisen JS, Westerfield M. Development and axonal outgrowth of identified motoneurons in the zebrafish. *J Neurosci* 1986;6:2278–2289.
28. Eisen JS, Pike SH, Romancier B. An identified motoneuron with variable fates in embryonic zebrafish. *J Neurosci* 1990;10:34–43.
29. Grunwald DJ, Kimmel CB, Westerfield, M, et al. A neural degeneration mutant that spares primary neurons in the zebrafish. *Dev Biol* 1988;126:115–128.
30. Liu DW, Westerfield M. The formation of terminal fields in the absence of competitive interactions among primary motoneurons in the zebrafish. *J Neurosci* 1990;10:3947–3959.
31. Myers PZ. Spinal motoneurons of the larval zebrafish. *J Comp Neurol* 1985;236:555–561.
32. Frost D, Westerfield M. Axon outgrowth of embryonic zebrafish neurons is promoted by laminin and inhibited by fibronectin. *Soc Neurosci Abstr* 1986;12:1114.
33. Phelan KA, Hollyday M. Axon guidance in muscleless chick wings: the role of muscle cells in motoneuronal pathway selection and muscle nerve formation. *J Neurosci* 1990;10:2699–2716.
34. Tosney KW. Proximal tissues and patterned neurite outgrowth at the lumbosacral level of the chick embryo: deletion of the dermamyotome. *Dev Biol* 1987;122:540–558.
35. Tosney KW. Proximal tissues and patterned neurite outgrowth at the lumbosacral level of the chick embryo: partial and complete deletion of the somite. *Dev Biol* 1988;127:266–286.
36. Kimmel CB, Kane DA, Walker C, et al. A mutation that changes cell movement and cell fate in the zebrafish embryo. *Nature* 1989;337:358–362.
37. Eisen JS., Pike SH. The *spt-1* mutation alters segmental arrangement and axonal development of identified neurons in the spinal cord of the embryonic zebrafish. *Neuron* 1991;6:767–776.

38. Ho RK, Kane DA. Cell-autonomous action of zebrafish *spt-1* mutation in specific mesodermal precursors. *Nature* 1990;348:728–730.
39. Eisen JS, Pike SH, Debu B. The growth cones of identified motoneurons in embryonic zebrafish select appropriate pathways in the absence of specific cellular interactions. *Neuron* 1989;2:1097–1104.
40. Pike SH, Eisen JS. Interactions between identified motoneurons in embryonic zebrafish are not required for normal motoneuron development. *J Neurosci* 1990;10:44–49.
41. Eisen JS. Determination of primary motoneuron identity in developing zebrafish embryos. *Science* 1991;252:569–572.
42. Kuwada JY, Goodman CS. Neuronal determination during embryonic development of the grasshopper nervous system. *Dev Biol* 1985;110:114–126.
43. Bixby JL, Pratt RS, Lilien J, Reichardt LF. Neurite outgrowth on muscle cell surfaces involves extracellular matrix receptors as well as Ca^{2+}-dependent and -independent cell adhesion molecules. *Proc Natl Acad Sci USA* 1987;84:2555–2559.
44. Dodd J, Jessell TM. Axon guidance and the patterning of neuronal projections in vertebrates. *Science* 1988;242:692–699.
45. Caudy M, Bentley D. Pioneer growth cone steering along a series of neuronal and non-neuronal cues of different affinities. *J Neurosci* 1986;6:1781–1795.
46. Lewis J, Al-Ghaith L, Swanson G, Khan A. The control of axon outgrowth in the developing chick wing. In: Fallon JF, Caplan AI, eds. *Limb development and regeneration*. New York: Alan R Liss, 1983;195–205.
47. Trevarrow B, Marks DL, Kimmel CB. Organization of hindbrain segments in the zebrafish embryo. *Neuron* 1990;4:669–679.

The Nerve Growth Cone, edited by P. C. Letourneau, S. B. Kater, and E. R. Macagno, Raven Press, Ltd., New York © 1992.

26

Tract Formation in the Brain of the Zebrafish Embryo

S. S. Easter, Jr., S. W. Wilson, L. S. Ross, and J. D. Burrill

Department of Biology and Neuroscience Program, University of Michigan, Ann Arbor, Michigan 48109-1048

Following the lead of the Oregon group, we have been studying the early development of the zebrafish, *Brachydanio rerio* (see chapter by Eisen and Pike). Although the fish is usually described as a "simple vertebrate," the mature brain is anything but simple. Its complexity is compounded by our ignorance of the detailed circuitry of any adult fish brain and by the huge number of species of fish, which makes one hesitate to extrapolate from one to another. This relative ignorance of the end point of development puts those of us who use fish to study developmental neurobiology at the systems level at a disadvantage relative to the students of mammalian development. Of course, we have advantages, too, particularly the rapid development (fertilization to hatching in 2½ days) and easy accessibility to the embryo at all stages.

Our aim was to understand the early development of circuitry in this vertebrate's CNS. We imposed two restrictions: one of time, the other of location. As for time— we could not possibly follow all development, so our first step was to pick one stage and concentrate on it. We carried out some preliminary studies on closely spaced stages from fertilization to hatching and examined 24 and 48 hr in detail. We concluded that the 48-hr CNS was already too complex to serve our purposes. We settled on 24 hr and described a "simple scaffold" of axon tracts that we believe serves as a substrate on which most axons grow during the next day or so, and probably beyond. For much of this chapter, the 24-hr brain will be the "end point," thus finessing the problem of not knowing much about adult circuitry. The space restriction was relatively unconventional—we attempted to study an anatomically defined region, the presumptive fore and midbrain (FMB), rather than a functionally defined one, such as the retinotectal projection. One of us (SE) had already attempted to study the early development of that projection in *Xenopus*, assuming that the optic fibers pioneered their pathway, and found that the first retinal axons were not only *not* the first ones in the diencephalon, but in fact, they seemed to follow others already in place (1). If one is to study the initial formation of tracts, one must know the milieu, and an important part of the milieu is other tracts, so it was important to try to learn all we could about a stage and region in which the tracts were few and well-separated. Others had already begun this sort of work on the hindbrain and spinal cord (2–4), so we could concentrate on the part of the CNS that they had not examined.

The FMB is derived from a neural tube that is underlain by prechordal mesoderm rather than the notochord, so its developmental history differs from the more caudal CNS. Its evolutionary history is probably different, too, as Gans and Northcutt (5) argued that the vertebrate head, including that part of the brain rostral to the noto-chord, was not an evolutionary *expansion* of the most rostral part of the protochor-date, but rather an *addition* to it. The FMB, with epaxial structures, lobes, and contorted ventricles, looks different from the more caudal parts even very early in development. Although Coghill, Herrick, and others of that generation had de-scribed its formation as best they could, most studies in the past 30 years or so had dealt with only a part, usually the visual system. So the time seemed ripe to use today's improved methods to describe the earliest axonal outgrowth in the FMB.

TECHNICAL CONSIDERATIONS

Herrick (e.g., ref. 6) described a relatively few tracts, 10 or so, in the presump-tive FMB of a salamander embryo. He used anatomical methods that we would consider inadequate today—paraffin sections, reduced silver stains, Golgi impreg-nations, and the like. Moreover, he reconstructed his sectioned material into three dimensions with wax models. Even so, his images are very informative, and in retrospect, accurate but incomplete.

Anatomical methods have improved considerably since Herrick's day, and we have applied some of the newly available techniques to reexamine early develop-ment. We have used electron microscopy, where appropriate, but most of our re-sults were obtained with light microscopy. In particular, we have used HRP and DiI for anterograde and retrograde axon tracing, immunocytochemical probes to mole-cules associated with early axons, and very importantly, whole-mounted brains rather than sections. The advantage of using whole-mounts is that one need not reconstruct—the brain and its labeled tracts appear in three dimensions. To be sure, a three-dimensional brain is difficult to photograph in a compound microscope, given the limited depth of focus, and the resolution is often less than what can be achieved with sections. But these limitations are not very severe when the brain is as small as the zebrafish embryo's—about 300 μm from the rostral tip to the boundary between the tectum and the cerebellum, and nowhere more than about 250 μm thick. (Note that the size of the CNS is relatively constant throughout the neuro-genic period of embryogenesis, because the embryo's total mass is limited by the mass of the zygote.) Moreover, the brain is quite transparent, a consequence of the fact that the yolk is in a single large sac rather than dispersed as platelets intra-cellularly where they can scatter light (as in amphibians). The microscopist is aided still further by the fact that all the early tracts develop superficially, directly beneath the presumptive pia, and are therefore separated from the microscope objective by just a few micrometers of neuroepithelial end feet.

THE SIMPLE SCAFFOLD

The 24-hr FMB has been described by Wilson and colleagues (7). The CNS has the shape of a dueling pistol: the FMB as the handle, the medulla and spinal cord as the barrel. The olfactory and trigeminal nerves are recognizable, but the optic nerve has not yet formed. Two immunocytochemical probes—the HNK-1 antibody and an antibody to α-acetylated tubulin (8)—reveal essentially similar images in whole-mounted brains. Most of the brain is free of label, indicating an absence of axons there, but five quite well-defined tracts and four commissures are evident. Figure 1 shows a summary of these structures. There are two dorsal tracts. The larger is the tract of the posterior commissure (TPC), made up of axons that contribute to the posterior commissure (PC). It courses from the commissure to the tract of the post-optic commissure (POC), which is described below. Slightly thinner than the TPC, the dorsoventral diencephalic tract (DVDT) originates from cells in or adjacent to the progenitor of the epiphysis (or pineal body) and courses down to intersect the TPOC about 50 μm rostral to the intersection of TPC and TPOC. The TPOC is the largest tract, measured either by length or by number of axons, in the FMB. It contains axons coursing in both directions and connects the postoptic commissure (POC) to the ventral longitudinal tract of the hindbrain and spinal cord. Numerous labeled axons emerge from telencephalic cells and course downward in a broad sweep, some forming the tract of the anterior commissure (TAC), so called because the axons form the anterior commissure (AC). Other telencephalic axons turn caudally into the supraoptic tract (SOT), so called because of its position above the optic stalk. The SOT intersects the TPOC. Finally, there is the ventral tegmental commissure (VTC), just caudal to the flexure. We think that these five tracts (TAC, SOT, TPC, DVDT, and TPOC) and four commissures (VTC, AC, PC, and TPOC) make up the entire circuitry of the presumptive FMB at 24 hr.

This conclusion is based on several independent lines of evidence. First, both antibodies gave essentially similar patterns of labeling (7,9). Second, microapplications of HRP or DiI that were made to a wide variety of sites only labeled axons associated with these tracts, or labeled none at all. Third, electron microscopic examination of midline sagittal sections showed commissures only at the four sites shown by the other methods (e.g., Fig. 2).

The HRP labeling not only confirmed the existence of the limited set of tracts and commissures, but also revealed the origins and destinations of some axons. Thus, we know that the DVDT axons all turn rostrally at their junction with the TPOC, that there are no ascending axons in the SOT, and other facts too numerous to mention here.

Similarly labeled whole-mounts of 48-hr embryos showed a huge increase in the

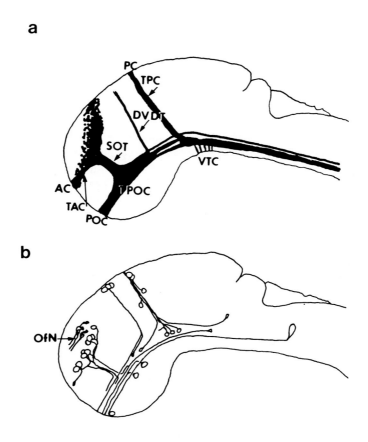

FIG. 1. Schematic lateral views of the 24-hr brain, skinned and with the eyes removed. Rostral is to the left; dorsal is up. **a:** "Simple scaffold" of five tracts and four commissures. **b:** Selected view illustrating the origins and directions of some of the axons in the network. AC, anterior commissure; DVDT, dorsoventral diencephalic tract; OfN, olfactory nerve fibers; PC, posterior commissure; POC, postoptic commissure; SOT, supraoptic tract; TAC, tract of the anterior commissure; TPC, tract of the posterior commissure; TPOC, tract of the postoptic commissure; VTC, ventral tegmental commissure. Calibration: 50 μm. (From ref. 7, with permission.)

number of axons. Figure 3 documents this for the commissures; the number grew by about 100-fold or more over the course of a day. In contrast, the number of pathways increased very slightly: only three new commissures and their associated tracts were added. Therefore, most axons added during the second day of embryogenesis joined established tracts and commissures rather than formed new ones. This implies that axons are the favored substrate for most other axons to grow on and prompted us to call the initial network a "scaffold."

Several features of this structure warrant comment. The best studies to date of early tract development have been those carried out on invertebrate preparations,

isogenic organisms: cellular interactions in the development of the optic lamina of *Daphnia. Proc Natl Acad Sci USA* 1973;70:433–437.

11. Bentley D, Keshishian H. Pathfinding by peripheral pioneer neurons in grasshoppers. *Science* 1982;218:1082–1088.

12. Bate CM. Pioneer neurons in an insect embryo. *Nature* 1976;260:54–56.

13. Bastiani MJ, du Lac S, Goodman CS. Guidance of neuronal growth cones in the grasshopper embryo. 1. Recognition of a specific axonal pathway by the pCC neuron. *J Neurosci* 1986;6:3518–3531.

14. McConnell SK, Ghosh A, Shatz CJ. Subplate neurons pioneer the first axon pathway from the cerebral cortex. *Science* 1989;245:978–982.

15. Holley JA, Silver J. Growth pattern of pioneering chick spinal cord axons. *Dev Biol* 1987;123:375–388.

16. Easter SS Jr, Purves D, Rakic P, Spitzer NC. The changing view of neural specificity. *Science* 1985;230:507–511.

17. Wilson SW, Easter SS Jr. A pioneering growth cone in a vertebrate brain. *Proc Natl Acad Sci USA* 1991;88:2293–2296.

18. Ross LS, Parrett T, Easter SS Jr. Axonogenesis, distortion, and segmentation in the embryonic brain of zebrafish. *J Neurosci (submitted.)*

19. Godement P, Vanselow J, Thanos S, Bonhoeffer F. A study in developing visual systems with a new method of staining neurones and their processes in fixed tissue. *Development* 1987;101:697–713.

20. Layer PG. Comparative localization of acetylcholinesterase and pseudocholinesterase during morphogenesis of the chick brain. *Proc Natl Acad Sci USA* 1983;80:6413–6417.

21. Hanneman E, Trevarrow B. Metcalfe WK, Kimmel CB, Westerfield M. Segmental pattern of development of the hindbrain and spinal cord of the zebrafish embryo. *Development* 1988;103:49–58.

22. Bentley D, Caudy M. Pioneer axons lose directed growth after selective killing of guidepost cells. *Nature* 1983;304:62–65.

23. Mendelson B. Development of reticulospinal neurons of the zebrafish. II. Early axonal outgrowth and cell body position. *J Comp Neurol* 1986;251:172–184.

24. Burrill JD, Easter SS Jr. Relationship of the developing retinofugal projection to other tracts in the embryonic zebrafish brain. *Invest Ophth Vis Sci* 1990;31:156.

The Nerve Growth Cone, edited by P. C. Letourneau,
S. B. Kater, and E. R. Macagno, Raven Press, Ltd.,
New York © 1992.

27

Growth Cone Form and Guidance in an Amphibian Spinal Cord

Ruth H. Nordlander

Department of Oral Biology, The Ohio State University, Columbus, Ohio 43210

Any adequate explanation of how the nervous system is assembled must account for the distinctive growth patterns of many diverse neuron types as and when they occur in the intact nervous system. Because the development of circuitry in the CNS is really the sum of choices made by growth cones of many different neuron classes, appreciation of the overall process will ultimately require knowledge of how growth cones of individual neuron types navigate their routes in the ever changing environment of the embryo.

The major thrust of work in my laboratory is aimed at determining the patterns and mechanisms by which early axon tracts are established in the spinal cord of *Xenopus*. The amphibian embryo offers a small and relatively simple nervous system that is ideal for studies of single or small groups of identified neurons in whole-mount preparations.

In the past we have taken several approaches in our studies. After first determining the sequence and distribution of developing tracts and identifying the neurons giving rise to them (1–4), we used anterograde horseradish peroxidase (HRP) fills to characterize growth cones of these early pathways (5). More recently, we have begun to look in detail at growth cone configurations and axon trajectories of several more precisely identified neuron types (6). Our focus on growth cone shapes is based on accumulating evidence that changes or differences in form may reflect developmentally significant interactions with the environment (7–10; see chapters by Kalil and Norris and by Mason and Godement).

In this chapter I will present (a) a brief account of the developmental anatomy of the early spinal cord, (b) a summary of some general patterns of growth cone configuration, (c) two pieces of evidence that uniquely identifiable pathways show distinctive growth cone morphologies, and finally, (d) some thoughts on the implications of these observations for axonal guidance.

DEVELOPMENTAL ANATOMY OF THE EARLY SPINAL CORD

Early attempts to correlate anatomical and behavioral events in the developing amphibian nervous system (11) revealed a basic scheme that has since been subjected to ongoing refinement using techniques such as HRP tracing (2,4,5,12,13), immunocytochemistry (13–16), and electrophysiology (17). Figure 1A shows a schematic view of the basic components of the early *Xenopus* spinal cord. The cord of the embryo is a simple tube of small diameter (30–80 μm) whose ventricular layer is surrounded by a mantle layer only a few cells thick. Like other lower vertebrates, *Xenopus* displays a distinct set of primitive neurons that develop very early and

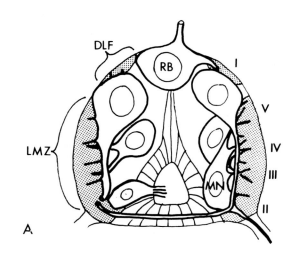

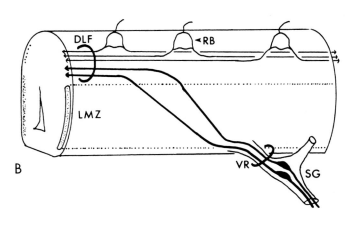

mediate the first coordinated movements of the embryo (17,18). Subsequently, other neurons add to the system, including a secondary set of sensory (Fig. 1B) and motor (not shown) cells distinct from the primary set. Secondary sensory neurons are located in ganglia outside of the spinal cord and eventually supersede the primary sensory system (19,20). The development of their central projections will be considered later in this chapter. Fiber areas of the cord at the stages examined here include a dorsal axon bundle, the dorsolateral fasciculus (DLF), in which travel longitudinal axons of RB and secondary sensory ganglion neurons and a lateral band of mostly longitudinal axons, the lateral marginal zone (LMZ).

OVERALL PATTERNS OF GROWTH CONE SHAPE AND DISTRIBUTION

By anterograde filling of developing axons with HRP, we were able to characterize growth cones belonging to early spinal neurons (5). As Ramón y Cajal recognized long ago (21), the shapes of growth cones of the developing spinal cord are quite variable (Fig. 2A). In *Xenopus* their size ranges from large (40 μm × 20 μm) to small terminal swellings representing a doubling or tripling of the axon's diameter. We recognized several forms ranging from complex (with filopodia and

---

FIG. 1. A: Schematic view of the early spinal cord of *Xenopus*. Bordering the central canal is the ventricular layer. Surrounding it is the mantle layer that contains differentiating neurons, several of which are illustrated here. Among them are the Rohon–Beard cells (RB) and motoneurons (MN), both of which send axons into the periphery. Also shown is an assortment of interneurons, including examples of commissural, circumferential neurons, cerebrospinal fluid–contacting neurons, and several other types. Fiber areas of the cord are stippled. The smaller dorsal fiber bundle is the dorsolateral fasciculus (DLF). Lateral and ventral to it is the lateral marginal zone (LMZ), which begins as a series of parallel longitudinal bundles that fuse to become the coherent band of fibers shown here. Roman numerals at right indicate the sequence of fiber development in the cord. The first long axons of the cord are the central RB axons, which initiate the DLF (I). Next axons appear ventrolaterally (II). New axon bundles add in a ventral to dorsal progression (III, IV, and V), but the LMZ also grows steadily in thickness by addition at the peripheral edge of the zone (28). Most axons whose development is described in this chapter travel through the LMZ after it has become a band. Axons of the ventral LMZ include those of motor neurons, spinal interneurons, and descending supraspinal pathways. Axons of other spinal interneurons join this bundle in more dorsal positions, finally. The LMZ contains primarily longitudinal fibers, with axons of some spinal neurons taking oblique courses across the cord (12,16). Deep to the long fibers of the cord are the circumferential and commissural axons (12,16), and intermingled with axons in the LMZ are dendrites of differentiating spinal neurons. There is a clear rostrocaudal development gradient in the spinal cord. **B:** Elements of the sensory ganglion (SG) system of the tail of *Xenopus*. Schematic view of the organization of the sensory ganglia and the path of their central projections. Sensory ganglion neurons form a loose cluster at the primary bifurcation point of the ventral root (VR). Central axons enter the cord via the ventral root and, once in the cord, take a diagonal pathway across the LMZ to reach the DLF where they join the RB axons and travel rostrally. Axons enter the cord as a group but cross the cord separately, joining again in the DLF. (Modified from ref. 6, with permission.)

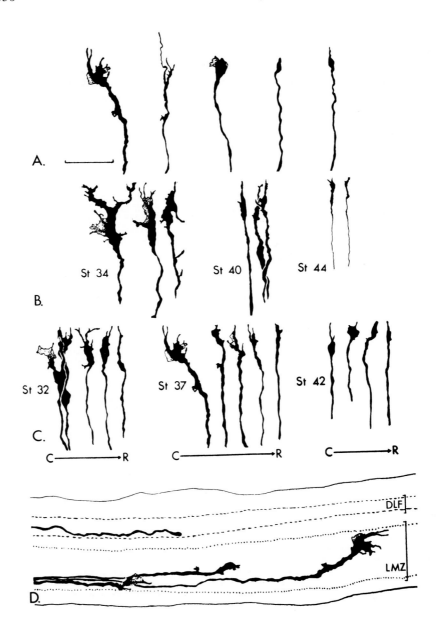

lamellipodia) to simple clavate or fusiform (Fig. 2A). Because growth cones are dynamic structures, some variations in configuration that we see in our fixed tissue probably represent a range of shapes typical of growth cones of each neuron type (22). But what emerged from these experiments were some clear differences in the spectrum of shapes characteristic for general neuron classes as they vary with age, position in the pathway, and other factors.

Growth Cones Are More Elaborate in Younger Animals

Growth cones of some neuron classes are larger and more complex in younger animals than in older ones (Fig. 2B). This is most obvious among descending supra-spinal axons of the ventrolateral LMZ. Growth cones of younger stages (before hatching) showed many processes, including filopodia and lamellipodia that spread widely over the LMZ and often reached its most dorsal extent. Such elaborate con-figurations are no longer seen after early larval stages; subsequent growth cones tend to be smaller and restricted to the fascicle occupied by their trailing axons. The gradual transition from elaborate to more simple growth cones occupies about 60 hr.

Leading Growth Cones Are More Elaborate in Some Pathways

If the shapes of growth cones in the descending ventrolateral axon bundles are compared at a number of positions along their route, it can be seen that the most distal (caudal) growth cones are generally larger and more elaborate than those at progressively more proximal (rostral) levels of the same bundle (Fig. 2C). This difference is apparent, although not as obvious, even at later stages when all growth cones are more simple than those of younger animals.

FIG. 2. Summary of general patterns of growth cone configurations seen in the developing spinal cord of *Xenopus* (5). **A:** Five growth cones presented as examples of the range of growth cone configurations seen in our preparations. **B:** Changes in growth cone shapes with age. Growth cones of descending supraspinal axons labeled from the hindbrain at three suc-cessive stages are illustrated. Trailing axons reside in the ventrolateral part of the LMZ. Note that growth cones are larger and more complex at younger stages and become progressively smaller and simpler with age. In all three groups the most caudal growth cone is at left. **C:** Differences in growth cone shape at successively more rostral positions along the ventrolateral descending pathway. For each of the three specimens illustrated, the most caudal growth cone is to the left with progressively more rostral ones to the right, as indicated. The most caudal growth cone is always more elaborate. The distance between the most caudal and rostral examples is 300 to 370 μm. Note also the decreasing complexity with age. **D:** Differences in growth cone shape and distribution with fiber region. Growth cones of the LMZ are more elaborate and may show wider spreads than those of the DLF. The growth cone shown here in the DLF is the clavate tip of a descending RB axon. In this and all other lateral views of the spinal cord, rostral is to the left. Scale bar, 20 μm. (Modified from ref. 5, with permission.)

Some Growth Cones Differ with Position in Cord Cross Section

Growth cones of some descending axons (and those of central SG axons in the tail, see below) traveling in the LMZ spread widely across the entire zone, even though their trailing axons consistently occupy a restricted part of it (Fig. 2D). In contrast, growth cones in the narrower DLF are never as elaborate and show restricted spreads (Fig. 2D).

What Is the Significance of These Variations in Growth Cone Shape?

Gradual shifts toward simplicity seen in growth cone shape over time and along a pathway can be related to the changing anatomy of the cord. Trends toward simpler growth cone structure among descending pathways in the LMZ may reflect, in part, the increasingly longitudinal orientation of elements, as the zone fills with fibers, and the accompaning decrease in available extracellular space (23). Leading growth cones navigate an environment dominated by radial and end foot processes of neuroepithelial cells. Later ones grow between end feet and longitudinal axons that have preceded them (23). The greater linearity of growth cones in the DLF throughout its development may be due to the presence there of these same features, beginning soon after DLF initiation in the embryo (16).

DISTINCTIVE GROWTH CONE MORPHOLOGIES IN IDENTIFIED PATHWAYS

Although we are able to recognize some very basic and distinctive patterns of growth cone behavior from HRP fills, growth cone identity can be precisely specified in only a few cases where axons or cell bodies are geographically isolated (e.g., sensory ganglion axons; see below). Some limitations of HRP can be overcome with the application of immunocytochemical methods, which can provide more precise identification of neuron types and can also mark intact neurons at earlier stages of outgrowth (14,15).

We have observed that growth cones belonging to some identifiable neurons display different forms that are attributable to intrinsic or environmental cues. In the spinal cord of *Xenopus* we have recognized differences—in one instance between growth cones from two different neuron types growing simultaneously through the same environment; in another, between growth cones of the same pathway as they move from one environment to another.

Two Neuron Types Show Differing Growth Cone Morphologies

Using antibodies to two neurotransmitters, we have recently observed that two descending supraspinal pathways growing side by side through the LMZ are lead by growth cones with distinctly different shapes (Fig. 3). These pathways are a se-

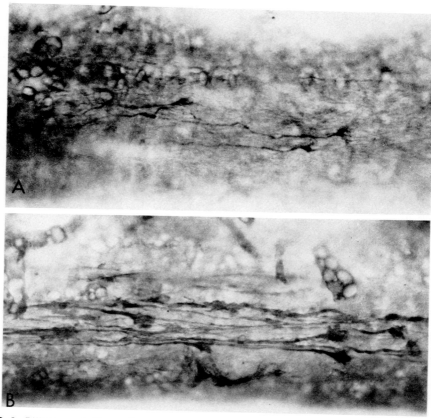

FIG. 3. Differences in the configuration of growth cones belonging to two different descending supraspinal pathways located in the same fiber zone of the cord. **A:** Growth cones labeled with anti-5HT and belonging to the early raphespinal pathway. Note that growth cones are small with a few fine processes running primarily longitudinally. **B:** Growth cones of reticulospinal axons labeled with anti-GABA. Growth cones of this pathway are flattened and have lobular outlines. Axons seem to be thicker here. Note that these growth cones are quite different than those shown above. Scale bar, 20 μm.

rotonin-immunoreactive (5HT-IR) raphespinal tract (15) and a mid-hindbrain reticulospinal tract, which is γ-amino butyric acid-immunoreactive (GABA-IR) (24). Axons of the former are ipsilateral and mostly concentrated in the ventral half of the LMZ. Those of the latter are bilateral and occupy only the ventral half of the LMZ (Fig. 3). Growth cones of the 5HT-IR neurons are generally slim with a few fine processes (Fig. 3A), whereas growth cones of the GABA-IR neurons are flattened in a plane parallel to the lateral surface of the cord and show lobular outlines (Fig. 3B). The implications of these differences are still unclear, but they do show that axons of two tracts developing simultaneously in the same region of the spinal cord have type-specific growth cone morphologies that imply differing interactions with a shared environment.

Growth Cone Shapes in Two Phases of the Same Pathway

Growth cones of the developing sensory ganglion (SG) system in the tail show striking differences in morphology as they move from one part of their route to another (6).

As indicated above, the secondary sensory system develops early in larval life. Trunk SG elements follow the classical form with dorsal root ganglia and central afferents entering the cord via dorsal roots. The pattern in the tail, however, is unusual (Fig. 1B) (3). Here, dorsal roots are absent and SG sit on the ventral roots, along which they send their central axons into the cord. From the ventral root entry point SG axons travel diagonally across the LMZ to reach the DLF where they course rostrally, along with the earlier-forming RB axons and central SG afferents of more rostral levels. In the established configuration of this pathway, SG axons are together in the ventral root, separate in the LMZ, and together again in the DLF (Figs. 1B and 4A).

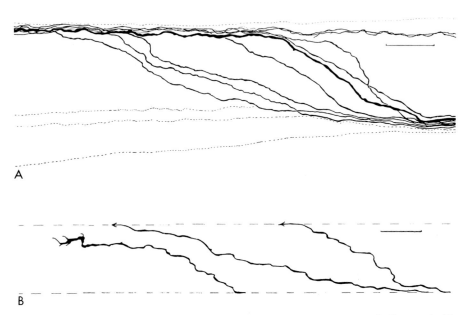

FIG. 4. Trajectories of sensory ganglion axons in the lateral marginal zone. **A:** Camera lucida drawing of a lateral view of seven labeled SG axons crossing the cord of a stage 46 larva. Axons are not fasciculated in this part of the route but travel independently of one another. Note also the range of slope patterns represented by these seven axons. (From ref. 3, with permission.) **B:** Camera lucida drawings of several diagonal SG axons in the LMZ, showing irregular trajectories that include step-like bends and plateaus. On the left is an axon tipped with a growth cone, which itself shows such a bend. Scale bars, 25 μm. (Modified from ref. 6, with permission.)

searching for whatever cues direct their diagonal course. Wide spreads and processes that explore even inappropriate routes are more compatible with diffuse and variable cues than with preformed and precisely laid out ones.

Although the diagonal pathways taken by central SG axons in the tail spinal cord is unusual, it is unlikely that the cues directing growth here are unique to this system. If anything, this pattern is likely to be a primitive condition. On the basis of growth patterns we have observed here, it seems that axons respond to two factors in their diagonal path, one directing them dorsally and another stronger one directing them rostrally (hence the low slopes of diagonal axons). It is possible that these factors are diffusible and work over a distance. There is now evidence of polarized and unique gene expression within the developing *Xenopus* nervous system in patterns corresponding to the major axes of the embryo (39,40) and thus to the two vectors of SG axon growth in the diagonal route. Although these products have not been implicated in axonal guidance, their distributions show that polarity-specific molecules are expressed by this tissue.

Irregularities and variations in axonal trajectories may result from stochastically fluctuating signals or from local features of the environment that deflect or cause detours in growth cone courses. Perhaps the step-like configurations of some diagonal axons result from temporary excursions along the longitudinal bundles of the DLF followed by periodic dorsal corrections (Fig. 4).

Many questions about the growth of these SG axons remain. Whether there are differences in substrate and contact patterns for growth cones in each of these two environments can be learned by subjecting material already available in our laboratory to high-resolution microscopy. Several other questions could be addressed by looking at SG axon growth in real-time (26). For example, how do growth rates in the DLF and LMZ compare, and might rate of growth relate to growth cone shape (7)? Do growth cones in the LMZ really explore actively as suggested by our fixed preparations? How closely do growth cone movements relate to final trajectories? In addition, *in vitro* tests could be set up to determine whether diffusible factors are at work here (32,41) and whether axons can recognize their proper position and direction of growth if isolated from their normal environment.

If there are unique contact and response patterns for identifiable growth cones, what are the mechanisms of their interactions with and selection of the substrata for their growth? Surely the study of mechanisms will move into the area of molecular biology, but study at this level must be grounded in a thorough understanding of the behavior in space and time of uniquely identified growth cones within the intact nervous system and how this behavior relates to the changing environment of the developing nervous system.

ACKNOWLEDGMENTS

The author is grateful to Dawn Awwiller Borror, Elizabeth Ullman Jaszczak, and Scott Watson for excellent technical assistance and to Drs. K.E. Alley, J.S. Edwards, and P. van Mier for discussion of the work discussed here. Support for research covered in this chapter came from NS-18773.

REFERENCES

1. Nordlander R. Developing descending neurons of the early *Xenopus* tail spinal cord. *J Comp Neurol* 1984;228:117–127.
2. Nordlander R. Motoneurons of the tail of young *Xenopus* tadpoles. *J Comp Neurol* 1986;253:403–413.
3. Nordlander RH, Awwiller DM, Cook H. Dorsal roots are absent from the tail of larval *Xenopus*. *Brain Res* 1988;440:391–395.
4. Nordlander RH, Baden ST, Ryba M. Development of early brainstem projections to the tail spinal cord of *Xenopus*. *J Comp Neurol* 1985;231:519–529.
5. Nordlander R. Axonal growth cones in the developing amphibian spinal cord. *J Comp Neurol* 1987; 263:485–496.
6. Nordlander R. Growth cones and axons trajectories of a sensory pathway in the amphibian spinal cord. *J Comp Neurol* 1991;307:539–548.
7. Bovolenta P, Mason CA. Growth cone morphology changes with position in the developing mouse visual pathway from retina to firs targets. *J Neurosci* 1987;7:1447–1460.
8. Bray D, Hollenbeck PJ. Growth cone motility and guidance. *Annu Rev Cell Biol* 1988;4:43–61.
9. Caudy M, Bentley D. Pioneer growth cone morphologies reveal proximal increases in substrate affinity within leg segments of grasshopper embryos. *J Neurosci* 1986;6:364–379.
10. Letourneau PC. Cell-substratum adhesion of neurite growth cones and its role in neurite elongation. *Exp Call Res* 1979;124:127–138.
11. Coghill GE. Correlated anatomical and physiological studies of the growth of the nervous system of amphibia. I. The afferent system of the trunk of *Amblystoma*. *J Comp Neurol* 1914;24:161–233.
12. Roberts A, Clarke JDW. The neuroanatomy of an amphibian embryo spinal cord. *Philos Trans R Soc Lond B* 1982;296:195–212.
13. van Mier P, ten Donkelaar HJ. Early development of descending pathways from the brain stem to the spinal cord in *Xenopus laevis*. *Anat Embryol* 1984;170:295–306.
14. Roberts A. The early development of neurons in *Xenopus* embryos revealed by transmitter immunocytochemistry for serotonin, GABA and glycine. In: *Developmental neurobiology of the frog*. Alan R. Liss, 1988;191–205.
15. van Mier P, Joosten HWJ, van Rheden R, ten Donkelaar HJ. The development of serotonergic raphespinal projections in *Xenopus laevis*. *Int J Dev Neurosci* 1986;4:465–476.
16. Nordlander R. HNK-1 marks earliest axonal outgrowth in *Xenopus*. *Devel Brain Res* 1989;50:147–153.
17. Roberts A. The neurons that control axial movements in a frog embryo. *Am Zool* 1989;29:53–63.
18. Hughes A. The development of the primary sensory system in *Xenopus laevis* (Daudin). *J Anat* 1957;91:323–328.
19. Hughes A, Tsumi P. The factors controlling the development of the dorsal root ganglion and ventral horn in *Xenopus laevis* (Daud). *J Anat* 1958;92:498–527.
20. van Mier P, ten Donkelaar HJ. The development of primary afferents to the lumbar spinal cord in *Xenopus laevis*. *Neurosci Lett* 1988;84:35–40.
21. Ramón y Cajal, S. *Studies on vertebrate neurogenesis* (trans. L Guth). Springfield, IL: Charles C Thomas, 1960.
22. Bray, D. Chapman K. Analysis of microspike movements on the neuronal growth cone. *J Neurosci* 1985;5:3204–3413.
23. Nordlander RH, Singer M. Spaces precede axons in *Xenopus* embryonic spinal cord. *Exp Neurol* 1982;75:221–228.
24. Roberts A, Dale N, Ottersen OP, Storm-Mathisen J. The early development of neurons with GABA immunoreactivity in the CNS of *Xenopus laevis* embryos. *J Comp Neurol* 1987;261:435–449.
25. Rathjen RG. A neurite outgrowth-promoting molecule in developing fiber tracts. *Trends Neurosci* 1988;11:183–184.
26. Harris WA, Holt CE, Bonhoeffer F. Retinal axons with and without their somata, growing to and arborizing in the tectum of *Xenopus* embryos: a time-lapse video study of single fibres *in vivo*. *Development* 1987;101:123–133.

27. Harris WA, Holt CE, Smith TA, Gallenson M. Growth cones of developing retinal cells *in vivo*, on culture surfaces and in collagen matrices. *J Neurosci Res* 1985;13:101–122.
28. Nordlander RH, Singer M. Morphology and position of growth cones in the developing *Xenopus* spinal cord. *Dev Brain Res* 1982;4:181–193.
29. Snow DM, Steindler DA, Silver J. Molecular and cellular characterization of the glial roof plate of the spinal cord and optic tectum: a possible role for a proteoglycan in the development of an axon barrier. *Dev Biol* 1990;138:359–376.
30. Lipton SA, Kater SB. Neurotransmitter regulation of neuronal outgrowth, plasticity and survival. *Trends Neurosci* 1989;12:265–269.
31. Goodman CS, Bastiani MJ, Doe CQ, et al. Cell recognition during neuronal development. *Science* 1984;235:1271–1279.
32. Lumsden AGS, Davies, AM. Chemotropic effect of specific target epithelium in the developing mammalian nervous system. *Nature (Lond)* 1986;323:538–539.
33. Connolly JL, Seeley RJ, Greene LA. Regulation of growth cone morphology by nerve growth factor: an comparative study by scanning electron microscopy. *J Neurosci Res* 1985;13:185–198.
34. Kapfenhammer PJ, Raper JA. Interactions between growth cones and neurites growing form different neural tissues in culture. *J Neurosci* 1987;7:1595–1600.
35. Bonhoeffer F, Huf F. Position-dependent properties of retinal axons and their growth cones. *Nature* 1985;315:409–410.
36. Bovolenta P, Dodd J. Guidance of commissural growth cones at the floor plate in embryonic rat spinal cord. *Development* 1990;109:435–447.
37. Godement P, Salaun J, Mason CA. Retinal axons pathfinding in the optic chiasm: divergence of crossed and uncrossed fibers. *Neuron* 1990;5:173–186.
38. Beattie MS, Bresnahan JC, Lopate G. Metamorphosis alters the response to spinal cord transection in *Xenopus laevis* frogs. *J Neurobiol* 1990;21:1108–1122.
39. Ruiz i Altaba, A. Neural expression of the *Xenopus* homeobox gene Xhox 3: evidence for a patterning neural signal that spreads through the ectoderm. *Development* 1990;108:595–604.
40. Sharpe CR, Gurdon JB. The induction of anterior and posterior neural genes in *Xenopus laevis*. *Development* 1990;109:765–774.
41. Tessier-Lavigne M, Placzek M, Lumsden AGS, Dodd J, Jessell TM. Chemotropic guidance of developing axons in the mammalian central nervous system. *Nature* 1988;336:775–778.

The Nerve Growth Cone, edited by P. C. Letourneau,
S. B. Kater, and E. R. Macagno, Raven Press, Ltd.,
New York © 1992.

28

Growth Cone Guidance in the Avian Limb: A Search for Cellular and Molecular Mechanisms

Lynn T. Landmesser

*Department of Physiology and Neurobiology, University of Connecticut,
Storrs, Connecticut 06269*

INNERVATION OF THE AVIAN LIMB: THE CASE FOR PRECISE PATHFINDING AND PERIPHERAL GUIDANCE CUES

Beginning with classical embryological studies some decades ago (1), the avian limb has proved to be an increasingly tractable system in which to study how vertebrate neurons make divergent pathway choices; this in turn has been shown to play an important, if not dominant, role in the formation of the specific motoneuron connectivity that underlies patterned motor behavior (2). Like the more complex central nervous system of higher vertebrates and in contrast to the simpler invertebrate systems that have been so elegantly exploited to determine the rules of neural development (3), we are confronted here with large numbers of neurons that are not uniquely identified (20,000 motoneurons per limb). However, the accessibility of the avian embryo and the application of increasingly modern techniques have allowed a number of experimental perturbations that directly test some of the hypotheses proposed to explain how motor specificity is achieved.

In contrast to the axial muscle system of the zebrafish where a simple segmental pattern is reiterated (4), the vertebrate limb is a multisegmental structure. Individual muscles are populated by somite-derived muscle precursor cells from two to four spinal cord segments, and these in turn are innervated by motoneuron pools stretching over the two-four corresponding segments (5). Thus although the axons of avian hindlimb motoneurons exit the spinal cord in eight separate spinal nerves (Fig. 1), they converge at the base of the limb in two plexuses (an anterior crural and a posterior sciatic) where they sort out into motoneuron pool–specific groups (6) and later diverge from common nerve trunks to project to their appropriate muscles (6–8). Midway through embryonic development there exists a precise pattern of connectivity between motoneurons and muscles, and the motoneuron pools are acti-

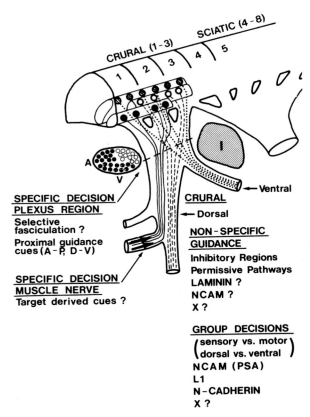

FIG. 1. Schematic view of the hindlimb innervation from a Stage 28 chick embryo. Three motoneuron pools that project into the crural plexus are shown. Their axons first sort out in the specific decision region of the plexus, where a cross section is indicated (A, anterior; V ventral), into ventral and dorsal crural trunks. Later the two dorsally projecting pools make divergent choices at the point of muscle nerve emergence. I, inhibitory region composed of precartilage; P, posterior; D, dorsal.

vated in a highly patterned manner as the embryo begins to move (6–10). How does this complex pattern of specific connections arise developmentally? As will be detailed below, it appears largely because of the guided growth of axons, emphasizing the importance of discovering the mechanism by which growth cones are able to detect and respond to an apparently complex array of environmental signals.

First through electrophysiology and retrograde HRP tracing (7,11), and later by orthogradely tracing the HRP-labeled axons of motoneurons from specific segmental levels (6,8,12), it was shown that chick motoneurons grow from the outset to their target muscles with few errors. Because this pattern was achieved by stage 30, before the onset of the motoneuron cell death period, axon guidance rather than subsequent correction by axon retraction and/or cell death was implicated. Early on, the tracing of retrogradely labeled axons projecting to specific muscles indicated another important point. As the axons of motoneurons exited the spinal cord, those destined to innervate different muscles were extensively intermingled; however, as they approached the base of the limb they began to sort out (see Fig. 1), grouping together in specific spatial locations within the plexus and proximal nerve trunks (6). Thus a simple system of passive deployment of axons to the nearest target could be excluded. Selective adhesion between axons belonging to a single motoneuron pool may contribute to this sorting out process, an idea that has yet to be adequately tested. However, because the axons also group into specific spatial locations within the nerve trunks (dorsal, anterior, etc.), the axons must also be responding to some extrinsic guidance cues. Further, because some degree of sorting out occurred even when the limb bud had been ablated (13), it was necessary to postulate the existence of some proximal guidance cues at the base of the limb, in addition to those possibly coming from the target muscles.

To test further the idea that limb motoneurons were responding to specific guidance cues, the normal spatial relationship between motoneurons and the limb was altered by *in ovo* surgery before motoneuron outgrowth (See Fig. 2). When motoneurons were displaced up to four segments by rotation of the neural tube about the anterior–posterior (A-P) axis, they invariably projected to their original muscle by making trajectory changes as they grew into the limb (14,15). We concluded that motoneuron pools possessed unique identities before axon outgrowth and that they were able to compensate for displacement by altering their direction of growth in response to environmental signals.

Additional perturbations [shifting or rotating the limb about the A-P (15) or D-V (16,17) axis] showed that motoneuron growth cones could make trajectory changes in response to signals along both axes of the limb. Finally, when an entire motoneuron pool was ablated, adjacent pools still projected to their own muscles, ignoring those that had been denervated (18). Apparently motoneurons were not constrained to their own territory by competing with each other. All these studies pointed strongly to the idea that motoneurons differed from one another in a way that allowed them to make divergent choices in response to environmental guidance cues. Although there have been some differences of opinion (16 vs. 19), the vast majority of data favors this basic interpretation not only for chicks, but for amphibians (20) and mammals (21) as well. In fact, in all major aspects these results are similar to those obtained on zebrafish, where the behavior of uniquely identified primary motoneurons has been determined after similar perturbations (4,22; see chapter by Eisen and Pike).

In contrast to these results, we found that when motoneurons were displaced greater distances and projected into the wrong plexus and a totally foreign limb environment, their growth cones often appeared unable to recognize specific guidance cues. The result was that they projected to a variety of foreign muscles, with no apparent pattern (10,15). Despite this, they followed the gross anatomical nerve pathways in the foreign region so that the shape of the plexus and major nerve

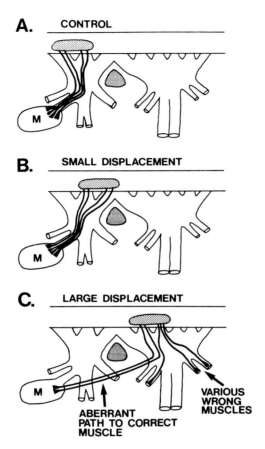

FIG. 2. Perturbations to study the mechanism of motoneuron pathfinding. **A:** A control moto-neuron pool is shown projecting to its muscle (M). **B:** Displacement of that motoneuron pool a short distance by early surgery results in axons making trajectory changes in the plexus region to reach their muscle. **C:** A larger displacement so that axons enter the wrong plexus results in many projecting to wrong muscles; however, some are apparently able to detect a specific cue and grow via an anatomically novel path directly to their muscle.

trunks was quite normal (Fig. 2C). This led us to make a distinction between specific guidance cues (signposts in the local language) and general guidance cues (permissive highways that any motoneuron could follow regardless of its ethnic identity).

Subsequent studies have further defined the highway system as being caused by inhibitory as well as permissive influences. The inhibitory regions, some of which correspond to precartilage (13) and also bind PNA (see chapter by Tosney), tend to channel axons into generally correct regions where they may then detect more specific cues (13). The role of such inhibitory influences in shaping neuronal circuitry

Never expressed on cell bodies or proximal axons, the 5E10 antigen first appears on the distal portion of some axons as they reach the plexus region. As can be seen in Fig. 3, it begins to be expressed by different subsets of motor as well as sensory axons at precise locations. These correspond to places where the axons in question would begin to respond to specific guidance cues (as inferred from our previous perturbation studies, refs. 6,8,15). Expression of this antigen, which appears to be a phosphorylated epitope, remains high along the course of these axons until they reach their targets, where it is down-regulated. In cultures of dissociated motoneurons, expression of this antigen could be induced by a variety of second-messenger activators (TPA, cyclicAMP, cyclicGMP, calcium ionophore) and tended to be confined to the base of the growth cone and immediately proximal axon (Fig. 3B), especially at places where axons tended to branch or make trajectory changes (S. Swain and L. Landmesser, *unpublished observations*). Its distribution (being confined to the core of the axon and growth cone and its abrupt and stable boundaries of expression) suggests that it may be associated with the cytoskeleton, although we have not yet identified the molecule. Much work reported in this volume (see chapters by Smith and Jahr, Bamberg et al., Gordon-Weeks and Mansfield, Diaz-Nido et al., and Goldberg et al.) has emphasized the importance of cytoskeletal assembly (tubulin, actin, etc.) in regulating axonal extension. It could also affect the direction of growth. In addition, the phosphorylation of cytoskeletal-associated proteins has been shown to be important in regulating cytoskeletal assembly. Thus although speculative, we postulate that detection of a specific guidance cue may result in the reorganization of the cytoskeleton of the growth cone, possibly mediated by second messengers and a phosphorylation event, so that axons grow toward the source of this cue, eventually reaching their target.

DO MOTONEURONS PROJECTING TO DIFFERENT TARGETS DIFFER FROM EACH OTHER?

In the spinal cord, two adjacent motoneurons that project to different muscles can have very different patterns of activation (35) because of differences in intraspinal connectivity; such motoneurons have also made divergent pathway choices during

---

FIG. 3. Expression of the 5E10 antigen. **A:** *In vivo* expression at Stage 28 shortly after axons have entered the limb. In both the crural and sciatic plexuses, the antigen is expressed (*shading*) at different spatial locations by different subsets of axons; these positions correspond to where axons are responding to specific cues. (A.D.T., anterior dorsal thigh; A.V.T., anterior ventral thigh; c., cutaneous nerve; m, muscle nerve; P.V.T., posterior ventral thigh; P.D.T.,posterior dorsal thigh; V.S., ventral shank; D.S., dorsal shank; F, foot. **B:** 5E10 expression on Stage 24 motoneurons dissociated and cultured for 2 days and evoked by TPA. *Left:* an antibody to NCAM stains the entire motoneuron uniformly; *right,* 5E10 expression is confined to distal axon and base of growth cone. Arrows indicate the same position in both left and right of **B.**

development. Clearly they must differ, presumably in the molecular composition of their cell surfaces. Yet numerous attempts by different laboratories to find such differences, mostly by generating monoclonal antibodies, have been disappointing. Although one cell surface antigen has been identified that is selectively and transiently expressed on all motoneurons during their period of outgrowth (36), none were found that distinguished subsets of motoneurons with a spatial pattern. Among the panel of antibodies that we recently generated are several that show quantitative spatial differences (i.e., higher levels of expression on crural as compared with sciatic axons), but overall the yield for this type of antigen was disappointing.

One possible explanation is that subsets are distinguished in some complex combinatorial manner so that a monoclonal against any given molecule fails to produce a meaningful pattern. We did obtain many monoclonals that recognized subsets of motoneurons but with no apparent spatial pattern. Alternatively, the molecules may be in low abundance or only weakly antigenic. Receptors for a chemotactic signal could be much less abundant than typical cell adhesion molecules such as L1, NCAM, or the fasciclins, which are fairly abundant membrane proteins.

Recently while studying another phenomenon, we discovered an unexpected difference between motoneurons. An antibody that recognizes the highly sialylated form of NCAM clearly distinguished motoneuron axons projecting to different limb regions. Axons projecting to dorsal thigh had high levels of polysialic acid (PSA), and those projecting to ventral thigh and shank had much lower levels (Fig. 4) (J. Tang, *unpublished observations*). What is the significance of this?

It is known that the degree of sialylation modulates the function of the NCAM molecule (37) and that levels of sialylation show complex spatial and temporal patterns of regulation during development (38). We recently demonstrated a strong correlation between PSA levels and the pattern of intramuscular nerve branching in chick muscle. More importantly, injection of an endosialidase that removed PSA produced changes in the branching pattern that were predicted by our hypothesis (38). In this and other studies, PSA has been shown to affect not only the function of NCAM, but that of other cell surface ligands such as L1 and laminin (37,38). This makes the point that the effective expression of a molecule can be modified without actually altering its genetic expression or even its concentration on the cell surface. The implications of this are rather frightening, especially when one is attempting to infer possible roles for a molecule based on its distribution. In addition, the fact that multiple cell surface ligands co-exist on the same cell and may interact in complex and as yet unknown ways (see chapter by Schachner) makes it difficult to predict the function of any given molecule in a complex developmental event even if a great deal is known about its structure and behavior in more simple tissue culture assays. Although the complexity is sobering, the approach of altering the function of specific molecules in intact tissue (*in vivo* or in slice preparations) by injection of antibodies or enzymes would seem to offer a useful approach.

What is the significance of the observed differences in PSA levels on limb axons during outgrowth? Based on previous work (37,38), it is likely that the differing levels of PSA will affect how these axons "see" their molecular world during out-

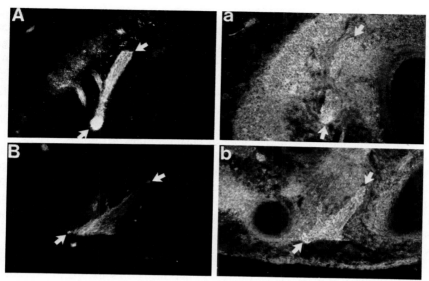

FIG. 4. Polysialic acid is differentially distributed in dorsal and ventral nerve trunks. The dorsal nerve trunk in this Stage 30 frozen cross section stains intensely with the 5A5 antibody that recognizes polysialic acid (**A**), whereas the ventral nerve trunk (**B**) stains only weakly. Adjacent sections (**a,b**) stained to reveal NCAM show no differences between trunks. Nerve trunks are indicated by arrows.

growth into the limb and might allow them to respond differently to a common signal. Further speculation is unwise in view of the complexities discussed above. We are now in the process of injecting endosialidase to remove the PSA during axon outgrowth and to determine its effect on the specificity of motor projections. It will also be interesting to determine how these differences in PSA levels (on motoneurons of the same age and similar spatial position) are brought about. In summary, however, the unexpected finding of such differences suggests the possibility that other carbohydrate modifications of known axonal cell surface molecules may occur and may play some role in axon guidance.

FUTURE DIRECTIONS

A pleasing consequence of the considerable work carried out in the past decade and reflected in this volume is that we are now able to pose questions on growth cone guidance in terms of known molecules and events whose cellular consequence cannot only be known but actually interfered with. For example, an increase in calcium caused by some contact-mediated event or second messenger may activate certain protein kinases, which alter specific molecules, which in turn affect a defined event such as cytoskeletal assembly. Advances in imaging technology now provide the potential to observe gowth cone behavior in intact tissue both normally and after precise perturbations.

With respect to the chick limb, the molecular nature of both the inhibitory and permissive signals that define the highway system is being elucidated. Additional studies, especially those involving perturbation of molecules in intact tissue, should greatly increase our understanding of these "nonspecific" cues. As for the specific cues, we have identified an antigen whose expression is a downstream consequence of a growth cone responding to a specific cue. Hopefully this can serve as a conduit to understanding the cellular basis of a growth cone turning in response to a specific cue (e.g., to gradients of known molecules such as cyclicAMP) (see chapter by Poo and Quillan) and eventually to those involved in guidance within the embryo. This will require determination of the molecular nature of the specific cues as well as the receptors on growth cones that detect them. Given the available tools, real progress in understanding growth cone guidance seems attainable, given one keeps in mind the probable real complexity that exists in the developing embryo and thereby avoids overly simplistic solutions.

ACKNOWLEDGMENTS

I would like to thank Steve Swain and Ji-cheng Tang, who allowed me to report some of their unpublished observations, and Liviu Cupceancu for his technical assistance and help with the artwork. This work was supported by NIH grant NS 10640 and a Wiersma Professorship from CalTech.

REFERENCES

1. Hamburger V. The development and innervation of transplanted limb primordia of chick embryos. *J Exp Zool* 1939;80:347–389.
2. Landmesser L, O'Donovan M. The activation patterns of embryonic chick motoneurons projecting to inappropriate muscles. *J Physiol Lond* 1984;347:189–204.
3. Bastiani MJ, Doe CQ, Helfand SL, Goodman CS. Neuronal specificity and growth cone guidance in grasshopper and *Drosophila* embryos. *Trends Neurosci* 1985;8:257–266.
4. Westerfield M, Eisen J. Neuromuscular specificity: pathfinding by identified motor growth cones in a vertebrate embryo. *Trends Neurosci* 1988;11:18–22.
5. Lance-Jones C. The effect of somite manipulation on the development of motoneuron projection patterns in the embryonic chick hindlimb. *Dev Biol* 1988;126:408–419.
6. Lance-Jones C, Landmesser L. Pathway selection by embryonic chick lumbosacral motoneurons during normal development. *Proc R Soc Lond B* 1981;214:1–18.
7. Landmesser L. The development of motor projection patterns in the chick hindlimb. *J Physiol Lond* 1978;284:391–414.
8. Tosney K, Landmesser L. Specificity of motoneuron growth cone outgrowth in the chick hindlimb. *J Neurosci* 1985;5:2336–2344.
9. Bekoff A. Ontogeny of leg motor output in the chick embryo: a neural analysis. *Brain Res* 1976; 106:271–291.
10. Landmesser L, O'Donovan M. Activation patterns of embryonic chick hindlimb muscles recorded *in ovo* and in an isolated spinal cord preparation. *J Physiol Lond* 1984;347:189–204.
11. Landmesser L, Morris DG. The development of the functional innervation in the hindlimb of the chick embryo. *J Physiol Lond* 1975;249:301–326.

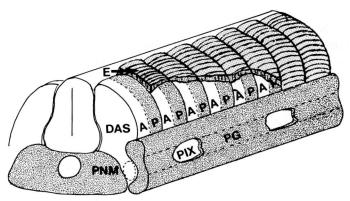

FIG. 3. Diagram of the spatial relations among tissues known to guide motor axons. Developing epaxial muscle (E) in each segment provides a specific cue that is essential only to the development of epaxial nerves. General cues that define the gross anatomical patterns of outgrowth are provided by paths (*white*) and barriers (*stippling*) such as the segmentally repeated anterior (A) and posterior (P) sclerotomes that dictate the anterior–posterior position of spinal nerves. The anterior sclerotome is subdivided into a path, dorsal–anterior sclerotome (DAS), and a barrier, perinotochordal mesenchyme (PNM), that dictate the dorsal–ventral position of spinal nerves. Beyond the somites, axons spread along the anterior–posterior axis in accord with the unsegmented distribution of a path tissue, the plexus mesenchyme (PIX; *dotted lines*), and then penetrate the barrier of the pelvic girdle (PG) through holes that dictate the positions where nerve trunks form. Anterior is to the left; dorsal is up.

rior sclerotome but not the more ventral sclerotome that surrounds the notochord, the *perinotochordal mesenchyme* (2,8) (Fig. 3). The barrier function of the perinotochordal mesenchyme was suggested by its position adjacent to the spinal nerve path and by its expression of markers typical of posterior sclerotome (2,10–12). Barrier function was experimentally established by rotating the neural tube to alter the initial direction of axon outgrowth to directly confront motor growth cones with perinotochordal mesenchyme (4). Under these conditions, growth cones turn to avoid the perinotochordal mesenchyme and project only through the dorsal–anterior sclerotome. Moreover, when the notochord is deleted, the perinotochordal mesenchyme does not develop barrier function or molecular markers for barrier function, and axons ramify within it (4).

As far as growth cones that extend into the limb are concerned, the role of the somites is limited. When somites are deleted, *only* the gross pattern of advance is disrupted (8). Growth cones still extend: Nothing essential to their outgrowth has been removed. Likewise, neural crest cells still advance and moreover condense to form sensory ganglia that are obviously abnormal only in their more extensive spatial distribution. Furthermore, because the specific projection of motor axons to limb muscles is normal in the complete absence of somites and of a segmented pattern of axon outgrowth, the specific cues can be dissociated from the general cues provided by the somites.

What, then, are the paths and barriers? Do all paths and all barriers have the same distinguishing features? A third set of tissues can be included when looking for such features; the plexus mesenchyme acts as a path, whereas the adjacent pelvic girdle precursor acts as a barrier (10) (Fig. 3). All path tissues (dorsal–anterior sclerotome, plexus mesenchyme, and limb paths) do appear to have a common developmental fate as connective tissue, differentially express butyrlcholinesterase and a 70-kDa membrane protein, and exhibit cell death and phagocytosis during axon outgrowth (4,12–15). Likewise, the three barrier tissues (posterior sclerotome, perinotochordal mesenchyme, and pelvic girdle precursor) all differentially express markers of early cartilage differentiation at the time growth cones and neural crest cells interact with them (4,16,17). Curiously, barriers as well as paths express molecules that are considered excellent substrata for axon advance including laminin, fibronectin, and NCAM (18–20). Therefore, paths are unlikely to be paths because they are the sole sites of suitable substrata. The differential fate of path and barrier tissues suggests that they may primarily assure that the gross anatomical nerve pattern is adapted to the developing architecture of the organism; growth cones will not advance through tissues that later form bone. Moreover, because many invasive populations respond independently and thus directly to the three sets of paths/barriers (e.g., refs. 4,19,21), it is reasonably likely that the mechanisms are the same in all cases.

A Developing Muscle Target that Provides a Specific Cue

The muscle targets within the proximal environment, the epaxial muscles, are innervated by epaxial motoneurons that lie medially in the spinal cord (2,3) (Fig. 1). Epaxial motor axons normally diverge from the spinal nerve path and extend directly toward their target (Figs. 2B and 4). Deletion of the dermamyotome shows that this muscle precursor is essential for the development of epaxial motor nerves (7). When the dermamyotome is deleted from a segment, the epaxial motor axons are deprived of target in that segment and form a nerve only when target is present in an adjacent segment. Moreover, these epaxial motor nerves are directed toward the closest target: Those with neighboring target to the anterior extend toward the anterior, and those with neighboring target to the posterior extend toward the posterior (Fig. 4, segments 2 and 4). In contrast, an epaxial nerve is never detected when dermamyotome has also been deleted in both adjacent segments (Fig. 4, segment 3), as though the epaxial growth cones were too distant from target to sense a diffusible cue required for their outgrowth. The dermamyotome is, however, irrelevant to the specific outgrowth of limb motor axons that continue to project to their appropriate muscles in the absence of dermamyotomes. Therefore, the dermamyotome provides a highly specific cue; it is essential only for the development of epaxial innervation. Likewise, there is less direct evidence that each muscle target in the limb exerts a short-range and specific attraction for the corresponding motor growth cones (e.g., refs. 22,23).

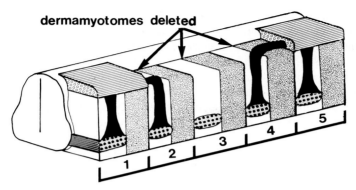

FIG. 4. Somites cut longitudinally in this diagram expose epaxial nerves and illustrate the effect of dermamyotome deletion on epaxial motor nerve formation. Epaxial motor axons (*black*) normally diverge from the spinal nerve path (*solid cylinders*) to enter muscle target (*hollow cylinders*) in the same segment, as shown in segments 1 and 5. Deletion of dermamyotomes before axon outgrowth has prevented development of target in segments 2, 3, or 4. Epaxial motoneurons in segments 2 and 4 extend into the closest target in an adjacent segment. Epaxial motor nerves do not form in segment 3, as though epaxial axons were too distant from target to detect an essential cue. Epaxial and limb motor axons traverse only anterior sclerotome (*white*) and avoid posterior sclerotome (*stippling*), regardless of the presence or absence of the dermamyotome. Anterior is to the left; dorsal is up.

The growth cones of epaxial motoneurons obey the constraints imposed by general cues even when they are responding to a specific cue simultaneously. For instance, when the only available target is in a posterior segment, epaxial growth cones do not take the most direct route toward it; they take a route that avoids the posterior sclerotome (Fig. 4, segment 4). The sclerotome is not, however, essential for the response to the target-related cue because the epaxial growth cones take the most direct route to target when sclerotome is deleted, even when the only available target is in an adjacent segment (8). Thus growth cones must normally respond independently and simultaneously to two classes of cues that are likely to be distinct molecular entities: general cues that determine where they can and cannot advance and more specific cues that determine the direction of travel.

THE PRESENT: IDENTIFICATION OF CELLULAR INTERACTIONS THAT MEDIATE GUIDANCE

Identification of the tissues that provide guidance cues opens abundant opportunities to investigate pathfinding mechanisms on cellular and molecular levels. Here I discuss the use of three *in vitro* assays to evaluate the roles of cellular interactions that may mediate both general and specific pathfinding in our system. This discussion is meant to exemplify the kinds of questions one can pursue—and, one hopes, answer—concerning cellular mechanisms of guidance once the relevant populations have been identified in any system. The potential success of each assay is predicated on the ability to view interactions directly and on the ability to make predictions about growth cone trajectory based on what we know of the cellular interactions that might mediate pathfinding.

Four classes of cellular interactions that are plausible candidates for guidance are first discussed for background. (a) Growth cones may respond to the physical organization of tissues, a mechanism termed *contact guidance*. However, extensive examination has failed to reveal obvious channels, alignments, or physical impediments in any path or barrier (2,24,25). The level of detection is sufficient to convince us to invest effort in defining differences at cellular and molecular levels. (b) All growth cone responses to diffusible substances will for simplicity be termed *chemotactic* interactions; these may be attractive or repulsive (see chapters by Lumsden and by Poo and Quillan). (c) Growth cone response to *direct contact* may be mediated by at least three different interactions. First, the reluctance of growth cones to enter barriers could be explained if their motility were actively inhibited by contact with barrier cells. We call this mechanism *contact paralysis*. It is a well-defined and obvious response to contact in which the growth cone collapses and transiently loses its ability to extend filopodia (26; see chapters by Raper et al. and Baier and Bonhoeffer). A second contact-dependent mechanism is *substratum preference*, defined by the growth cone's ability to discriminate among different substrata that all support outgrowth. When in contact with two such substrata, the growth cone exhibits a preference by ultimately extending only on one (27; see chapter by Letourneau, Bentley and O'Connor, Eisen and Pike, and Boloventa et al.). This mechanism is distinct from a third contact-dependent mechanism in which a substratum is *totally nonpermissive* and simply does not support outgrowth. (d) One cellular mechanism is not a reaction of growth cones to their environments but rather an action of growth cones on their environments. Proteolytic enzymes released by the growth cone could contribute to path/barrier function if paths were more susceptible to *proteolysis* and thus to growth cone penetration than were barriers (28; see chapter by Seeds et al.). We have yet to assess this possible mechanism in this system. I emphasize that there may be no single right answer; more than one of these mechanisms may contribute to pathfinding. In fact, the current work on cellular interactions strongly suggests that multiple mechanisms mediate general pathfinding.

Somite Strip Assay

An ideal assay to determine which of the cellular interactions described above are relevant to guidance would allow the researcher to watch growth cones as they interacted with the critical tissues. Unfortunately, when a somite is placed in culture it soon spreads out and forms a confusing pile of cells. We have surmounted this difficulty by developing an assay in which sclerotomes are exposed to view and yet retain their physical relationships and molecular characteristics in culture. We remove the viscera, notochord, and spinal cord from stage 17 embryos and cut strips of several somites. These *somite strips* are cultured ectoderm-side down on laminin. The ectoderm spreads on the laminin, but the somites do not spread on the ectoderm and the borders between and within somites remain visible. Because the notochord is essential for the development of barrier function in perinotochordal mesenchyme (4), omission of the notochord assures that the entire anterior sclerotome is functionally a path in culture and makes this assay highly suitable for investigating mechanisms of axonal segmentation. Motoneurons are labeled by injection of DiI (see ref. 29) into stage 21–24 spinal nerves, dissociated, and sprinkled over the exposed sclerotomes where they land at random. At present, we have analyzed neurite lengths and trajectories after 18 to 24 hr in culture (30).

A number of the cellular interactions that could mediate axonal segmentation predict that neurites would be longer on anterior than on posterior sclerotome halves in this assay, and this is clearly evident (Fig. 5). The ability to detect robust differences in neurite outgrowth on anterior and posterior sclerotome validates the use of this assay. Moreover, several of the possible interactions make unequivocal predictions concerning the trajectory of axons, as detailed below. This assay is thus particularly useful in identifying the most likely candidates for the vital cellular interactions, which may then be investigated more fully in assays designed particularly to document them.

1. If posterior sclerotome were the source of a diffusible, repellant molecule, we would expect neurites from motoneurons on anterior sclerotome to turn away from posterior sclerotome and to do so before contacting it. Such behavior is rarely seen, suggesting that there is no repellent molecule or that a gradient of such a molecule cannot be maintained in our cultures.

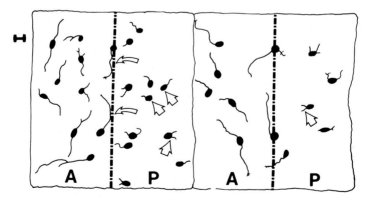

FIG. 5. Typical patterns of outgrowth from motoneurons labeled with DiI and deposited on somite strips. Motor neurites are consistently longer on anterior (A) than on posterior (P) sclerotome halves. Neurites from motoneurons on anterior sclerotome halves turn to avoid posterior halves and do so only after contact (*curved arrows*). In addition, neurites from motoneurons on posterior halves tend to be oriented toward the closest anterior half (e.g., *straight arrows*). Calibration bar, 10 μm.

2. If anterior sclerotome released a diffusible, attractive molecule, we would expect that neurites from motoneurons on posterior halves of sclerotomes would be oriented toward the closest anterior half, and such a preferential orientation is common [Fig. 5 (straight arrows)]. A long-distance cue may thus contribute to axonal segmentation. A substance may normally diffuse from anterior sclerotome in the embryo, or it may diffuse only under our culture conditions. We will follow-up this observation using the assay devised by Lumsden and Davies (31; see chapter by Lumsden), which is designed to maintain putative chemotactic gradients in culture.

3. If the posterior sclerotome were a completely nonpermissive substratum we would expect that few if any motoneurons would extend axons on posterior sclerotome. Because motoneurons consistently extend axons on posterior sclerotome (Fig. 5), we can confidently rule out the possibility that the posterior sclerotome is simply unable to support outgrowth.

4. This assay provides strong evidence for a contact-mediated mechanism. Neurites from motoneurons on posterior halves always cross to the anterior if they contact a border. Conversely, neurites from somata on anterior halves invariably turn to avoid posterior halves and only do so after contact [Fig. 5 (curved arrows)]. This behavior is consistent either with contact paralysis or with substratum preference, which may be distinguished using a dissociated cell assay (see below).

Furthermore, a comparison of neurite lengths on sclerotome populations and on other substrata in the same dish reveals differences that have intriguing implications for pathfinding. Despite a clear preference for extending on anterior rather than on posterior sclerotome, neurites grow much more robustly on the laminin substratum than on any portion of the somite strip. Moreover, neurite outgrowth is extensive on any remnants of the spinal cord's basal lamina and on the myotome. The rather reluctant growth of neurites even on anterior sclerotome suggests that this path tissue is a relatively hostile environment for motor axon extension and that the posterior sclerotome is more hostile than the anterior. The real choice confronting the growth cone is between awful (path) and worse (barrier).

Why would growth cones colonize an environment that appears to have so little to recommend it? First, life is hard. The choices facing a growth cone are limited, and awful is better than worse. Second, the growth cone may get a little help from its friends (see also ref. 2). The actual choice confronting a growth cone on its exit from the spinal cored is not merely between barrier and path; the choice is between barrier, path, and axon. To simplify, consider those growth cones that exit the spinal cord at a distance from anterior sclerotome. Their choice is limited to posterior sclerotome cells and axons. Because axons appear to be the very most favored substratum for growth cones (2), such growth cones are likely to turn along the anterior–posterior axis to fasciculate with their neighbors and to advance distally only on axons that have penetrated the more supportive anterior sclerotome. Moreover, fascicles of motor axons exiting the cord are larger in posterior than in anterior sclerotome (25), suggesting that fasciculation is enhanced in a barrier environment, possibly because posterior sclerotome is such a poor substratum. Fasciculation may therefore contribute to the avoidance of barrier tissues and construct an axonal scaffolding that aids in penetration of the path environment. The fasciculation would, however, only amplify rather than create path/barrier differences, and the functional differences in these environments must still be explained.

A second implication of the meager encouragement for advance offered by paths concerns the relationship between general and specific cues. If, as seems likely, even the paths are near the bottom of any hierarchy of substratum preference, specific cues may be provided by any one of an abundance of features that are more stimulatory to specific growth cone populations, such as more preferred substrata or population-specific diffusible cues. Because the basic path environment is so hostile, a wide range of more positive interactions is possible. Conversely, a cue that would cause a growth cone to exit from a common path could be provided by rendering the common path even more hostile for one specific population. There is evidence for such an interaction. Moorman and Hume (32) have shown that preganglionic sympathetic axons are specifically paralyzed on contact with sensory neurites that they would normally encounter in the region where they turn ventrally from the common path and travel toward the sympathetic ganglion.

Dissociated Cell Assay

Analysis of interactions using the somite strip assay suggests that substratum preference or contact paralysis is important to motor axon segmentation (see also ref. 33). To distinguish between these mechanisms, analysis of fixed cultures is insufficient; the interactions must be directly monitored over time. The initial results of such a study more strongly supports substratum preference (34). Typically, a motor growth cone will readily extend onto an anterior sclerotome cell even when grown on laminin, which is itself an excellent substratum (Fig. 6A,B,C). In contrast, a motor growth cone that contacts a posterior sclerotome cell remains on the laminin substratum and does not extend onto the surface of the cell (Fig. 6D,E,F). Motor growth cones in such video sequences exhibit a substratum preference for laminin = anterior sclerotome cells > posterior sclerotome cells. Moreover, the growth cone continues to extend filopodia enthusiastically after contact with the posterior sclerotome cell (Fig. 6E,F), a result inconsistent with a contact paralysis mechanism.

This culture system will make it possible to correlate the morphology of growth cones with their pathfinding behavior as they respond to these physiologically relevant choices. Do motor growth cones show consistent alterations in size, shape, or in protrusion and retraction of cell processes during the period when they are selecting a path over a barrier cell? Further, a more detailed analysis should show whether contact paralysis contributes in a less obvious way to barrier function. Molecules that elicit paralysis may be nonuniformly localized on barrier cells (35) and only inhibit individual filopodia that contact them. Such partial inhibition could slow rather than stop the forward movement of growth cones and might be sufficient to encourage growth cones to turn and avoid further contact with barrier cells. We are addressing this possibility by monitoring the rate of filopodial extension after contact with path versus barrier cells.

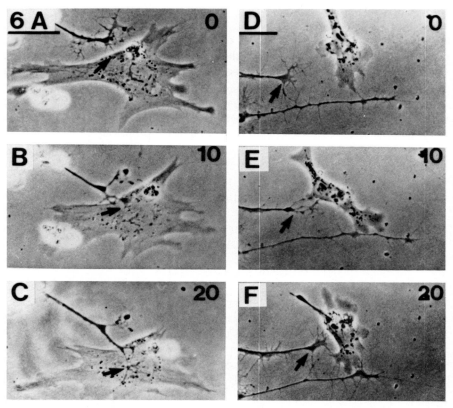

FIG. 6. Interactions between growth cones of motoneurons (*arrows:* identified as such by prior DiI label) and anterior (A,B,C) and posterior (D,E,F) sclerotome cells in dissociated culture. Elapsed time in minutes is shown at upper right. Growth cones exhibit a substratum preference by advancing readily onto anterior sclerotome cells and by failing to extend onto the surface of posterior sclerotome cells. Growth cones are not paralyzed by contact with posterior sclerotome cells and instead continue to extend processes (E,F). The identity of the bottom growth cone in D,E,F is not known. Calibration bars, 10 μm.

Slice Assay

Landmesser developed a most promising assay in which a 200- to 300-μm thick section or "slice" of an embryo can be maintained with apparently normal development for 2 days in culture, giving a time window sufficient for the examination of elements important to axon guidance (36). This slice assay is particularly suitable for monitoring *de novo* growth cone extension and thereby to documenting changes in the morphology and trajectory of growth cones as they proceed through a relatively unperturbed environment.

We have begun to use this assay to define interactions that mediate the specific response of epaxial motoneurons to their developing target. The surgical evidence favors chemotaxis but does not rule out a contact-mediated mechanism since epaxial nerves may have been absent in operated embryos because axons had retracted when they failed to contact target. The target may thus be essential because it supplies a diffusible cue or because it stabilizes those epaxial growth cones that contact it, similar to the stabilization by specific targets in the leech (see chapter by Wolszon and Macagno).

Epaxial growth cones are identified in a slice by their dorsal trajectories following injection of DiI into the ventral spinal cord (Fig. 7A), and individual growth cones can be monitored as they extend through the sclerotome toward the target (Fig. 7B).

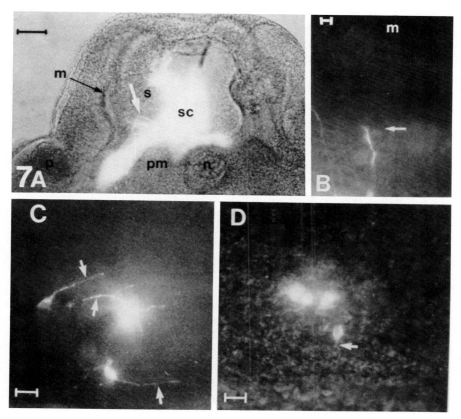

FIG. 7. A: A "slice," a 250-μm thick section through 3-day chick embryo, after 18 hr in culture. DiI injected into the spinal cord (sc) has labeled epaxial motor axons (*white arrow*) and motor axons in the spinal nerve path. m, myotome; n, notochord; p, pelvic girdle precursor; pm, perinotochordal mesenchyme; s, sclerotome. **B:** Epaxial growth cone (*arrow*) labeled with DiI extends toward the myotome (m) in a slice. **C:** Motoneurons labeled with DiI and deposited on an unlabeled slice have extended lengthy neurites (*arrows*) on dorsal–anterior sclerotome after 18 hr in culture. **D:** In contrast, motoneurons have extended only stubby neurites (*arrow*) on adjacent perinotochordal mesenchyme during the same time period. Calibration bars, **(A)** 50 μm; **(B,C,D)** 10 μm.

Moreover, it is much easier to surgically delete tissues from a slice than from an intact embryo. We plan to delete all but a few myotubes and thereby obtain a tiny, spatially localized target that we know to be sufficient for epaxial outgrowth in the organism (7). This surgery assures that a putative cue would diffuse from a highly localized source. If the target supplies a diffusible cue, we would predict that epaxial axons would extend directly toward the remaining myotubes. In contrast, if the target is essential because it stabilizes rather than attracts axons, we would expect random outgrowth and withdrawal or continued wandering of those growth cones that do not happen to contact target. Analysis of the axonal trajectories will thus allows us to define the mechanism of specific guidance for the epaxial population.

Once the mechanism is known, we should be able to document the dynamic alterations in growth cone form and correlate these with the behavior of the growth cone as it responds to the specific cue (for similar analyses in another system, see chapter by Bentley and O'Connor). For instance, if the cue is chemotactic, do the growth cones extend more processes toward the source of the cue, is the lifetime of processes enhanced on the side of the growth cone that is closest to the cue, do filopodia closest to the target become preferentially engorged to form the dominant growth cone, and does the size of the growth cone vary in a systematic way as it travels up the diffusion gradient? What is the morphological and behavioral consequence of a complete loss of target? If direct contact is important, is the growth cone prevented from wandering away because it becomes paralyzed on contact with its target (as suggested by its morphology *in vivo*; see ref. 3)?

The slice preparation can also be used to investigate directly growth cone interactions with various tissues that provide general guidance cues, regardless of the normal timetable of outgrowth, by sprinkling labeled, dissociated neurons on a slice. Using this approach, Landmesser has shown that the early limb is an inhospitable environment for axon advance (36) in accord with the global distribution of markers for barrier function in the early limb, which gradually disappear in paths before growth cones enter (12). We are using this method to address the cellular interactions that may mediate the function of a variety of paths and barriers. We find that motoneurons on dorsal–anterior sclerotome readily extend neurites (Fig. 7C) in contrast to those on perinotochordal mesenchyme, which extend wimpy neurites in the same slice (Fig. 7D). As in the somite strip assay, analysis of neurite lengths, trajectories, and behavior at borders between paths and barriers, both in fixed slices and with time-lapse video, should allow us to distinguish relevant mechanisms and to determine whether the mechanisms are the same for all sets of paths and barriers.

THE FUTURE: IDENTIFICATION OF MOLECULAR MECHANISMS

The cellular interactions that may mediate pathfinding each predict that different types of molecules are important and thus focus research toward particular classes of molecules. For instance, if a path, a barrier, or a target provides a diffusible cue, it would be reasonable to assess the contribution of known tropic molecules and to search for novel factors. A contact paralysis mechanism implies that there is a single ligand in a barrier tissue and a common receptor on the responding populations. The most likely candidate for a common ligand is one of the molecules that binds to peanut agglutinin lectin, as recently reviewed in more detail elsewhere (37; see also ref. 35). Substratum preference is thought to be caused by the cellular averaging of all the substratum contacts that a growth cone makes and therefore implies that all the potential substratum molecules within a path/barrier set of tissues could contribute to guidance. If substratum preference is shown to contribute to general guidance, it would be important to determine the hierarchy of growth cone preference for the various molecular substrata within each path and barrier and to ask if some molecules typical of barriers mask molecular binding sites that would otherwise provide preferred substrata. In addition, systematic analysis of the susceptibility of path components to enzymes released by growth cones could be informative.

If the sets of cellular interactions that mediate the response of a variety of growth cones turn out to be the same sets for all three sets of paths/barriers, it will then be vital to determine whether the mechanisms are the same or different at the molecular level. A likely starting point would be to investigate molecules that are typical of early cartilage differentiation and of all three of the experimentally defined barriers (including molecules that bind peanut agglutinin lectin), many of which are known to discourage neurite advance in culture (see ref. 4). Such markers have also been found to be transiently expressed in several other cell populations during the periods when these are also suspected to act as barriers (see ref. 4) such as the dermis (17), the roof plate (38), the barrel cortex (39), and oligodendrocytes (40). This raises the intriguing possibility that the molecular mechanisms of general guidance may turn out to be widely applicable.

The bioassays that have been developed to define the cellular mechanisms of guidance can be easily adapted to the job of assessing the functional significance of various molecular species. For instance, application of enzymes, addition of lectins or sugars, and use of function-blocking antibodies could implicate particular molecular species if they abolished the ability of growth cones to respond to guidance cues. Initial efforts to do so are now underway. Ultimately, one would like to know how physiologically relevant molecular signals are transduced at the growth cone surface to alter the form and trajectory of the growth cone. Once the molecular mechanisms of guidance are identified, we should be able to make excellent use of the parallel work on transduction mechanisms that are reviewed in Section 2 of this volume.

ACKNOWLEDGMENTS

Work in the author's laboratory is supported by NIH grants NS-21308 and NS-27634. Robert Oakley is thanked for his usual useful discussions and for the use of his unpublished figures (Figs 2B and 5).

REFERENCES

1. Lance-Jones CJ, Landmesser LT. Pathway selection by chick lumbosacral motoneurons during normal development. *Proc R Soc Lond B* 1981;214:1–18.
2. Tosney KW, Landmesser LT. Development of the major pathways for neurite outgrowth in the chick hindlimb. *Dev Biol* 1985;109:193–214.
3. Tosney KW, Landmesser LT. Growth cone morphology and trajectory in the lumbosacral region of the chick embryo. *J Neurosci* 1985;5:345–358.
4. Tosney KW, Oakley RA. Perinotochordal mesenchyme acts as a barrier to axon advance in the chick embryo: implications for a general mechanism of axon guidance. *Exp Neurol* 1990;109:75–89.
5. Detwiler SR. An experimental study of spinal nerve segmentation in *Amblystoma* with reference to the plurisegmental contribution to the brachial plexus. *J Exp Zool* 1934;67:395–441.
6. Keynes RJ, Stern CD. Segmentation in the vertebrate nervous system. *Nature* 1984;310:786–789.
7. Tosney KW. Proximal tissues and patterned neurite outgrowth at the lumbosacral level of the chick embryo: deletion of the dermamyotome. *Dev Biol* 1987;122:540–588.
8. Tosney KW. Proximal tissues and patterned neurite outgrowth at the lumbosacral level of the chick embryo: partial and complete deletion of the somite. *Dev Biol* 1988;127:266–286.
9. Stern CD, Keynes RJ. Interactions between somite cells: the formation and maintenance of segment boundaries in the chick embryo. *Development* 1987;99:261–272.
10. Tosney KW, Landmesser LT. Pattern and specificity of axonal outgrowth following varying degrees of chick limb bud ablation. *J Neurosci* 1984;4:2158–2527.
11. Oakley RA, Tosney KW. Peanut agglutinin (PNA) binds to tissues that act as barriers to axon advance in the chick embryo. *Soc Neurosci Abstr* 1988;14:870.
12. Oakley RA, Tosney KW. Peanut agglutinin and chondroitin-6-sulfate are markers for tissues that act as barriers to axon advance. *Dev Biol (in press)*.
13. Layer PG, Alber R, Rathjen FG. Sequential activation of butyrul-cholinesterase in rostral half somites and acetylcholinesterase in motoneurons and myotomes preceding growth of motor axons. *Development* 1988;102:387–396.
14. Tanaka H, Agata A, Obata K. A new membrane antigen revealed by monoclonal antibodies is associated with motoneuron axonal pathways. *Dev Biol* 1989;132:419–435.
15. Tosney KW, Schroeter S, Pokrzywinski JA. Cell death delineates axon pathways in the hindlimb and does so independently of neurite outgrowth. *Dev Biol* 1988;130:558–572.
16. Oakley RA, Tosney KW. Evidence for the delineation of axon pathways by inhibitory boundaries. *Soc Neurosci Abstr* 1991;16:1006.
17. Schroeter S, Lasky C, Oakley RA, Tosney KW. Evidence for the delineation of neural crest migration pathways by inhibitory boundaries. *Soc Neurosci Abstr* 1990;16:313.
18. Rogers SL, Edson KJ, Letourneau PC, McLoon SC. Distribution of laminin in the developing peripheral nervous system of the chick. *Dev Biol* 1986;113:429–435.
19. Rickmann M, Faucet J, Keynes R. The migration of neural crest cells and the growth of motor axons through the rostral half of the chick somite. *J Embryol Exp Morphol* 1985;90:437–455.
20. Tosney KW, Watanabe M, Landmesser L, Rutishauser U. The distribution of NCAM in the chick hindlimb during axon outgrowth and synaptogenesis. *Dev Biol* 1986;114:437–452.
21. Landmesser L, Honig MG. Altered sensory projections in the chick hind limb following the early removal of motoneurons. *Dev Biol* 1986;118:511–531.
22. Lance-Jones CJ, Landmesser LT. Pathway selection by embryonic chick motoneurons in an experimentally altered environment. *Proc R Soc Lond B* 1981;214:19–52.
23. Lance-Jones CJ. Motoneuron axon guidance: development of specific projections to two muscles in the embryonic chick limb. *Brain Behav Evol* 1988;31:209–217.
24. Tosney KW. Somites and axon guidance. *Scan Microsc* 1988;2:427–442.
25. Dehnbostle D, Tosney KW. Initial axon outgrowth. *Soc Neurosci Abstr* 1990;16:1006.
26. Kapfhammer JP, Raper JA. Collapse of growth cone structure on contact with specific neurites in culture. *J Neurosci* 1987;7:201–213.
27. Letourneau P. Cell-to-substrate adhesion and guidance of axonal elongation. *Dev Biol* 1975;44:92–101.
28. Kryostosek A, Seeds NW. Peripheral neurons and Schwann cells secrete plasminogen activator. *J Cell Biol* 1984;98:773–776.
29. Honig MG, Hume RI. Fluorescent carbocyanine dyes allow living neurons of identified origin to be studied in long-term culture. *J Cell Biol* 1986;103:173–187.

during navigation to both sides of the neuraxis, and the arrest of elongation on encountering target cells in target regions. With the optic chiasm in the mouse retinal axon pathway as a model for axon divergence and the mouse cerebellum as a model for target cell interactions and selection, we have investigated how the different shapes of growth cone that develop during these phases mirror behavior and cell–cell interactions. Second, we have begun to examine the cellular and molecular basis of cues that instigate changes in trajectory and cessation of extension.

DIVERGENCE OF CROSSED AND UNCROSSED FIBERS IN THE OPTIC CHIASM: GROWTH CONE INTERACTIONS AT THE MIDLINE

In the development of pathways in the CNS, the mechanisms underlying the bilateral distribution of fibers, or decussation, in the visual system and other partially crossed paths are poorly understood. In the visual system of higher vertebrates, most axons, generally deriving from nasal retina, cross through the optic chiasm to targets on the opposite side of the brain, whereas a smaller proportion, in mouse deriving from inferior temporal retina, remain on the same side of the brain (26). We therefore examined whether growth cones mediating these trajectories have different configurations, especially where they grow apart from each other within the optic chiasm.

Labeling neurons in fixed brain with lipophilic dyes (27) provided an experimental approach to this issue in embryonic brain at the time the retinal axons were extending toward their targets. Localized injections of the carbocyanine dye DiI were made in various parts of the retina, yielding labeling of a small number of fibers. The results of this study (28) supported our previous observations (11) that the majority of growth cones from both populations became more complicated, with filopodial appendages and more spread bases, as fibers entered the chiasm (Fig. 2).

The most striking difference between the two populations was the trajectory of the uncrossed fibers. Ipsilateral-projecting axons from inferior temporal retina do not travel directly into the ipsilateral optic tract, nor do they travel separately or at different times than the contralaterally projecting fibers (29,30). Instead, these fibers travel with crossing fibers toward the midline, then make a sharp turn back toward the ipsilateral side, generally within 150 to 200 μm proximal to the midline. As they turn, these fibers develop elaborate growth cones, spreading and extending along an unseen barrier, as though they are unable to penetrate it (Fig. 2 and 3). The form of these elaborate growth cones closely resembles those seen *in vitro* along the border of a preferred and nonpreferred substrate (31).

Real-time video recordings of the behavior of living retinal ganglion cell axons have confirmed the existence of the different morphologies of growth cones (32). After DiI is injected into selected ganglion cells in a semi-intact preparation including the eye, optic nerves, and ventral slab of brain, the axons are viewed in the chiasm with fluorescence optics and an image-intensifier video camera. Time-lapse recordings are made over 3 to 20 hrs at both low and high power. These experiments

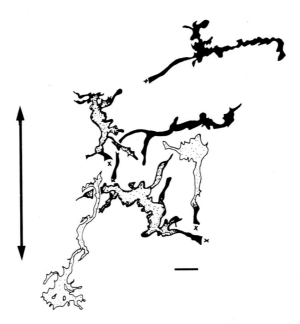

FIG. 3. Drawing of highly complex retinal axon growth cones at midline of the optic chiasm. Retinal ganglion cells were labeled in inferior temporal retina of fixed brain with DiI, at E16. Static and real-time observations suggest that most axons from this part of the retina will grow to a zone along the midline, retract and advance a number of times, then make a sharp turn. Three forms are evident: spread forms, which advance and retract (see Fig. 4) (*lightly stippled*); more complex and branched forms (*darkly stippled*), the topmost one extending along the axis of the midline (*arrow*); more slender forms, having already turned (*filled*). Bar, 10 μm.

show, first, that within the chiasm, axons that grow relatively straight ahead, including fibers that have already turned or those that are crossing, grow rapidly, up to 100 μm/hr. Second, even during straight growth, growth cones constantly change their form. These observations match the recent characterization of growth cone behavior in other intact or semi-intact vertebrate nervous systems (33–36).

The form and behavior of growth cones at the midline mimics a "soft battering ram," as Ramón y Cajal described the behavior of growth cones that he viewed in static preparations (37). Growth cones of fibers labeled in the inferior temporal retina, presumably destined to remain ipsilateral, extend up toward the midline and hesitate. They advance, pause, and retract several times, all the while having a spread shape (Fig. 4). After several hours of this behavior, Y-shaped and branched growth cones develop, extending along the contours of a line parallel to the midline (28). Finally, a filopodium forms, pointing toward the ipsilateral optic tract; a new growth cone develops at the tip of the "backward" filopodium and rapidly extends. The establishment of a new growth direction by a single filopodium has also been observed in the grasshopper (see chapter by Bentley and O'Connor).

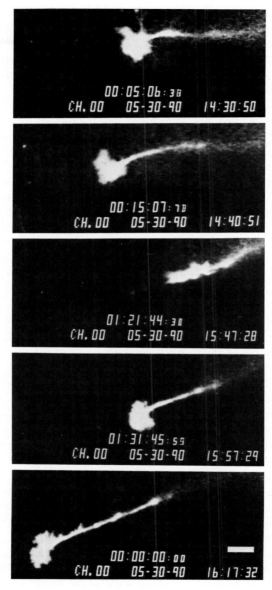

FIG. 4. Repeated advance and retraction of retinal axon growth cones of the optic chiasm, recorded in real-time. The behavior of DiI-labeled growth cones was observed with an intensified video camera and an optical disc recorder. Bar 10 μm.

To understand what cues might be present at the midline, the point in the path where the most dramatic shape transformations occur as fibers turn back, we investigated the cellular composition of this locale by immunohistochemistry and antisera to a variety of glial and neuronal surface antigens (38). These studies revealed a palisade of radial glia-like cells that curves from the bottom of the third ventricle around the midline, spanning 100 to 200 μm to either side of the midline and corresponding to the zone near the midline that uncrossed fibers never penetrate. The principal marker that has demarcated this midline structure is RC2, which stains radial glia in the mouse CNS (39). In sections double-labeled for RC2 and DiI, crossing axons pass through the RC2-positive palisade, and ipsilaterally projecting axons make their turn at the border of the palisade.

Examination of identified dye-labeled growth cones in the electron microscope (Fig. 5) suggests that cells of the chiasm provide cues for the turning of uncrossed fibers (38). As we saw earlier in the optic nerve, growth cones with straight trajectories within the chiasm have more streamlined and long forms, which signifies fasciculation with other axons (11) (Fig. 5A). Growth cones captured in the act of turning contact many other neurites and interdigitate with numerous small profiles, candidates for the fibers comprising the glial palisade (Fig. 5B). These analyses have provided strong support for cues in the midline region that might be comprised of glial cells bearing molecules that inhibit growth of fibers destined to remain ipsilateral but not those that cross. In addition to the glial palisade, dye-filled turning growth cones course around cells with scant cytoplasm that appear to be RC2-negative. The identity of these cells is currently under investigation.

The occurrence of a palisade of radial glia at the midline has precedent in the spinal cord. The floor plate of the chick and mouse spinal cord acts as a permissive site for crossing of the commissural axons (20,21,41; see chapter by Lumsden). In zebrafish, whereas the commissural axons traverse the floor plate, other populations are inhibited from entering it (40). The floor plate of the mouse spinal cord shares some antigenic determinants with the midline palisade in the chiasm (C. Mason, P. Godement, and J. Dodd, *unpublished*). Other midline structures (e.g., the dorsal roof plate) apparently play only an inhibitory role (42). All these midline structures occur at sites where axon populations change their direction of growth.

The midline glial structure is one possible cue for the turning of uncrossed fibers. A second is fiber–fiber interactions, suggested by removal of one eye. If enucleation is performed before the period of axonal outgrowth, at E13, the fibers from inferior temporal retina that would normally cross grow toward the midline and stall here (28). This confirms that the midline region contains an inhibitory cue for fibers with an uncrossed destination. Because these fibers do not aberrantly cross or grow back normally in the absence of crossing fibers from the other eye, a two-step mechanism for guidance of uncrossed fibers is implicated, a cue at the midline impeding growth and a cue for growth with fibers from the other eye once the turn is made. Additional support comes from ultrastructural observations, that turning growth cones contact numerous fascicles of fibers, each oriented at different angles (Fig. 5B).

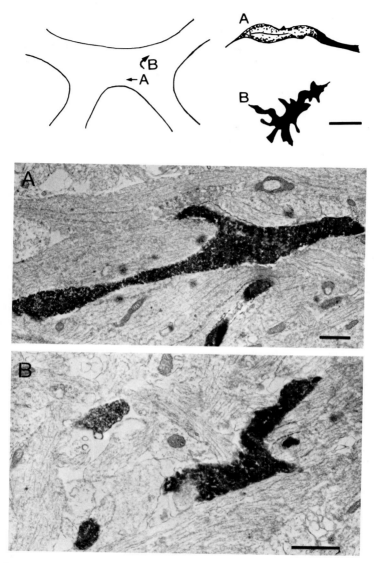

FIG. 5. Cellular relations of a straight-growing and a turning growth cone in the optic chiasm. Axons were labeled with DiI and preparations were photoxidized to render the DiI electron-dense. **Inset** shows the optic chiasm at low power, and right-hand drawings show detail of growth cones A and B. Growth cone A aims straight and is more streamlined. In the electron micrograph, it is interposed with other axons in a fascicle, the common relationship for such a shape of growth cone. Growth cone B has a more complex shape and appears to be in the act of turning. This growth cone contacts many axonal and radial glial fibers (cut in different planes of section). Bar in drawing, 10 μm, in micrographs, 1 μm.

Thus, in these studies, we have defined two cues, one glial and the other axonal, manifested by the highly complex growth cones seen at the midline of the optic chiasm on fibers that will remain on the same side of the brain. From static DiI-labeled material, we deduced that the complex spread and branched growth cones effected a turn, verified by the observations of living growth cones in real-time. Immunocytochemical and electron microscopical studies have implicated a midline structure composed of immature glia as a candidate cue for the turning back of uncrossed fibers. *In vitro* studies are in progress to characterize the resident molecules and to test the role of the midline glial palisade and of fiber–fiber interactions as cues for the growth of uncrossed fibers within the chiasm.

AFFERENT GROWTH CONE–TARGET CELL INTERACTIONS IN THE CEREBELLUM

Whereas the retinal pathway provides information on guidance in pathways, the developing cerebellum provides a model for axon–target interactions. Target cells are readily identified, and their genesis, migration and differentiation are well-characterized. Moreover, cell-specific markers, particularly for Purkinje cells, are available, and *in vitro* methods have been developed to purify and culture target cells.

Coordination of Afferent Axon Ingrowth and Target Cell Development

A first step in unraveling growth cone–target cell interactions was to define the temporal and spatial features of afferent axon growth into this target region. In most regions of the CNS, even though axons can now be labeled in fetal brain with the carbocyanine dyes, their target cells are difficult to localize. Thus, the coordination of afferent ingrowth and target cell migration is generally not well understood. To accomplish this, we examined the ingrowth of the climbing fiber afferents from the inferior olivary nuclei and the time course of migration of their target Purkinje cells in embryonic mouse cerebellum (43–45). Climbing fibers were selectively labeled by injecting DiI into the inferior olivary nucleus in the brainstem, and Purkinje cells

---

FIG. 6. Three stages of cerebellar axon–target interactions: growth cone forms and position and interaction-specific. **A:** At E15, Purkinje cells (*arrow*), labeled with antisera to calbindin, are clustered near the ventricular zone. **B:** DiI-labeled olivocerebellar fibers, the future climbing fibers, arrive at the borders of the cerebellar anlage (*arrow*). **C:** Their axons are tipped with large tapered growth cones (*arrows*) similar to those in tracts in other systems. **D:** At E16–17, Purkinje cells are migrating away from the ventricular zone (*arrow*); **E:** olivocerebellar axons enter the anlage (*arrow*) and mingle with migrating cells, rather than "waiting." **F:** Complex growth cones, typical of those in other decision regions are common; **G:** many axons bear small tapered growing tips, near the entry zone and in the zones near the pia where Purkinje cells have settled. **H:** By E19, Purkinje cells have settled into a wide band 5–8 Purkinje cells thick (*arrow*). **I:** Olivocerebellar fibers project into this band (*arrows*). **J:** All axons in this zone have small tapered tips. Bar in **A, B, D, E, H, I,** 100 mm; in **C, F, G, J,** 10 mm.

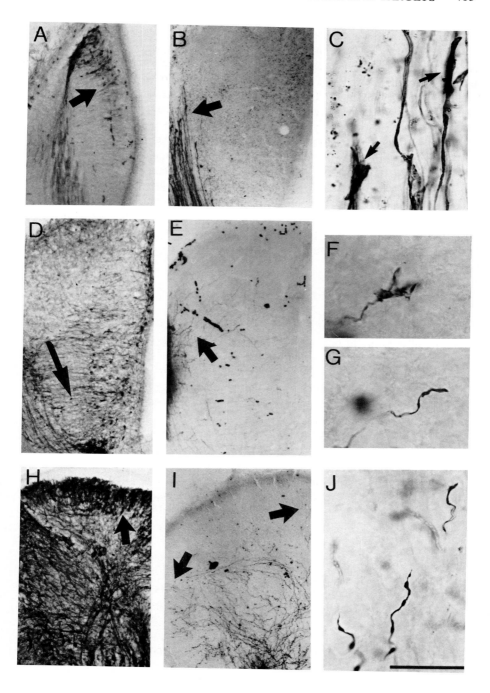

were localized with a Purkinje cell–specific antigen, calbindin 28-K, in the same or age-matched preparations (Fig. 6).

The schedule of events is as follows: Purkinje cells arise in the proliferative zone lining the fourth ventricle between E11 and E13 and migrate out into the cerebellar cortical plate from E15–17. By E15, the olivocerebellar afferents are positioned to enter the anlage in a broad tract at the border of the cerebellar anlage (Fig. 6 A,B). From E16–17, these axons exit the tract into the anlage, growing toward lanes of migrating Purkinje cells and toward zones of settled Purkinje cells beneath the developing external granule layer (Fig. 6D,E). By E18–19, all olivocerebellar axons project into the Purkinje cell settling zones, by now several cells thick (Fig. 6 H,I). Thus, climbing fiber afferents enter the cerebellar cortex just after target cell generation and contact target Purkinje cells during their migration and positioning. Climbing fibers, therefore, do not "wait" in zones before contacting targets, but rather contact targets straightaway after their migration and maintain simple terminations on the soma for several days before arborizing (43,44).

Growth Cone Form Within Targets Is Position- and Interaction-Specific

Having defined the timing of ingrowth of climbing fiber afferents and of migration and positioning of target Purkinje cells, we investigated whether the form of growing tips on olivary axons during the three phases of growth within targets is position-specific (45). When axons arrive at the boundaries of the cerebellar anlage at E15–16 but are still located within the tract, their growth cones are large, long (up to 30–40 μm), and foliate (Fig. 6C), similar to those in the optic nerve and tract of the retinal axon pathway during outgrowth (11). On exit from the tract and entry to the cerebellum at E16–17, growth cones become more complex (Fig. 6F): The base becomes foreshortened (10–15 μm), and filopodia develop. Distal to the entry zone, axons enter two regions: zones of settled Purkinje cells, and lanes of migrating Purkinje cells. In the settled zones, axon endings diminish considerably in size (1–5 μm), to small buds, beads, or unitary stick-like endings (Fig. 6G). By E19, when all olivocerebellar fibers project among the settled Purkinje cells, axons are relatively unbranched and still end in the bud-like endings seen at E17 in Purkinje cell zones (Fig. 6J).

To clarify whether these shapes of growth cone reflected different cell–cell relationships in each of these phases, we examined identified dye-filled growth cones in the electron microscope (45). The growth cones in tracts that are large and foliate relate primarily to fascicles of other axons that populate the tracts, as we saw in the retinal axon pathway. The complex growth cones in the entry zone and in regions where targets are migrating contact different profiles and other fascicles, either of radial glia and other axons (45; see chapter by Kalil and Norris), and profiles of unidentified cells. The simple, bud-like growth cones were invariably apposed to the soma of Purkinje cells in the zones where Purkinje cells settled. In the early part of the contact period (E17), a few specializations were seen, primarily postsynaptic.

35. O'Rourke NA, Fraser SE. Dynamic changes in optic fiber terminal arbors lead to retinotopic map formation: an *in vivo* confocal microscopic study. *Neuron* 1990;5:159–171.
36. Sretavan DW. Axon navigation at the mammalian optic chiasm: direct observation using fluorescent time-lapse video microscopy. *Soc Neurosci Abstr* 1990;16:1125.
37. Ramón y Cajal S. *Recollections of my life* (trans. E. Craigie). *Mem Am Philos Soc*, 1937; vol. 8. (Repr. MIT Press, 1989).
38. Mason CA, Misson JP, Blazeski R, Godement P. Retinal axon navigation in the mouse optic chiasm: midline cues and cell–cell relations (*Abstr*). *Soc Neurosci Abstr* 1990;16:1125.
39. Misson JP, Edwards M, Yamamoto M, Caviness, V. Identification of radial glial cells within the developing murine central nervous system: studies based upon a new immunohistochemical marker. *Dev Brain Res* 1988;44:95–108.
40. Kuwada JY, Bernhardt RR, Chitnis AB. Pathfinding by identified growth cones in the spinal cord of zebrafish embryos. *J Neurosci* 1990;10:1299–1308.
41. Dodd J, Jessell TM. Axon guidance and the patterning of neuronal projections in vertebrates. *Science* 1988;242:692–699.
42. Snow DM, Steindler DA, Silver J. Molecular and cellular characterization of the glial roof plate of the spinal cord and optic tectum: a possible role for a proteoglycan in the development of an axon barrier. *Dev Biol* 1990;138:359–376.
43. Mason CA, Christakos S, Catalano SM. Early climbing fiber interactions with Purkinje cells in the postnatal mouse cerebellum. *J Comp Neurol* 1990;297:77–90.
44. Mason CA, Christakos S, Blazeski R. Axon–target interactions in developing cerebellum: I. Afferent climbing fibers contact Purkinje cells during migration and positioning. (*submitted.*)
45. Mason CA, Blazeski R. Axon–target interactions in developing cerebellum. II. Growth cone shape in targets is position and interaction-specific. (*submitted.*)
46. Catalano S, Killackey HP. Early ingrowth of thalamocortical afferents to the neocortex of the prenatal rat. *Proc Natl Acad Sci USA* 1991;88:2999–3003.
47. Sperry RW. Chemoaffinity in the orderly growth of nerve fiber patterns and connections. *Proc Natl Acad Sci USA* 1963;50:703–710.
48. Baird DH, You Y, Friedman L, et al. Cerebellar afferent interactions with target and non-target cells *in vitro* (*Abstr*) *Soc Neurosci Abstr* 1989;15:1263.
49. Baird DH, Hatten ME, Mason CA. Target neurons and astroglia have opposing roles in modulating afferent neurite outgrowth. (*submitted.*)
50. Hatten ME. Neuronal regulation of astroglial morphology and proliferation *in vitro*. *J Cell Biol* 1985;100:384–396.
51. Wang L-C, Baird DH, Hatten ME, et al. Astroglial differentiation, not "age," is critical for neurite outgrowth (*Abstr*). *Soc Neurosci Abstr* 1990;16:1005.
52. Baptista CA, Hatten ME, Mason CA. Survival and differentiation of purified Purkinje cells from mouse cerebellum (*Abstr*). *Soc Neurosci Abstr* 1990;16:1150.
53. Baird DH, Baptista CA, Hatten ME, et al. Cerebellar mossy fiber, but not climbing fiber, elongation is interrupted by target neurons *in vitro* (*Abstr*). *Soc Neurosci Abstr* 1990;16:1127.
54. Kapfhammer JP, Raper JA. Collapse of growth cone structure on contact with specific neurites in culture. *J Neurosci* 1987;7:201–212.
55. Schwab ME, Caroni P. Oligodendrocytes and CNS myelin are non-permissive substrates for neurite outgrowth and fibroblast spreading *in vitro*. *J Neurosci* 1988;8:2381–2393.
56. Moorman SJ, Hume RI. Growth cones of chick sympathetic preganglionic neurons *in vitro* interact with other neurons in a cell-specific manner. *J Neurosci* 1990;3158–3164.
57. Cox EC, Muller B, Bonhoeffer F. Axonal guidance in the chick visual system: posterior tectal membranes induce collapse of growth cones from the temporal retina. *Neuron* 1990;4:31–37.
58. Furley AJ, Morton SB, Manalo D, Karagogeos D, Dodd J, Jessell TM. The axonal glycoprotein TAG-1 is an immunoglobulin superfamily member with neurite outgrowth promoting activity. *Cell* 1990;61:157–170.
59. Jessell TM. Adhesion molecules and the hierarchy of neural development. *Neuron* 1988;1:3–13.
60. Abercrombie M, Heaysman JM. Observations on the social behavior of cells in tissue culture. *Exp Cell Res* 1954;6:293–306.
61. Reichardt LF, Bossy B, Carbonetto S, et al. Neuronal receptors that regulate axon growth. *Cold Spring Harbor Symp Quant Biol* 1991;55 (*in press*).

anteroposterior plane. Rather, axons from contiguous areas of cortex that are closely bundled as they grow out of the cortex begin to diverge widely in the callosum as they approach the midline. Nor are axons projecting from opposite cortical hemispheres spatially segregated. Axons have highly individual undulations over broad areas of the callosum and do not fasciculate with their neighbors (Fig. 2). These results are consistent with ultrastructural studies showing that individual axons can continually change their relationships within fascicles (7,17). Second, we found that growth cones in the callosal tract assume a variety of complex morphologies (Fig. 3) that in size and shape are independent of their age and position in the corpus callosum. Growth cones are spread out with complex filopodial and lammellipodial extensions at all points along their trajectories. Given the tight packing of axons in the callosum and the straight unbranched trajectory of this tract, we expected that callosal axons would grow straight. Because previous studies had shown that the morphology of growth cones is roughly correlated with the architecture of their environment and the challenges they encounter (38), we expected that callosal growth cones would be simple and slender, rather than large and complex. In decision regions of various vertebrate pathways, where neurites alter their direction, such as the motor nerve plexus of the chick hindlimb (10), and the mouse optic chiasm (11,12), growth cones have elaborate morphologies. Although the corpus callosum lacks decision regions for the pathway as a whole, the complexity of individual growth cones could mean that each is acting as an independent decision-making entity, consistent with observations of independent navigation of growth cones in the visual pathway of *Xenopus* (8).

At the ultrastructural level, we found that growth cones do not make obligatory contacts with specific cells in the corpus callosum and therefore do not use cell-specific contacts as a means to navigate along this pathway (37). Electron microscopy revealed no specialized contacts between growth cone processes and other

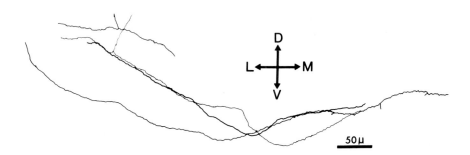

FIG. 2. Camera lucida drawing of callosal axons labeled with HRP injected into the sensorimotor cortex of a hamster at 38 hr postnatal. Fibers converge and diverge from one another in different regions of the callosum without fasciculating with neighboring axons. Note branching axons make right angle turns from different depths of the white matter toward cortex. Midline (M) to the right; contralateral cortex was injected.

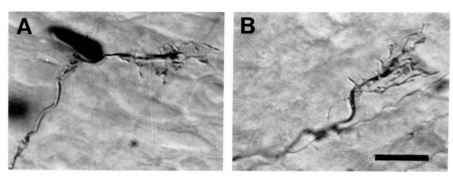

FIG. 3. Examples of HRP-labeled growth cones in the newborn hamster corpus callosum, illustrating complex lamellipodial (**A**) and filopodial (**B**) morphologies. Scale bar, 10 μm. Nomarski optics.

cellular elements, such a filopodial insertion into guidepost cells observed in the insect nervous system (39,40). The observation that individual growth cones could touch a large number of diverse cellular elements suggests that they are responding to broadly distributed molecular cues rather than to cues restricted to specific cell surfaces.

DECISION REGIONS

For both callosal and corticospinal pathways, an important decision region for individual axons is the point at which they leave the axon pathway and enter specific target regions. In the corpus callosum, axons can make turns at any dorsal–ventral depth. Callosal axons enter specific cortical regions in several ways. First, the main growth cone trailing its axon can make sharp right-angle turns toward cortical targets. Alternatively, a parent axon and its growth cone can continue along the callosal pathway while a side branch is directed at right angles toward the cortex (see Fig. 2). Side branches may be formed by bifurcation of growth cones within the white matter with one branch orienting toward the target and the second branch continuing to extend within the callosum (Fig. 4) or by back-branching.

By labeling corticospinal axons with DiI *in vivo*, we have examined the choice points at which corticospinal axons leave the dorsal column and enter the spinal target (R. Kuang and K. Kalil, *submitted*). As in the adult, topography of corticospinal connectivity during development is specific, and axons destined for lumbar segments never extend inappropriate branches into the cervical cord. Thus, as in the establishment of callosal connections, although modifications in arbor morphology and number of axons in the tract may occur later in development (31,32), the initial decisions to branch into targets are correct. As illustrated in Fig. 5 showing parasagittal views of the developing corticospinal pathway, several branches may

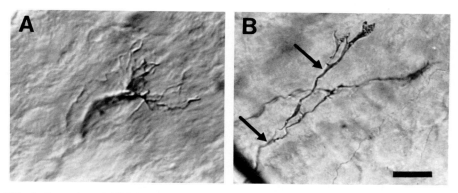

FIG. 4. Examples of HRP-labeled growth cones in the newborn hamster corpus callosum, showing bifurcation of growth cones within the tract. Growth cone in **B** contains two branches as indicated by *arrows*.

bud from a single axon that, as indicated by the presence of a growth cone at its tip, is still elongating. As in the adult hamster (41), such collateral branches innervate several consecutive segments of the spinal cord. In some instances, axons can also enter the spinal gray matter and extend longitudinally over several segments emitting collateral branches along the way. These observations suggest that decisions to enter targets need not be made by the growth cone of the primary axon but may, as previously demonstrated by O'Leary and Terashima (21), involve budding of side branches, sometimes tipped with small growth cones.

WAITING PERIODS

Previous studies have concluded that axons, before entering a target, may "wait" outside targets before growing into them. Waiting of afferent axons outside the rodent cortex, for example, can last for as long as 1 week (19). In contrast, our results obtained with the sensitive DiI label describe growth of callosal axons into the hamster sensorimotor cortex (C. Norris and K. Kalil, *submitted*) and show that axons wait no more than a few hours before entering the cortex. Thus, there is no significant temporal delay between the arrival of callosal axons at the opposite hemisphere at 36 hr and their actual invasion of the cortical gray matter beginning at 2 days postnatal. Further evidence against waiting of callosal afferents in the white matter was the slow and steady growth of callosal axons toward the cortical plate once they had entered the cortical gray matter (C. Norris and K. Kalil, *submitted*). The formation of interstitial axon collaterals from corticospinal fibers (R. Kuang and K. Kalil, *submitted*) may mean that, as in development of corticopontine projections (21), the actual "waiting period" is a delay between the growth of the main axon past the target and the interstitial budding of collaterals. Whether branching occurs interstitially or by splitting of the major growth cone, waiting periods by

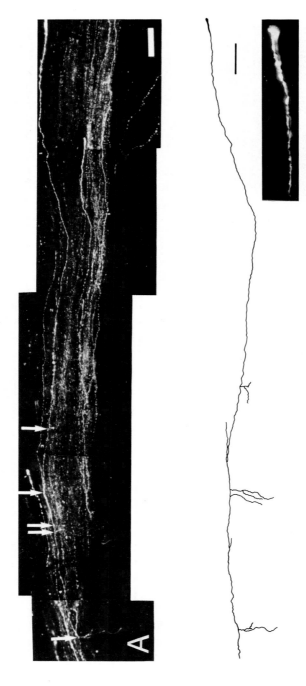

FIG. 5. Parasagittal views of the developing hamster corticospinal tract labeled with DiI. *Arrows* in photomicrographs show points at which branches extend from the axon, as illustrated in matching camera lucida drawings. Scale bars, 200 μm. **A:** Growth cone (shown at higher power in **inset**) with branching from its axon occurring about 2 mm proximal to the growth cone. Figure shows five segments of the lumbar enlargement at 8 days postnatal. **B:** Multiple branching of collaterals from a single axon into multiple spinal segments of the cervical cord at 7 days postnatal. Figure shows four segments of the cervical enlargement.

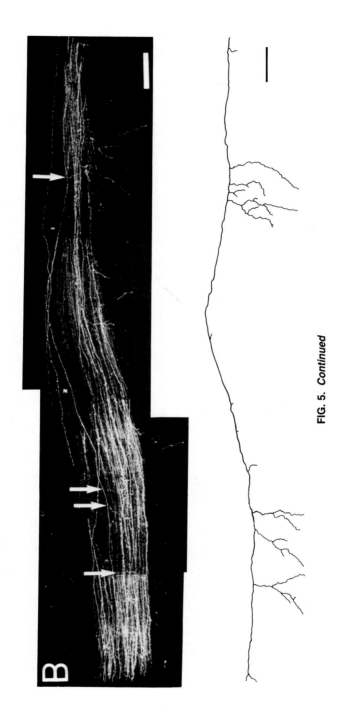

FIG. 5. *Continued*

corticospinal axons outside spinal targets appear to be no more than a few hours. Observations of corticospinal axon outgrowth in hamster littermates sacrificed at half-day intervals show that as axons reach a given level of the cord, branching into targets begins to occur (R. Kuang and K. Kalil, *unpublished observations*). In some cases branching occurs a few millimeters behind the major growth cone (Fig. 5). This revised notion of waiting periods, however, may be more applicable to the rapid neural development of the rodent in contrast to the prolonged embryonic growth of the primate brain.

ESTABLISHMENT OF TERMINAL DOMAINS BY CALLOSAL AND CORTICOSPINAL GROWTH CONES

Growth cones in the corpus callosum exhibit a variety of large and complex morphologies, whereas those that have entered the cortex become dramatically smaller and simpler (37) (Fig. 6) and more uniform in morphology and size, averaging about one-third the length of those in the callosum. Moreover, calculations of the speed of extension by growth cones in the callosum (60 μm/hr) versus those in the cortex (5–6 μm/hr) showed at least a 10-fold difference in speed of growth cone extension in these two environments. What accounts for the dramatic decrease in the size and speed of callosal growth cones once they enter the cortex? One possibility is that in the cortex, growth cones are responding to a vastly different environment, and these responses are manifested by morphological shape changes. To examine the relationship of growing callosal afferent axons with the cellular elements of the developing cerebral cortex, we carried out an ultrastructural study in which

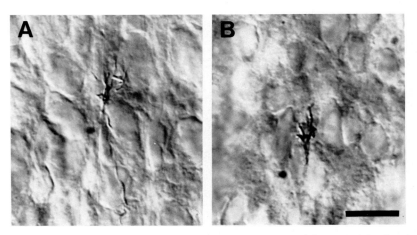

FIG. 6. Examples of HRP-labeled growth cones that have entered the contralateral cortex at 2.5 days postnatal. Note smaller, simpler morphologies. (Magnification is the same as in Fig. 3). Scale bar, 10 μm. Nomarski optics.

HRP-labeled axons and their growth cones that had entered the contralateral cortex were serial thin-sectioned in their entirety for electron microscopic analysis and then reconstructed (41a).

At 3 days postnatal, when these experiments were performed, the hamster sensorimotor cortex is extremely immature. Ultrastructurally, the developing cerebral cortex is organized in a pattern of "radial units" as defined by Rakic (26). In the coronal plane, a radial unit is bounded on either side by migrating cortical neurons and their associated fascicle of radial glia, which spans the cerebral wall from the ventricular to the pial surface and along which the neurons migrate (23,24). The region between two glial fascicles contains primarily small axons oriented perpendicular to the radially oriented glial fascicles. Radial glial processes were identified first by ultrastructural criteria such as their size, regular arrays of microtubules, and electron-lucent cytoplasm, and second, by the close association of migrating neurons with these processes.

An examination of the relationship of growing callosal axons and their growth cones to developing radial units revealed that, in all cases, the afferent axon was apposed to a continuous fascicle of radial glial fibers and that growth cones were associated with the same glial fascicle as their axon (Fig. 7). Growth cone processes often extended into the neuropil surrounding the radial glial fascicle with which its axon associated, but they never extended beyond glial fascicles bordering adjacent radial units. These observations suggest that radial glia, in addition to providing a scaffold for migration of cortical neurons, also provide a guidance mechanism for callosal growth cones and their axons as they extend through the developing neocortex. Tracking of callosal growth cones along radial glia could explain why callosal growth cones in the cortex have smaller, simpler morphologies and grow more slowly. A correlation between simple growth cone morphologies and tracking behaviors along other cellular processes has been noted in a variety of vertebrate and invertebrate neural pathways (38; see chapter by Mason and Godement). The guidance of afferent axons by radial glia could provide a mechanism for connecting callosal axons with their appropriate "ontogenetic columns" in the contralateral cortex. Neurons that become organized into functional cortical columns by migrating along the same radial glia would also become innervated by topographically appropriate afferent axons extending along these same glia (Fig. 8). This mode of axon guidance necessitates the presence on glial fascicles of molecular cues recognized by topographically appropriate callosal afferents. At present the nature of such cues is unknown.

Although the HRP techniques did not fill growth cones beyond 3 days postnatal, we were able to follow the further radial growth of callosal axons at later stages of development by labeling them with DiI *in vivo* at 3 to 8 days postnatal or in fixed brains (C. Norris and K. Kalil, *submitted*). These observations provided further evidence that before branching laterally, axons first establish their radial territory by growing through the cortex along glial processes. Growth of axons proceeded slowly but steadily with no significant pauses. The majority of axons are unbranched as they extend through the cortex, and their trajectory is radial (i.e., per-

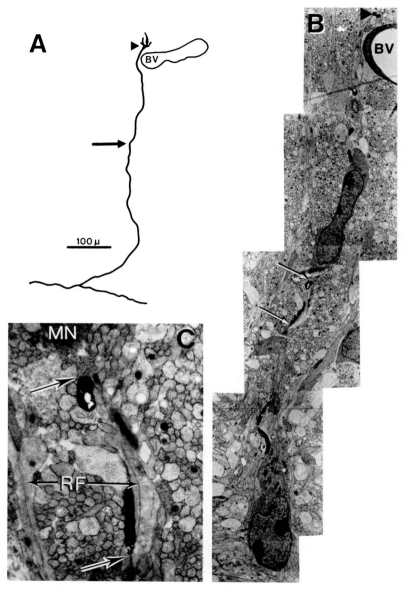

FIG. 7. Relationship of growing callosal axon and its growth cone to a continuous fascicle of radial glial fibers in hamster cortex at 2.5 days postnatal. **A:** Camera lucida drawing of HRP-labeled callosal axon and its growth cone extending through layer 6 beneath the cortical plate. Reference blood vessel (BV) is the same as in the mcirograph in **B**. *Arrowhead* in **A** and **B** points to base of growth cone. *Arrow* indicates region of axon shown in **C**. **B:** Low-magnification photomontage (300X) of the axon shown in **A**. The HRP-labeled callosal axon weaves in and out of the plane of the thin section. Note relationship between afferent axon, filled with black HRP reaction product, and column of electron-dense migrating neurons. **C:** Photomicrograph of region (between arrows in **B**) of the callosal axon at higher magnification (5,000X). Part of the HRP-labeled axon is apposed to the trailing process of a migrating neuron (MN); the majority of the axon is apposed to electron-lucent radial glial fibers (RF).

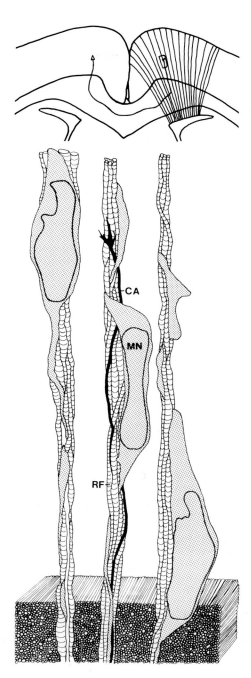

FIG. 8. Schematic drawings illustrating the relationship between callosal afferents (CA) and radial glial fascicles (RF) and their associated migrating neurons (MN). At top schematic illustration of callosal axon that has entered contralateral cortex and is growing parallel to the radial glia fibers spanning from the ventricular to the pial surface. Box in cortex represents region shown below. At bottom, a composite drawing made from tracings of photomicrographs of serial sections from the developing cortex, schematized to illustrate growing callosal axon in relation to radial units. A radial unit is bounded on either side by a fascicle of radial glial fibers. Bottom of figure shows axons in cross section between radial glia. (Modeled after ref. 24.)

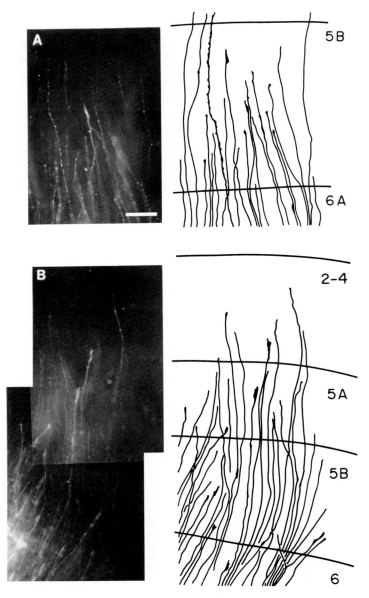

FIG. 9. Callosal afferents in cortex at 6 days postnatal labeled with DiI in fixed tissue (*at left*) and matching drawing with numbered cortical layers (*at right*). Note straight unbranched radial trajectories of callosal axons that, at this age, have extended as far as layers 2–4. Scale bar, 100 μm.

pendicular to cortical layers) (Fig. 9). Callosal axons rarely branch until 8 days postnatal, the age when the cortical plate completes differentiation and many axons arrive at the outer layer of cortex (Fig. 10). Thus, callosal afferents do not branch until relatively late in their extension through the cortex. In this way they could first establish their important radial or columnar territory by extending along radial glia in register with their appropriate columnar target neurons before branching laterally to arborize in cortical layers.

In addition to following the radial mode of growth of callosal axons, we were also able to establish that the initial innervation of cortex by these axons is topographically appropriate and in overall distribution resembles the patchy distribution of the adult sensorimotor cortex (C. Norris and K. Kalil, *submitted*). Previous reports

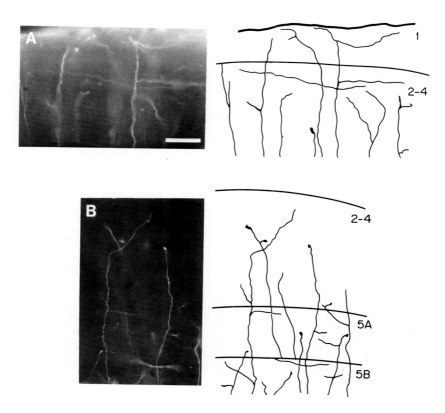

FIG. 10. Callosal afferents in cortex at 8 days postnatal labeled with DiI in fixed tissue (*at left*) and matching drawing with numbered cortical layers (*at right*). Note beginning of numerous side branches in all layers from radially oriented callosal axons. In **A**, some axons have extended to pial surface, but others, as indicated by the presence of growth cones, are still growing toward layer 1. Scale bar, 100 μm.

based on retrograde labeling techniques have concluded that the patchy distribution of adult callosal connectivity derives from an initial homogeneous pattern of continuous callosally projecting neurons throughout the sensorimotor cortex (20,42). Our results with anterograde labeling methods show that only cytoarchitecturally appropriate areas of cortex are innervated. Thus, it is likely that callosal axons destined to be eliminated do not actually enter the cortex. Within areas of cortex that do receive callosal input, the topography of the connections is reciprocal and point to point (i.e., homotopic) as in the adult. Topography would therefore develop as a result of directed axonal outgrowth.

Observations of growing corticospinal axons labeled with DiI *in vivo* show that as in the corpus callosum, initial growth of axons into spinal targets is remarkably precise (R. Kuang and K. Kalil, *submitted*) (Fig. 11) and resembles the adult pattern of projections (41). Axons project only to one side of the cord and only to the dorsal or ventral horn, but never to both. Although extensive fiber loss occurs in the developing corticospinal tract (31,32), axon elimination does not seem to be a mecha-

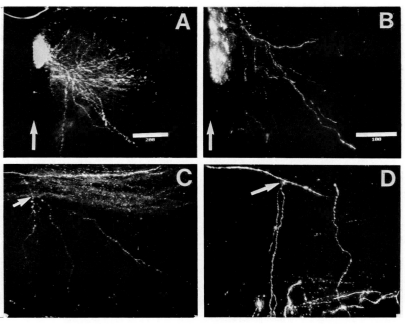

FIG. 11. Examples of DiI-labeled (*in vivo*) corticospinal axons during initial growth into spinal targets, showing appropriate projection patterns. **A:** Axons arborizing only in one side of the spinal cord. Transverse section taken from lumbar cord of 12-day animal. **B:** A single axon extending and branching only into the ventral horn. Transverse section taken from cervical cord of 6-day animal. *Arrows* in **A** and **B** indicate the midline. **C, D:** Single axons branching immediately as they leave the corticospinal tract. Parasagittal sections from cervical cord of 7–8 day animals. *Arrows* indicate branch points. Magnification is the same as in **B**.

nism for *(handwritten: leave white matter, arborizn)* .ons leave the white
matter, t dorsal or ventral horn
where th ill growing across the
gray m ation is underscored
by resu corticospinal pathway
(42a). I on one side early in
develop *(handwritten: interstitial collateral)* osite side of the cord
sproute c specificity as normal
arbors *(handwritten: sprouting)* is crossing the midline
often p ed underneath it, mak-
ing sh ese results suggest that
putati sprouting must be quite
powei ng the axon, even on a
branc ay occur without the involve
In rgent target cell groups is
in marked contrast ctory of growing callosal
axons, suggesting that the mode of growth of axons their subsequent development into arbors is strongly dictated by the configuration of the target tissue. This
conclusion is exemplified by recent findings on development of intramuscular nerve
branching patterns in chick hindlimb (43). Branching to slow muscle occurs interstitially behind the major growth cone, whereas branching to fast muscle occurs by
branching of the major growth cones as it traverses the muscle.

CONCLUSIONS

In mammalian CNS tracts, the major role of growth cones may be rapid extension
of axons toward the vicinity of target regions. Except for decision regions, positions
of growth cones within pathways and contacts by growth cone processes with specific axons or other cell types do not seem to be critical. Many axon tracts such as
the corpus callosum and corticospinal pathway can accommodate large numbers of
supernumerary axons, some of which are inappropriate. These errors are eliminated
by withdrawal of axons during development. Unlike axon tracts in which gross
errors can be corrected later in development, target regions exclude inappropriate
afferents from the beginning. Guidance cues for growth cones navigating within
targets ensure that individual axons can contact a specific set of target neurons, such
as a cortical column. Thus, in contrast to growth cone guidance in tracts, growth
cones in target regions need to use precise guidance mechanisms to decide which
neurons to innervate. Remarkably, even in complex targets such as the cerebral
cortex, the establishment of initial terminal domains is appropriate and is not
achieved by error correction. In the cortex, growth cones of afferent callosal axons
extend along radial glia in register with columnar arrays of migrating cortical neurons and may thereby establish appropriate radial territories. In the spinal cord,

immediate and divergent branching of developing corticospinal arbors reflects the configuration of widely divergent sets of target neurons. Initial entry of axons into CNS targets may occur without significant waiting periods. Further, establishment of terminal domains need not always involve turning behaviors or bifurcation of the major growth cone but can occur by collateral branching. In summary, the large and complex targets of the mammalian brain necessitate precise sets of guidance cues to ensure that growth cones of afferent axons establish appropriate territories. In different regions of the brain, these cues (such as radial glia in the developing cortex) could serve to keep the trajectory of the growing axon in register with the organization of its target neurons.

FUTURE DIRECTIONS

Guidance mechanisms in the mammalian brain have been largely inferred by observations in fixed tissue of consistent morphological differences among growth cones captured in different regions of a given neural pathway. In the translucent nervous systems of simpler vertebrate embryos (see, e.g., refs. 15,44,45), it has been possible to make direct observations of growth cone behaviors *in situ* by labeling growth cones with fluorescent dyes and observing them under low light–level conditions. Unless axon tracts and their targets are located near the brain surface, such experiments are difficult to carry out in the mammalian CNS. However, recent experiments (46; see chapter by Mason and Godement) suggest that slice preparations of the mammalian brain can be used to observe growth cone behaviors as axons extend in real-time within the slice. Laser confocal microscopy, by reducing out-of-focus light, makes it possible to see details of growth cones in thick tissue sections. Slices through the developing callosal pathway are advantageous for studies of pathway development because the entire pathway and its target are contained in a single slice, and individual axons remain in a narrow (100-μm) rostral–caudal plane. Preliminary results (M. Halloran, C. Norris, and K. Kalil, *unpublished observations*) suggest that confocal microscopy of DiI-labeled callosal growth cones in living slices of newborn hamster sensorimotor cortex will provide a means of directly observing growth cone shape changes in real-time *in situ*. Of special interest will be the turning behavior of growth cones as they change direction and grow toward the cerebral cortex. Do growth cones pause at these decision regions? How frequently do they change shape, and are shape changes correlated with changes in direction? Do growth cones change shape and speed as they extend through cortex? How do axon branches form as arbors begin to develop in the cerebral cortex?

Another useful strategy for studying growth cone behaviors of mammalian CNS neurons responding to putative guidance cues in different regions of the CNS is to observe dissociated CNS neurons in culture as they grow on cryostat sections of the brain. In recent experiments, for example, Covault and colleagues (47) found that embryonic chick ciliary ganglion neurons would extend neurites on sections of rat muscle, peripheral nerve, and cerebral cortex. Patterns of axon outgrowth reflected specific molecular interactions as opposed to purely mechanical factors and were based on active choices by growth cones among potential pathways. Various peripheral ganglionic neurons from newborn rats and embryonic chick have also been cultured on sections from rat CNS and PNS (48,49). Results from these studies, although obtained from fixed preparations, demonstrate that growth cones of neurons on tissue sections make meaningful choices resembling those *in vivo* about where to grow. However, to understand what cellular elements influence growth

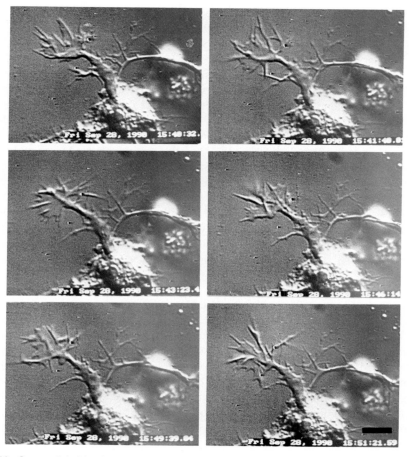

FIG. 12. Sequential video images of growth cones extending from cortical neurons. Neurons were dissociated from E15 (1 day before birth) hamster sensorimotor cortex and grown on a poly-L-lysine substrate. Images were acquired with video-enhanced contrast-differential interference contrast (VEC-DIC) microscopy over a 10-min time period. Note rapid shape changes in growth cone extending at left as regions of lamellipodia protrude between filopodial extensions. Photographs were obtained directly from the videomonitor. Scale bar, 10 μm.

cone steering, it will be important to make direct observations with high-resolution video techniques [i.e., video-enhanced contrast-differential interference contrast (VEC-DIC) microscopy] of living CNS growth cones navigating on relevant CNS substrates. By observing growth cones of dissociated hamster cortical neurons interacting with brain tissue sections, it may be possible to determine whether growth cones respond differently to tracts versus target regions with respect to trajectory and speed of extension. Such experiments with tissue sections from brains of different ages can also ask whether significant differences exist at different developmental ages in cell surface cues to which growth cones respond. Growth cones of living cultured neurons from the mammalian CNS have been little studied with high-resolution video techniques. Images of cortical growth cones in culture obtained with VEC-DIC microscopy (M. Halloran and K. Kalil, *unpublished observations*) suggest that cortical growth cones exhibit dynamic morphological shape changes (Fig. 12) similar to those of neurons from simpler invertebrate systems (see, e.g., refs. 50,51). Studies of cortical neurons *in vitro* may thus provide detailed information about how growth cones of CNS neurons respond to relevant CNS guidance cues.

In vitro preparations will also be important in identifying the cues that underlie formation of specific connectivity during development. Recently, explants of developing co-cultured neural tissue have provided an important way to address this question in the mammalian CNS (28–30,52,53; see chapter by Mason and Godement). Yamamoto and co-workers (53), for example, found that DiI-labeled axons from explanted embryonic rat lateral geniculate nucleus co-cultured with visual cortex targets arborized within the visual cortex in patterns similar to geniculo-cortical arbors *in vivo*. Thus, in future, co-cultured explants of developing cortical systems will be useful in evaluating the specificity of axon–target interactions in the absence of normal intervening pathways, the distances over which targets elicit directed axon outgrowth, and the role of targets in shaping developing arbors.

ACKNOWLEDGMENTS

We are grateful to Cheryl Adams for assistance with photography and histology and to Art Lies for expert help with the electron microscopy. We thank Rong zhen Kuang and Mary Halloran for permission to use unpublished data. This work was supported by NIH grant NS-14428 and Training Grant T32G 07507.

REFERENCES

1. Bentley D, Keshishian H. Pathfinding by peripheral pioneer neurons in grasshoppers. *Science* 1982;218:1082–1088.
2. Bentley D, Caudy M. Pioneer axons lose directed growth after selective killing of guidepost cells. *Nature (Lond)* 1983;304:62–65.
3. Goodman CS, Bastiani MJ, Doe CQ, et al. Cell recognition during neuronal development. *Science* 1984;225:1271–1279.
4. Bastiani MJ, Goodman CS. Guidance of neuronal growth cones in the grasshopper embryo. III. Recognition of a specific glial pathway. *J Neurosci* 1986;6:3542–3551.

The Nerve Growth Cone, edited by P. C. Letourneau,
S. B. Kater, and E. R. Macagno, Raven Press, Ltd.,
New York © 1992.

32

Introduction

Kenneth J. Muller

*Department of Physiology and Biophysics, University of Miami School of Medicine,
Miami, Florida 33136*

Ramón y Cajal recognized that regenerating axons are tipped by growth cones that are fundamentally the same as those on developing fibers, but he also knew that the injured nervous system poorly restores its original complement of connections (1). This section presents data that address concerns that Cajal might have had regarding the role of the growth cone and its interactions with its environment during regeneration, and it examines issues that are at the heart of development and regeneration as we understand them today. Thus, one can consider that successful regeneration requires both a vigorous, directed extension of the growth cone toward those cells or structures that are the axons' normal targets and an accurate, effective reconnection with those targets.

It is humbling to realize that so much of the groundwork of our understanding of regeneration was laid by Cajal. Major topics, from plasticity and sprouting to progressive degeneration and regeneration, were the objects of his investigations. Today we sometimes lose sight of his observations on the variability as well as similarity of axon and growth cone responses to axotomy. The shape of the growth cone itself varies with its position relative to other growth cones. During development the lead or pioneer growth cone can have extensive veils and filopodia that are commonly considered to be the growth cone's hallmarks, whereas growth cones of cells in the same population following a short distance behind are typically quite compact (2). Whether there are such shape variations during regeneration is less clear. There are differences in regenerative ability. Not only do central and peripheral axons respond quite differently to axotomy, but even within a nerve the response might not be uniform. At least one special case is of particular interest, namely, those sensory axons that have peripheral *and* central components (3).

Cajal was, of course, aware that the environment faced by regenerating growth cones is different than during maturation. An important question has been whether successful regeneration requires the presence or reappearance of certain developmental features of the cell and its environment, and this is addressed and answered by chapters in this section and elsewhere in this volume. The techniques of tissue culture were developed in Cajal's day (4), and regeneration *in vitro* as a tool has typically been considered separately from regeneration *in vivo*, even in this volume, but it is decidedly regeneration. Regenerating preparations offer advantages and opportunities to the experimentalist interested in broader aspects of development. Thus, from studies on growth cones of neurites in tissue culture to examination of sprouting axons *in situ*, it has been possible to determine what guides growth cones and triggers them to start and to stop growing.

Any investigation of growth-promoting substances and substrates must now consider opposing influences that are nonpermissive or inhibitory. Added to these are features of the environment that may guide the axon, such as topographical and mechanical properties of the substrate, that can be placed in a separate category because they fundamentally neither impede nor promote growth. In some cases, however, it may be difficult to draw distinctions between categories. The chapter by Bovolenta and colleagues examines growth promoting and inhibiting effects on central neurons of astrocytes and their membranes. It evaluates the inhibitory action of surface molecules in certain types of reactive astrocytes and in myelin and shows that the type of injury may be of critical importance in repair. The experiments of Bray and co-workers show in adult mammals, too, that both the substrate and type of injury can be critical. The inhibitory properties of CNS oligodendrocytes are only part of what impedes regeneration. The optic nerve must be severed close to its head, where it emerges from the eye, if the axons are to regenerate. This, Skene points out, may indicate that the proximal stump of the optic nerve may inhibit growth, perhaps through an interaction of axons and oligodendroglia. Skene and Bray and colleagues discuss regeneration of optic axons in terms of growth triggers and the appearance and transport of the growth-associated protein GAP-43.

A component of the environment that is conducive to growth cone extension is laminin. Bray and co-workers and Muller and colleagues point out that this molecule that promotes growth *in vitro* is also associated with regeneration *in vivo*, so long as it is not present with a nonpermissive or inhibitory substrate. There must, however, be a match between the growing neurons and their substrate. Axons that grow on laminin during development express integrins that are laminin receptors only during outgrowth, and these receptors must be reexpressed for laminin to be effective during regeneration (5). Sotelo and co-workers use a different tack to examine this question, having discovered that embryonic cerebellar neurons transplanted into their adult environment will extend toward their normal targets, at least for short distances. It may be that such axons have growth-promoting receptors that are lacking in adults, or instead that they are not impeded as are adult axons, or perhaps both are factors.

The chapters in the section on regeneration show that there is little directed growth at a distance, save for the direction afforded by the nerve or sheath along which the growth cones extend. Whether the appropriate target is present or not, axons can grow along a suitable pathway. However, axons in the vicinity of their targets do appear to be specifically directed by those targets, as discussed by Bray and colleagues, Sotelo and co-workers, and Muller and associates.

It is particularly encouraging that in the mammalian brain those axons that find themselves in the vicinity of their usual targets form synapses with them. There is an interaction in which the targets as well as growing axons are participants. Whether the new connections are precise and, in that sense, specific is unclear in the mammalian brain, but in lower vertebrates functionally appropriate connections are restored; in invertebrates connections are made with precisely those cells that are the usual targets. The role of target denervation is also unclear. It might be, for example, that denervation makes the target more receptive to reinnervation, but denervation can also result in inappropriate collateral sprouting or in transsynaptic degeneration. A major goal for the future is to discover those conditions that can foster vigorous and functionally accurate regeneration without cell death in mammals as occurs in some invertebrates and lower vertebrates.

Cajal did not know about axonal transport and the synthesis of growth-associated proteins, but he knew there were phases of growth, some of which are dependent on the cell body and others not. The chapter by Skene points out that effective growth may not begin until the synthetic machinery in the soma begins operating. However, within hours of axotomy, axons and axon segments will sprout and begin to grow, even if they have been quiescent. For axon segments the growth is abortive, but in invertebrates and vertebrates in which axon segments may be long-lived, it might be linked to an interesting and perhaps ultimately useful phenomenon discussed in the chapter by Muller and colleagues. This is the ability of regenerating axons to synapse on or, for certain types of axons, to fuse with their severed distal segment, which acts as a splice, thereby rapidly and fully restoring connections with the original complement of targets.

Work on diverse systems has shown that considerable function can be restored when only a fraction of fibers reconnect with targets. The chapters in this section reveal surprising and encouraging progress in assisting neurons to grow axons and connect with targets in the adult nervous system. With a combined effort to stimulate directed growth, neutralize factors that impede growth, and maintain targets and growing neurons it should be possible to focus on assuring the precise regeneration of connections established during development and aid the mammalian nervous system, even that of humans, in its successful repair.

REFERENCES

1. Cajal S Ramón. *Degeneration and regeneration of the nervous system*. New York: Hafner, 1928.
2. LoPresti, V, Macagno ER, Levinthal C. Structure and development of neuronal connections in isogenic organisms: cellular interactions in the development of the optic lamina of *Daphnia*. *Proc Natl Acad Sci USA* 1973;70:433–437.
3. Richardson PM, Issa VM. Peripheral injury enhances central regeneration of primary sensory neurones. *Nature* 1984;309:791–793.
4. Harrison, RG. The cultivation of tissues in extraneous media as a method of morphogenetic study. *Anat Rec* 1912;6:181–193.
5. Reichardt LF, Bixby JL, Hall DE, Ignatius MJ, Neugebauer KF, Tomaselli KJ. Integrins and cell adhesion molecules: neuronal receptors that regulate axon growth on extracellular matrices and cell surfaces. *Dev Neurosci* 1989;11:332–347.

The Nerve Growth Cone, edited by P. C. Letourneau,
S. B. Kater, and E. R. Macagno, Raven Press, Ltd.,
New York © 1992.

33

The Growth Cone: Sprouting and Synapse Regeneration in the Leech

*Kenneth J. Muller, *,**Xiaonan Gu, *Ellen McGlade-McCulloh, *†Adrian Mason, and *‡Steven R. Young

*Department of Physiology and Biophysics, University of Miami School of Medicine, Miami, Florida 33136; **Department of Biology, University of California at San Diego, LaJolla, California 92093; †University Department of Pharmacology, Oxford, England; ‡Department of Pharmacology, SUNY Downstate Medical Center, Brooklyn, New York 11203

Ramón y Cajal argued that the growth cone is under local control and is, in that sense, an independent entity. One convincing demonstration of this was his observation of sprouting at the proximal ends of axon segments isolated by cutting them from their cell bodies (1). For example, after cutting the sciatic nerve in the cat he found that the proximal end of the severed distal segments grew for several days before the axons began to degenerate—a separate process that occurred after about 1 week. Thus, phenomena of regeneration and degeneration were used by Cajal to understand developmental events, for he recognized that regeneration and embryonic development share basic mechanisms.

A fresh perspective on these and many of Cajal's other fundamental observations on sprouting and regeneration of axons and synapses has emerged from studies of invertebrate nervous systems including the leech. The leech offers the advantages of identifiable, manipulable cells that regenerate synapses in the adult. The axon and synapse regeneration of mature neurons can be compared with their development in the embryo and their performance in tissue culture. This chapter focuses on the leech as it examines triggers for growth cone sprouting, extension, and stopping in regeneration and development. It considers (1) the sprouting of surgically isolated axons, (2) sprouting of intact axons in response to denervation, (3) ionic currents in the growth cone, and (4) the role of substratum in axon sprouting and regeneration. Although many mechanisms appear to be shared in regeneration and development, their balance may shift with maturation of the nervous system.

It is worthwhile first describing several basic aspects of the leech nervous system to place the work in context. The segmented nervous system of the leech, an annelid, consists of a chain of similar segmental ganglia, each containing 400 cells, many of which have been identified as to function as well as location and size of soma, electrical characteristics, and embryonic lineage (2,3). Certain neurons are mechanosensory cells, others are motoneurons, and others are interneurons that are neither sensory nor motor but may receive synaptic input from sensory neurons and themselves synapse on motoneurons. Although neurons in the leech CNS cannot regenerate if they are lost, just as most vertebrate neurons cannot, leech neurons can regenerate their synaptic connections accurately after their axons have been severed, thereby restoring apparently normal function after injury. The plain visibility of leech neurons, the large glia, their basic resemblance to their mammalian counterparts, and the manageable size of its neatly wired CNS have made the leech nervous system particularly fruitful for study.

GROWTH OF ISOLATED AXON SEGMENTS

Cajal's observation that isolated stumps, particularly those of unmyelinated fibers, can grow at the site of the lesion has been repeated for isolated neurites growing in tissue culture by Bray, Shaw, Wessells, Levi, and others (4–7). This independent property of growth cones in tissue culture is a feature of interest discussed in several other chapters of this volume. Curiously, the phenomenon and its potential importance have received little additional attention in nerves *in vivo*. Of course, Cajal recognized that the growth was basically abortive. But *in vivo* was it unique to his preparations, and what are other capabilities of isolated segments?

A few years ago we began to use the leech to reexamine such cell-independent growth, in part to learn whether isolated axon segments could grow at both ends (8). Individual pressure-sensory cells in the leech were filled with fluorescent tracers not degraded within the cell. After the dye had filled the axon, segments were isolated and their growth tracked by low-light fluorescence microscopy similar to that used in other systems (9). The results were reminiscent of Cajal's. Axon segments sprouted at both end. Their growth was tracked for at least a week, and the sprouts were observed to retract as well as extend. Because the marker was fluorescent, processes finer than the resolution of the microscope and video system were detectable, as confirmed by electron microscopy. To demonstrate that similar sprouting could occur *in vivo* and without injecting the cell with markers, nerve cords were cut within the animal, and axons containing catecholamines were stained using glyoxylic acid (10) (Fig. 1).

What might be the significance of such sprouting for regeneration? In contrast with isolated axon segments in the peripheral nerves of mammals, many axons in invertebrates can survive independently of the neuron soma for weeks or months (11) and can act as a splice linking the regenerating axon with its target, either by making an electrical synapse (12) or by direct fusion (13,14) of an axon with its distal segment. In either case, if the distal segment sprouts into the lesion toward the regenerating fiber, the probability of an encounter between the regenerating fiber and its distal segment would seem to be increased. Whether regeneration is normally enhanced by proximal sprouts of distal segments remains speculative.

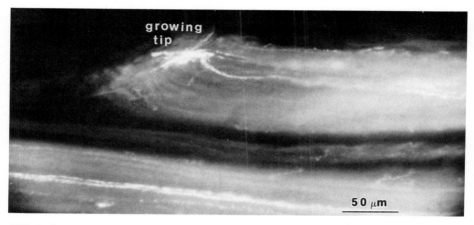

FIG. 1. Sprouting of an axon segment 5 days after isolation within the leech. The nerve cord was cut in two places between a pair of ganglia, removed from the animal, processed with glyoxylic acid (10), and viewed under epifluorescence with a Zeiss 18 filter set. The sprouted axon was that of a dopamine-containing cell, its soma located in the periphery in the segmental nerve (68). Each end of the axon (one end not shown) had sprouted.

Important problems for the future are how isolated segments are maintained, where their components for the growth cone and trailing axon originate, and how such segments are specifically recognized by the regenerating fiber, in some cases to form a reciprocal synapse. There is evidence that temperature plays a major role in axon segment survival in vertebrates (15–18), and axons that survive months at room temperature in a tropical leech (*Haementeria ghilianii*) degenerate (and regenerate) within days at a tropical temperature (19). The role of metabolism in long-term survival is not clear, but its significance is already evident.

SPROUTING OF INTACT AXONS

Although a severed axon will typically reseal and sprout, it is not necessary to injure an adult axon to prompt sprouting. A prime example of this is in the vertebrate peripheral nervous system, where both sensory (20) and motor (21–23) neurons sprout when a suitable target is denervated. But denervation-induced sprouting has also been amply demonstrated in the adult mammalian CNS (24–26). Such sprouting often reflects an active competition between fibers for a potential target. For nociceptive neurons in the leech CNS, the competition can be lopsided, so that one neuron apparently excludes another from contacting a suitable target—the soma of another sensory cell in its own ganglion (27). Selective denervation of the target prompts sprouting by the uninjured neuron within weeks. This growth is distinct from the apparently ongoing sprouting and remodeling visible within certain autonomic ganglia of mammals (28), but what triggers it is unclear.

It is believed that a neuron's synaptic contact with its targets can inhibit growth, thus target death might be expected to induce sprouting. A nice example of this is the single S interneuron in each segmental ganglion of the leech. The S cell has two giant axons, each extending halfway along the connectives linking adjacent ganglia. Midway between ganglia each axon makes an electrical synapse with its target, the axon of the homologous S cell in the adjacent ganglion. When the S cell axon is crushed and thus severed, it regenerates along its usual path, taking about a month, and stops growing when it forms a synapse with the target (29). During regeneration a fine axon that thickens as function is restored trails the growth cone (Fig. 2), as Cajal described for his peripheral nerve preparations. If the target is selectively destroyed by intracellular injection of protease, the S-cell axon neither extends nor retracts, but if the cell's other axon is severed, causing it to regenerate, the axon that lost its target sprouts and extends a growth cone toward the ganglion of its usual target as shown in Fig. 3 (30,31). Experiments confirmed that it is the contact at the synapse and not connection with the ganglion that prevents growth (30). It is interesting that in the cerebellum of the *nervous* mutant mouse, after Purkinje cells die, there is no extension or retraction by granule cell axons once they have stopped growing (32). Perhaps granule cell axons respond as do S-cell axons. For S-cell axons, contact with the target inhibits sprouting, but that inhibition is manifest only when the neuron is otherwise triggered to grow, as occurs when the S cell's other axon is injured.

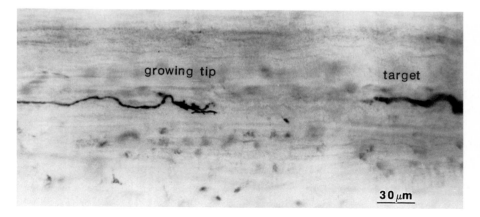

FIG. 2. Growth cone at the tip of a regenerated S-cell axon 3 weeks after it was severed. Before fixation the fine regenerating axon had grown to within 150 μm of the uninjured target S cell, and both regenerate and target were injected with horseradish peroxidase, stained, and mounted whole. After reconnection and formation of an electrical synapse, by 1 month, the regenerated axon increases in caliber. (From ref. 29, with permission.)

32. Sotelo C, Triller A. Fate of presynaptic afferents to Purkinje cells in the adult nervous mutant mouse: a model to study presynaptic stabilization. *Brain Res* 1979;175:11–36.
33. McGlade-McCulloh E, Muller KJ. Developing axons continue to grow at their tip after synapsing with their appropriate target. *Neuron* 1989;2:1063–1068.
34. Lamoureux P, Buxbaum RE, Heidemann SR. Direct evidence that growth cones pull. *Nature* 1989; 340:159–162.
35. Heidemann SR, Buxbaum RE. Tension as a regulator and integrator of axonal growth. *Cell Motil Cytoskeleton* 1990;17:6–10.
36. Bray D. Axonal growth in response to experimentally applied mechanical tension. *Dev Biol* 1984; 102:379–389.
37. Young SR, Stewart RR, Liu Y, Muller KJ, Ross WN. Non-inactivating K⁺ channels on growth cones, neurites, and somata of leech Retzius cells in culture (*Abstr*). *Soc Neurosci Abstr* 1989;15:74.
38. Sigurdson WJ, Morris CE. Stretch-activated ion channels in growth cones of snail neurons. *J Neurosci* 1989;9:2801–2808.
39. Morris CE, Sigurdson WJ. Stretch-inactivated ion channels coexist with stretch-activated ion channels. *Science* 1989;243:807–809.
40. Grinvald A, Farber IC. Optical recording of calcium action potentials from growth cones of cultured neurons with a laser microbeam. *Science* 1981;212:1164–1167.
41. Cohan CS, Connor JA, Kater SB. Electrically and chemically mediated increases in intracellular calcium in neuronal growth cones. *J Neurosci* 1987;7:3588–3599.
42. Ross WN, Arechiga H, Nicholls JG. Influence of substrate on the distribution of calcium channels in identified leech neurons in culture. *Proc Natl Acad Sci USA* 1988;85:4075–4078.
43. Ross WN, Arechiga H, Nicholls JG. Optical recording of calcium and voltage transients following impulses in cell bodies and processes of identified leech neurons in culture. *J Neurosci* 1987; 7:3877–3887.
44. Grumbacher-Reinert S. Local influence of substrate molecules in determining distinctive growth patterns of identified neurons in culture. *Proc Natl Acad Sci USA* 1989;86:7270–7274.
45. Harrison RG. The reaction of embryonic cells to solid structures. *J Exp Zool* 1914;17:521–544.
46. Harrison RG. The cultivation of tissues in extraneous media as a method of morphogenetic study. *Anat Rec* 1912;6:181–193.
47. Letourneau PC, Shattuck TA, Roche FK, Takeichi M, Lemmon V. Nerve growth cone migration onto Schwann cells involves the calcium-dependent adhesion molecule, N-cadherin. *Dev Biol* 1990;138:430–442.
48. Letourneau PC. Cell-to-substratum adhesion and guidance of axonal elongation. *Dev Biol* 1975; 44:92–101.
49. Letourneau PC, Shattuck TA. Distribution and possible interactions of actin-associated proteins and cell adhesion molecules of nerve growth cones. *Development* 1989;105:505–519.
50. Carbonetto S, Gruver MM, Turner DC. Nerve fiber growth in culture on fibronectin, collagen, and glycosaminoglycan substrates. *J Neurosci* 1983;3:2324–2335.
51. Hammarback JA, Palm SL, Furcht LT, Letourneau PC. Guidance of neurite outgrowth by pathways of substratum-adsorbed laminin. *J Neurosci Res* 1985;13:213–220.
52. Toyota B, Carbonetto S, David S. A dual laminin/collagen receptor acts in peripheral nerve regeneration. *Proc Natl Acad Sci USA* 1990;87:1319–1322.
53. Tawil NJ, Houde M, Blacher R, et al. α₁β₁ Integrin heterodimer functions as a dual laminin/collagen receptor in neural cells. *Biochemistry* 1990;29:6540–6544.
54. Nakatsuji N, Nagata I. Paradoxical perpendicular contact guidance displayed by mouse cerebellar granule cell neurons *in vitro*. *Development* 1989;106:441–447.
55. Edgar D. Neuronal laminin receptors. *Trends Neurosci* 1989;12:248–251.
56. Cohen J, Burne JF, Winter J, Bartlett P. Retinal ganglion cells lose response to laminin with maturation. *Nature* 1986;322:465–467.
57. Cohen J, Nurcombe V, Jeffrey P, Edgar D. Developmental loss of functional laminin receptors on retinal ganglion cells is regulated by their target tissue, the optic tectum. *Development* 1989; 107:381–387.
58. Liesi P, Kaakkola S, Dahl D, Vaheri A. Laminin is induced in astrocytes of adult brain by injury. *EMBO J* 1984;3:683–686.
59. Liesi P. Laminin-immunoreactive glia distinguish regenerative adult CNS systems from non-regenerative ones. *EMBO J* 1985;4:2505–2511.
60. Garzino V, Berenger H, Pradel J. Expression of laminin and of a laminin-related antigen during early development of *Drosophila melanogaster*. *Development* 1989;106:17–27.

61. Masuda-Nakagawa L, Beck K, Chiquet M. Identification of molecules in leech extracellular matrix that promote neurite outgrowth. *Proc R Soc Lond B* 1988;235:247–257.
62. Chiquet M, Masuda-Nakagawa L, Beck K. Attachment to an endogenous laminin-like protein initiates sprouting by leech neurons. *J Cell Biol* 1988;107:1189–1198.
63. Chiquet M, Nicholls JG. Neurite outgrowth and synapse formation by identified leech neurones in culture. *J Exp Biol* 1987;132:191–206.
64. Masuda-Nakagawa LM, Muller KJ, Nicholls JG. Accumulation of laminin and microglial cells at sites of injury and regeneration in the central nervous system of the leech. *Proc R Soc Lond B* 1990; 241:201–206.
65. Morgese VJ, Elliott EJ, Muller KJ. Microglial movement to sites of nerve lesion in the leech CNS. *Brain Res* 1983;272:166–170.
66. McGlade-McCulloh E, Morrissey AM, Norona F, Muller KJ. Individual microglia move rapidly and directly to nerve lesions in the leech central nervous system. *Proc Natl Acad Sci USA* 1989; 86:1093–1097.
67. Krause TL, Bittner GD. Rapid morphological fusion of severed myelinated axons by polyethylene glycol. *Proc Natl Acad Sci USA* 1990;87:1471–1475.
68. Lent CM, Mueller RL, Haycock DA. Chromatographic and histochemical identification of dopamine within an identified neuron in the leech nervous system. *J Neurochem* 1983;41:481–490.

GAP-43 Responds to Primary Retrograde Signals

An alternative possibility (24) is that synthesis or transport of GAP-43 and other GAPs might be blocked in abortively regenerating neurons, not because they respond directly to the influence of degenerating distal stump but because their induction is a secondary response to successful axon elongation. In successful regeneration, for example, either the biochemical action within advancing growth cones or access of the growth cones to specific cues in the distal nerve environment might activate signals that are relayed to the neuron cell body to induce secondary responses. Two observations argue that the induction of GAP-43 is not a secondary response that depends on axon outgrowth. First, the response of the GAP-43 gene precedes axon outgrowth in successful regeneration. This is most clearly resolved in cold-blooded vertebrates, in which regenerative events take place on a slower time scale than in the mammalian PNS. After interruption of fish optic nerve, for example, regenerating axons first cross the lesion site and enter the distal nerve stump approximately 4.5 days after injury (33), and the earliest indications of axon sprouting can be detected at the electron microscope level 2 days after a lesion (34). Under similar circumstances, the GAP-43 mRNA is elevated more than fourfold within 1 day after axotomy and is fully induced by 4 days (35). More direct evidence that GAP-43 induction does not depend on axon outgrowth comes from experiments in which axon outgrowth is directly prevented after interruption of mammalian peripheral nerves. We injected colchicine into rat sciatic nerves at the time of crush lesion to depolymerize microtubules at the lesion site, blocking both growth cone activity and productive axon elongation. Although the colchicine treatment was effective in preventing axon outgrowth, it had no effect on the induction of GAP-43 mRNA in the cell bodies of dorsal root ganglia projecting axons to the lesion site (36). The failure of GAP-43 induction in the mammalian CNS after distal axotomy, therefore, is not simply a secondary consequence of the failure of axons to elongate.

A second explanation for the failure of GAP-43 induction in certain distally axotomized CNS neurons is that the GAP-43 gene in these cells is unable to respond to the retrograde signals that trigger GAP-43 induction in other systems. Recent evidence from other laboratories, however, shows that GAP-43 can be induced by proximal axotomy in two different CNS tracts that fail to induce the protein after more distal lesions. Willard, Aguayo, and their colleagues (37) showed that proximal lesions of rat optic nerve induced an increase in GAP-43 immunoreactivity and axonal transport of newly synthesized GAP-43 in retinal ganglion cells. Consistent with earlier results, more distal lesions failed to induce these responses. Tetzlaff and co-workers (38,39) also reported an increase in GAP-43 mRNA in rubrospinal neurons after axotomy in the cervical spinal cord, a lesion site that permits regeneration of rubrospinal axons into PNS grafts (32), but no such induction after more distal lesions. These reports show that the primary impediment to GAP-43 induction in more distally axotomized neurons does not reside in the nucleus or cell soma but arises along the surviving axons of the long proximal stump.

Retrograde Repression Versus Impairment of an Active Inducer

The failure of GAP-43 induction after distal axotomy in the mammalian CNS indicates that the presence of a long CNS proximal stump prevents or interferes with some step in the retrograde signaling that leads to GAP-43 induction after axon interruption in peripheral nerves. One possible explanation is that GAP-43 induction in the periphery results from the generation at the site of injury or in the degenerating distal nerve stump of a positive cue for induction, and the subsequent relay of this signal through the surviving proximal stump (Fig. 1A). This would invite the interpretation that elements of a long CNS proximal stump interfere with the relay of such a positive inductive signal from either the endogenous CNS pathway distal to an injury site or from an exogenously supplied segment of peripheral nerve. To test this possibility, we examined whether induction of GAP-43 mRNA after peripheral axotomy depends on positive signals relayed from the injury site or distal nerve stump. Induction of GAP-43 mRNA in rat dorsal root ganglia after sciatic nerve lesions was not altered by nerve resection to remove the distal nerve stump, in

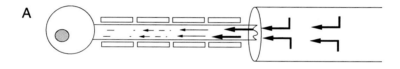

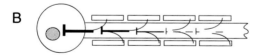

FIG. 1. Models for the impairment of GAP-43 induction by a long proximal nerve stump remaining after distal axotomy in the mammalian CNS. **A:** GAP-43 expression depends on an active induction by signals originating at the site of injury or in the degenerating distal nerve stump, relayed retrogradely through the surviving proximal axons. The distal stump depicted could represent either the degenerating distal segment of the injured CNS tract itself or a segment of peripheral nerve grafted into a CNS lesion site. In this model a long CNS proximal stump interferes with the retrograde relay of a positive signal, so that the effectiveness of the signal progressively dissipates with increasing length of the proximal stump. **B:** In this model, elements of the mature axons and glia in the surviving CNS proximal stump initiate a retrograde signaling pathway that directly represses expression of GAP-43. The repressive influence is depicted as summing over the length of the axons. Because the axonal and glial structure and cellular interactions in the proximal nerve stump are largely the same as in an uninjured adult tract, the signaling events preventing induction of GAP-43 after distal axotomy would be assumed to maintain the chronic repression of GAP-43 expression in many neurons of the intact adult CNS.

growth restrictions imposed by the down-regulation of GAP-43 or other growth cone components remains to be elucidated. Even if these developmentally regulated growth cone components are required for frank axon elongation of the sort that characterizes the initial outgrowth or regeneration of long axon tracts, it remains possible that retrograde repression of specific subsets of these proteins in mature neurons can restrict certain forms of axon growth in mature neurons while permitting more restricted modes of remodeling and synaptic plasticity.

If retrograde regulation restricts some modes of growth in most neurons, do neurons that retain high levels of GAP-43 expression in adult life also retain a capacity for more extensive axonal growth? Not necessarily. Some neurons, such as interneurons, might initiate GAP-43 expression during their early differentiation but never express some of the other proteins required to extend a long projection-type axon. In such a case, the continued expression of GAP-43 could result from the failure to extend long axons and establish the specific sets of glial or other interactions that trigger down-regulation in most projection neurons. Thus, continued expression of GAP-43 would be a byproduct of the *in*ability of those neurons to carry out some forms of axon growth. It appears, however, that at least some of the neurons that maintain high levels of GAP-43 expression in the adult CNS do maintain long axons (2–6). Neurons of this sort might be proposed as a population of neurons that retain capacities for axon growth and remodeling lost in the majority of mature neurons. An interesting question is whether the same cells that maintain high levels of GAP-43 expression in adults also coordinately express other genes repressed in the majority of mature neurons, especially those encoding axonal or growth cone proteins. The answer would shed light on whether those neurons are likely to retain many of the growth capacities of developing neurons or only a more circumscribed set of "immature" properties.

ACKNOWLEDGMENTS

Work from this laboratory was supported by NIH grants NS-20178 and EY-07397. I am grateful to Kate Kalil, Mark Willard, Albert Aguayo, and Guriq Basi for many helpful discussions of the ideas considered here.

REFERENCES

1. Skene JHP. Axonal growth-associated proteins. *Annu Rev Neurosci* 1989;12:127–156.
2. Benowitz LI, Apostolides PJ, Perrone-Bizzozero NI, Finklestein SP, Zwiers H. Anatomical distribution of the growth-associated protein GAP-43/B-50 in the adult rat brain. *J Neurosci* 1988;8:339–352.
3. Benowitz LI, Perrone-Bizzozero NI, Finklestein SP, Bird, ED. Localization of the growth-associated phophoprotein GAP-43 (B-50,F1) in the human cerebral cortex. *J Neurosci* 1989;9:990–995.
4. De la Monte SM, Federoff HJ, Ng SC, Grabczyk E, Fishman MC. GAP-43 gene expression during development: persistence in a distinctive set of neurons in the mature nervous system. *Dev Brain Res* 1990;46:161–168.
5. Neve RL, Finch E, Bird ED, Benowitz LI. Growth-associated protein GAP-43 is expressed selectively in associative regions of the adult human brain. *Proc Natl Acad Sci USA* 1988;85:3638–3642.

6. Oestreicher AB, Gispen WH. Comparison of the immunocytochemical distribution of the phospho-protein B-50 in the cerebellum and hippocampus of immature and adult rat brain. *Brain Res* 1986; 375:267–279.
7. Jacobson RD, Virag I, Skene JHP. A protein associated with axon growth, GAP-43, is widely distributed and developmentally regulated in rat CNS. *J Neurosci* 1986;6:1843–1855.
8. Kalil K, Skene JHP. Elevated synthesis of an axonally transported protein correlates with axon outgrowth in normal and injured pyramidal tracts. *J Neurosci* 1986;6:2563–2570.
9. Basi GS, Jacobson RD, Virag I, Schilling J, Skene JHP. Primary structure and transcriptional regulation of GAP-43, a protein associated with nerve growth. *Cell* 1987;49:785–791.
10. Karns LR, Ng SC, Freeman JA, Fishman MC. Cloning of complementary DNA for GAP-43, a neuronal growth-related protein. *Science* 1987;236:597–600.
11. Maness PF, Aubry M, Shores CG, Frame L, Pfenninger KH. C-*src* gene product in developing rat brain is enriched in nerve growth cone membranes. *Proc Natl Acad Sci USA* 1988;85:5001–5005.
12. Stein R, Mori N, Matthews K, Lo LC, Anderson DJ. The NGF-inducible SCG10 mRNA encodes a novel membrane-bound protein present in growth cones and abundant in developing neurons. *Neuron* 1988;1:463–476.
13. Ramos P, Sanfei R, Kayalar C, Ellis L. Isolation and sequence of lambda gt11 cDNA clones encoding the 5B4 antigen expressed on sprouting neurons. *Mol Brain Res* 1989;5:297–303.
14. Wallis I, Ellis L, Suh K, Pfenninger KH. Immunolocalization of a neuronal growth-dependent membrane glycoprotein. *J Cell Biol* 1985;101:1990–1998.
15. Kalil K, Perdew M. Expression of two developmentally regulated brain-specific proteins is corre-lated with late outgrowth of the pyramidal tract. *J Neurosci* 1988;8:4797–4808.
16. Farmer SR, Robinson GS, Mbangkollo D, et al. Differential expression of the beta-tubulin multi-gene family during rat brain development. *Ann NY Acad Sci* 1984;466:41–50.
17. Miller FD, Naus CCG, Durand M, Bloom FE, Milner RJ. Isotypes of a-tubulin are differentially regulated during neuronal maturation. *J Cell Biol* 1987;105:3065–3073.
18. Matus A. Microtubule-associated proteins: their potential role in determining neuronal morphology. *Annu Rev Neurosci* 1988;11:29–44.
19. Simkowitz P, Ellis L, Pfenninger KH. Membrane proteins of the nerve growth cone and their developmental regulation. *J Neurosci* 1989;9:1004–1017.
20. Goslin K, Schreyer DJ, Skene JHP, Banker G. Development of neuronal polarity: GAP-43 distin-guishes axonal from dendritic growth cones. *Nature* 1988;336:672–674.
21. Skene JHP, Willard M. Axonally transported proteins associated with axon growth in rabbit central and peripheral nervous systems. *J Cell Biol* 1981;89:96–103.
22. Miller FD, Tetzlaff W, Bisby MA, Fawcett JW, Milner RJ. Rapid induction of the major embryonic a-tubulin, Ta1, during nerve regeneration in adult rats. *J Neurosci* 1989;9:1452–1463.
23. Hoffman PN. Expression of GAP-43, a rapidly transported growth-associated protein, and class II beta tubulin, a slowly transported cytoskeletal protein, are coordinated in regenerating neurons. *J Neurosci* 1989;9:893–897.
24. Redshaw JD, Bisby MA. Fast axonal transport in central nervous system and peripheral nervous system axons following axotomy. *J Neurobiol* 1984;15:109–117.
25. Reh TA, Redshaw JD, Bisby, MA. Axons of the pyramidal tract do not increase their transport of growth-associated proteins after axotomy. *Mol Brain Res* 1987;2:1–6.
26. Ramón y Cajal S. *Degeneration and regeneration of the nervous system.* London: Oxford University Press, 1928.
27. Caroni P, Schwab ME. Two membrane protein fractions from rat central myelin with inhibitory properties for neurite growth and fibroblast spreading. *J Cell Biol* 1988;106:1281–1288.
28. Benfey M, Aguayo AJ. Extensive elongation of axons from rat brain into peripheral nerve grafts. *Nature* 1982;296:150–152.
29. David S, Aguayo AJ. Axonal elongation into peripheral nervous system "bridges" after central nervous system injury in adult rats. *Science* 1981;214:931–933.
30. Villegas-Perez MP, Vidal-Sanz M, Bray GM, Aguayo AJ. Influences of peripheral nerve grafts on the survival and regrowth of axotomized retinal ganglion cells in adult rats. *J Neurosci* 1988;8:265–280.
31. Richardson PM, Isaa VMK, Shemie S. Regeneration and retrograde degeneration of axons in the rat optic nerve. *J Neurocytol* 1982;11:949–966.
32. Richardson PM, Issa VMK, Aguayo AJ. Regeneration of long spinal axons in the rat. *J Neurocytol* 1984;13:165–182.

33. McQuarrie LG, Grafstein B. Effect of a conditioning lesion on optic nerve regeneration in goldfish. *Brain Res* 1981;216:253–264.
34. Lanners HN, Grafstein B. Early stages of axonal regeneration in the goldfish optic tract: an electron microscopic study. *J Neurocytol* 1980;9:733–751.
35. LaBate ME, Skene JHP. Selective conservation of GAP-43 structure in vertebrate evolution. *Neuron* 1989;3:299–310.
36. Basi GS, Skene JHP. Regulation of GAP-43 gene expression during axonal regeneration in sensory neurons. *Abstr Soc Neurosci* 1988;14:803.
37. Doster SK, Lozano AM, Aguayo AJ, Willard M. Expression of the growth-associated protein GAP-43 in adult retinal ganglion cells following axon injury. *Neuron* 1991;6:1–13.
38. Tetzlaff W, Alexander SW, Miller FD, Bisby MA. Response of facial and rubrospinal neurons to axotomy: changes in mRNA expression for cytoskeletal proteins and GAP-43. *J. Neurosci.* 1991 *(in press)*.
39. Tetzlaff W, Tsui BJ, Balfour JK. Rubrospinal neurons increase GAP43 and tubulin mRNA after cervical but not after thoracic axotomy *(Abstr)*. *Abstr Soc Neurosci* 1990;16:338.
40. Baizer L, Fishman MC. Recognition of specific targets by cultured dorsal root ganglion neurons. *J Neurosci* 1987;7:2305–2311.
41. Bisby MA. Dependence of GAP43 (B50,F1) transport on regeneration in rat dorsal root ganglion neurons. *Brain Res* 1988;458:157–161.
42. Woolf CJ, Reynolds ML, Molander C, O'Brien C, Lindsay RM, Benowitz LI. The growth-associated protein GAP-43 appears in dorsal root ganglion cells and in the dorsal horn of the rat spinal cord following peripheral nerve injury. *Neuroscience* 1990;34:465–478.
43. Reh T, Kalil K. Development of the pyramidal tract in the hamster. II. An electron microscopic study. *J Comp Neurol* 1982;205:77–88.
44. Perrone-Bizzozero NI, Irwin N, Lewis SE, Fischer I, Neve RL, Benowitz LI. Posttranscriptional regulation of GAP-43 mRNA levels during process outgrowth *(Abstr)*. *Abstr Soc Neurosci* 1990;16:814.

The Nerve Growth Cone, edited by P. C. Letourneau,
S. B. Kater, and E. R. Macagno, Raven Press, Ltd.,
New York © 1992.

35

Central Neurite Outgrowth over Glial Scar Tissue *In Vitro*

Paola Bovolenta, Francisco Wandosell, and
Manuel Nieto-Sampedro

Neural Plasticity Laboratory, Instituto Cajal, 28002 Madrid, Spain

CELLULAR EVENTS AFTER CNS INJURY IN MAMMALS

Damage to the CNS breaks the physical and functional boundaries of the nervous tissue, disrupts the interactions between neural cells, and destroys both the neurons and the connections in which they are involved. Cajal showed at the beginning of the century that, on its own, damaged CNS was unable to regenerate (6). Subsequent morphological studies confirmed Cajal's observations while, at the same time, revealing that injury "rejuvenates" adult CNS, causing it to replay many of its developmental capabilities.

Severe CNS trauma evokes the following major cellular events. Immediately after the lesion, the blood–CNS barrier breaks down at the injury site. Local ischemia/hypoxia/hypoglycemia occur as a consequence of both vascular spasm and vascular disruption. Blood cells and serum proteins invade the injury area (9,27). Edema, resulting from both extracellular fluid accumulation and astrocyte swelling, is obvious 24 hr later (17,20). Ultrastructural abnormalities in the axons in both gray and white matter can be observed immediately after a contusive injury and uniform necrosis and myelin degeneration follow 8 to 24 hr later (2). Many blood-derived macrophages and activated microglial cells accumulate 48 hr after an open wound and engulf degenerating myelin and other cell debris (14). Groups of neurons not killed immediately after injury begin to die 1 to 2 days later and gradually enlarging cysts develop and coalesce to form cavities within the CNS parenchyma (19) that separate previously connected neurons. Astrocytes close to the lesion site also begin to proliferate, and their enlarged fibrous processes form a web that isolates the surfaces of the injury from the surrounding tissue (9,27). At about the same time, fibroblasts from the proximal connective tissue invade the injury site and overlay the injury surfaces with a layer of collagen (21,47), completing the formation of a new *glia limitans*, the so-called glial scar.

Although the glial scar was classically accepted as the major obstacle to axon regeneration *in vivo* (29,37), it has been shown recently that two proteins present in CNS myelin and oligodendrocyte membranes are strongly inhibitory for neurite outgrowth (7,8,40,45). Monoclonal antibodies against these proteins partly neutralize their inhibitory effect and permit regrowth of a small proportion of damaged corticospinal axons in rat spinal cord (39). This finding indicates that inhibitory molecules present on CNS oligodendroglial cells may indeed inhibit axonal regeneration. However, not all the inhibition seems accounted for by myelin. Growth across glial scars that contain no myelin and few if any oligodendrocytes does not occur (C. Sotelo, *personal communication*). Furthermore, in damaged myelinated tracts, regrowth in the presence of an excess of neutralizing antibodies to the inhibitors was only partial (39).

To summarize, it is still unclear at present why injured axons do not regenerate successfully in the adult mammalian CNS. Central neurons can extend long neurites through a segment of peripheral nerve (1,38,43); hence the environment of the regenerating axon (i.e., CNS glia) must be involved in growth success or failure. The major components of the glial scar are "reactive" astrocytes (9). The usual meaning of *reactive* is that (a) the astrocytes are larger than the resting form, (b) they express increased amounts of intermediate filaments, immunoreactive with antibodies to glial fibrillary acidic protein (GFAP), and (c) they are capable of responding to mitogens. Reactive astrocytes also express a number of molecules absent in resting astrocytes that are potential "reactivity" markers. Such are epidermal growth factor receptor immunoreactivity (EGFR-IR), laminin (LN), and β-amyloid precursor proteins (APP) (22,30,31,42). We suspect that other functional properties change in parallel with the observed morphological alterations, but whether the changes are connected with neurite outgrowth promotion or inhibition shall at present be ignored.

IN VITRO MODEL OF REACTIVE ASTROCYTES

Although regenerative axonal sprouts do not cross a reactive astrocyte boundary, during development growth cones often associate with astrocytes (4,41). The detailed comparison of neurite outgrowth over developing, resting, and reactive astrocytes would be greatly facilitated by *in vitro* models of resting and reactive astrocytes. Neonatal rat brain astrocytes, maintained in culture for 15 to 20 days, have an epithelioid, polygonal morphology. Despite their very different morphology, these cells are generally assimilated to resting protoplasmic astrocytes.

Cultured polygonal astrocytes are always a preferred substrate for CNS axons (12,32,34,44). After treatment with dibutyryl cychic AMP (dBcAMP), purified polygonal astrocytes assume a stellate morphology (15), and stellate cells have been proposed as a model of reactive astrocytes in culture (13). However, CNS neurite outgrowth over dBcAMP-treated astrocytes was similar to that on untreated cells. Neurite outgrowth elicited by dBcAMP-treated type 1 astrocytes from explants of embryonic rat retina, septum, hippocampus, and spinal cord was often undistinguishable from that evoked by polygonal astrocytes (5).

Because type 2 astrocytes and oligodendrocytes share a common precursor (26,35), it was thought that they may be better *in vitro* models of inhibitory reactive, astrocytes. However, astrocytes type 2, treated or not with dBcAMP, also promoted neurite outgrowth from explants of embryonic rat retina, spinal cord, septum, and hippocampus. When comparing neurite outgrowth over cultured type 1 and type 2 astrocytes, the only difference consistently observed was the growth of fewer and more fasciculated neurites over type 2 astrocytes (5). Treatment with dBcAMP did not affect neurite outgrowth or induce the expression of reactive markers such as LN and EGFR-IR (46). Both forms of cultured astrocytes, polygonal and stellate, are capable of division and have, in total, more properties in common with astroblasts than with reactive astrocytes.

Because astrocytes treated with dBcAMP did not seem a good model of reactive astrocytes, we searched for an alternative approach. Astrocytes from the brain of uninjured adult rats survive in culture very poorly or not at all (33), but astrocytes from gliotic tissue survive comparatively well (24). However, the surviving cells, from both injured and uninjured adult brain, grow in culture as flat, epithelioid blast-like cells. In view of these results, we have used a totally different approach to recreate a "glial scar" in culture. In the experiments presented here, we used purified membranes from reactive astrocytes generated *in vivo* as substrate for central neurite outgrowth.

MEMBRANE PURIFICATION FROM ANISOMORPHIC AND ISOMORPHIC GLIOTIC TISSUE

Two types of reactive gliosis, called *anisomorphic* and *isomorphic*, are distinguished based on whether or not gliosis is elicited by an open injury (16). In both cases, the lesion site is highly enriched in reactive astrocytes (3,18). Electrolytic ablation of the entorhinal cortex of adult rats evokes (a) anisomorphic gliosis on the damaged cortical area and (b) isomorphic gliosis in the deafferented ipsilateral hippocampus. Anisomorphic gliosis was also achieved by aspiration of the parietal cortex, and isomorphic gliosis was achieved in the hippocampus by intraventricular injection of kainic acid (0.8 μg/ventricle). The region immediately adjacent to the cortical injury and the deafferented or lesioned hippocampi at 3, 10, and 20 days postlesion were dissected, homogenized in HEPES buffer (20 mM, pH 7.2) and plasma membranes purified by a combination of differential and sucrose gradient centrifugation (27). Purified membranes were washed once in PBS, resuspended in sterile PBS, and protein concentration determined; aliquots (0.2 mg/ml) were stored at -80°C and thawed only once. A similar method was used to purify membranes from adult rat liver, lung, cortex, and hippocampus. Rat brain myelin was used as inhibitory control.

Suspensions of membranes or myelin (0.1 mg/ml, 5-μl drops) were absorbed overnight at 4°C on Petriperm dishes (Heraeus) pre-coated with poly-L-lysine (PLL) (20 μg/ml). Usually, nine different spots were deposited on each dish, and two explants were placed on each spot. For substrate choice experiments, dishes prepared as above were overlayered with laminin (BRL; 10 μg/ml), and the explants were placed on LN a small distance from the drop. Membranes (1 mg protein/ml) were heat-treated (100°C, 30 min), trypsinized (0.025% trypsin w/v, 37°C, 20 min), or homogenized at room temperature sequentially with 0.2%, 0.5%, and 2% CHAPS. Pellet and supernatant were separated by centrifugation (TL100.3, 30,000 rpm, 45 min) and used in adhesion, neurite promoting, and substrate choice tests, as described below.

EXPLANT ADHESION

Explants from embryonic rat retina (E15), septum (E17), and hippocampus (E17) were dissected in HBSS on ice, cut in small fragments and plated on test membranes in DMEM/F12 medium, supplemented with N2 and 5% FCS. Six hours after plating, explant adhesion was evaluated under phase contrast. Purified membranes from uninjured or injured tissue did not interfere with explant adhesion with one exception. Membranes from hippocampus, 3 days after open injury, deafferentation, or kainic acid injection, completely prevented explant attachment to PLL-treated cell culture plastic. In the presence of LN, explants attached to the membrane-treated substrate, but no outgrowth was observed. After treatment with 0.2% CHAPS, the membrances no longer prevented explant attachment.

NEURITE OUTGROWTH OVER PURIFIED MEMBRANES

Plasma membrane fractions purified from normal brain and from areas of isomorphic gliosis or anisomorphic gliosis attached well to the PLL-treated culture dish and were used as substrates for central neurite outgrowth. Neurite outgrowth was evaluated 24, 48, and 72 hr after plating, using an inverted microscope equipped for phase contrast and fluorescence (Axiovert, Zeiss). Purified myelin and type 1 astrocyte membranes were used as negative and positive controls, respectively.

Embryonic explants from septum (unmyelinated axons) or hippocampus (potentially myelinated axons) showed profuse neurite outgrowth after 24 hr of culture over LN or type 1 astrocyte membranes (Fig. 1A). Neurite outgrowth was also observed over purified anisomorphic reactive astrocytes membranes (ARAM) col-

———————————————————————————————▶

FIG. 1. Neurite outgrowth over gliotic membranes. Neurites from septal explants (**A**) grew well over cultured type I astrocyte membranes. **B:** Explants showed no outgrowth over purified myelin or (**C**) purified membranes from isomorphic gliotic tissue. **D:** Anisomorphic gliotic tissue membranes were much less inhibitory than isomorphic. (× 125.)

Septal or hippocampal growth cones extended close to these membranes, touching them but finally turning away. The result was a thick bundle of neurites surrounding, at a distance, the membrane spot but never invading it. Neurites encountering ARAM showed a somewhat different behavior. Thick bundles of neurites surrounded the boundary of the membrane spot but in close apposition to it (Fig. 3D); occasionally, fasciculated axons invaded the ARAM spot.

DISCUSSION AND PERSPECTIVES

The major conclusions from our results are that the glial scar contains actively inhibitory component(s) that (a) prevent central neurite outgrowth and (b) repel already growing neurites, and (c) these inhibitory molecules are most likely present in reactive astrocyte membranes.

Membranes from isomorphic gliosis did not allow neurite outgrowth, most probably because of inhibitory component(s) present in the membrane. It has been reported that a hyaluronate-binding protein is present on isomorphic but not on anisomorphic reactive astrocytes (25), perhaps underlying the difference in permissiveness between these two types of cells. We found that inhibitory component(s) could be removed by detergent, uncovering the neurite-promoting activity concomitantly present. Membranes from anisomorphic gliotic tissue allowed some neurite growth, but detergent extraction further improved neurite extension, suggesting that growth promoters and inhibitors were also simultaneously present. At present, we believe that isomorphic and anisomorphic glial membranes have similar components and that their individual surface properties are determined by their unique relative proportion of growth-promoting and growth-inhibiting components. In the case of anisomorphic membranes, the proportion of neurite-promoting and inhibitory molecules is more favorable to growth. Future work is necessary to test this hypothesis and examine the presence of other inhibitors as well as growth promoters. Glucuronic acid containing carbohydrates may be good candidates. Carbohydrate polymers, in general, seem very appropriate and economical as growth regulators, because it is conceivable how small modifications of structure may lead to very different, even opposite, activities. These small modifications may only require regulation of specific enzyme activities or compartmental location, without new protein expression.

Two myelin components (mol. wt., 250 kDa and 35 kDa) inhibit neurite outgrowth (40). Hybridomas against these proteins, implanted in spinal cord after cor-

---

FIG. 3. Substrate preference of growing neurites. Neurites growing from septal explants were asked to cross from a laminine substrate (LN) on the left of the figure to a membrane substrate (M) on the right. A: Neurites show no preferences and invade the membranes (*arrowheads* define the boundary) when these derived from cultured type 1 astrocytes. B: Thick bundles of neurites remain at a distance from myelin or (C) IRAM. D: Neurites encountering ARAM grow in close apposition to the boundary. (X400.)

ticospinal transection, seemed to favor regeneration of these fibers (39). Recently, other inhibitory components (growth cone–collapsing activities) have also been partially purified (10,11,36). The same or similar inhibitory molecules could be responsible for the inhibitory activity(ies) present in our membrane preparations. However, plasma membranes from gliotic tissue are unlikely to be contaminated with myelin, because they were purified in a sucrose gradient that separates these fractions very well. In addition, a comparison of SDS-PAGE of purified myelin and ARAM or IRAM gave different profiles, and myelin-associated inhibitors do not seem to be present in our membrane preparation. However, a strict comparison of these molecules awaits their purification and characterization.

Is the neurite inhibitory activity really associated to reactive astrocytes? Several reasons suggest so. Soon after a lesion, the tissue immediately adjacent is filled with activated microglial cells (and blood-derived phagocytes in the case of anisomorphic gliosis), which, with time, are replaced by reactive astrocytes. Membrane collected at 3 days postlesion might, therefore, contain both microglia and reactive astrocytes. However, at 10, and more so at 20, days postlesion, gliotic tissue contains mostly reactive astrocytes. The fact that no differences were observed between membranes prepared from tissue 10 and 20 days postlesion suggests that reactive astrocytes are indeed responsible for neurite inhibition. The greater proportion of microglial cells at 3 days postlesion could account for the lesser adhesivity of the membranes from that tissue.

In the past few years the studies on growth regulation are shifting from a period dominated by positive growth regulation (growth factors) to the present period in which the accent is placed on negative growth regulation. Certainly, simultaneous positive and negative regulation of growth seems natural, efficient, and capable of fast response to changes such as injury. As we acquire data on growth inhibitors, the similarities between adult plasticity and developmental processes again become obvious. It seems that some developmental processes are maintained during the lifetime of the organism and activated when conditions make it necessary. Knowing the molecular details of these processes may provide the key to CNS injury repair.

ACKNOWLEDGMENTS

This work was supported by grant FAR 89-0683 from the National Program for Pharmaceutical Research and Development and a fellowship from the Department of Education and Science (PB).

REFERENCES

1. Aguayo AJ. Axonal regeneration from injured neurons in the adult mammalian central nervous system. In: Cotman CW, ed. *Synaptic plasticity*. NY: Guildford, 1985;457–484.

2. Balentine JD. Pathology of experimental spinal cord trauma. II. Ultrastructure of axons and myelin. *Lab Invest* 1978;39:254–266.

3. Bignami A, Ralston HJ. The cellular reaction to Wallerian degeneration in the CNS of the cat. *Brain Res* 1969;13:444–461.

4. Bovolenta P, Mason CA. Growth cone morphology varies with position in the developing mouse visual pathway from the retina to first targets. *J Neurosci* 1987;7:1447–1460.

5. Bovolenta P, Wandosell F, Nieto-Sampedro M. Neurite outgrowth over resting and reactive astrocytes. *Restor Neurol Neurosci* 1991; (*in press*).

6. Cajal, S Ramón y. *Degeneration and regeneration in the nervous system.* New York: Haffner, 1928.

7. Caroni P, Schwab ME. Antibodies against myelin associated inhibitor of neurite growth neutralizes non-permissive substrate properties of CNS white matter. *Neuron* 1988;1:85–96.

8. Caroni P, Schwab ME. Two membrane protein fraction from rat central myelin with inhibitory properties for neurite growth and fibroblast spreading. *J Cell Biol* 1988;106:1281–1288.

9. Clemente CD. Structural regeneration in the mammalian CNS and the role of neuroglia and the connective tissue. In: Windle WF, ed. *Regeneration in the central nervous system.* Springfield, IL: Charles Thomas, 1955:147–161.

10. Cox EC, Müller B, Bonhoeffer F. Axonal guidance in the chick visual system: posterior tectal membranes induce collapse of growth cones from temporal retina. *Neuron* 1990;4:31–37.

11. Davies JA, Cook GMW, Stern CD, Keynes RJ. Isolation from chick somites of a glycoprotein fraction that causes collapse of dorsal root ganglion growth cones. *Neuron* 1990;4:11–20.

12. Fallon J. Preferential outgrowth of central nervous system neurites on astrocytes and Schwann cells as compared with nonglial cells *in vitro. J Cell Biol* 1985;100:198–207.

13. Fedoroff S, McAuley WAJ, Houle JD, Devon RM. Astrocyte cell lineage. V Similarity of astrocytes that form in the presence of dBcAMP in culture to reactive astrocytes *in vivo. J Neurosci Res* 1984;12:15–27.

14. Fujita S, Kitamura T. Origin of the brain macrophages and the origin of the microglia. *Prog Neuropathol* 1976;3:1–50.

15. Goldman JE, Chiu FC. dBcAMP causes intermediate filament accumulation and actin reorganization in astrocytes. *Brain Res* 1984;306:85–95.

16. Greenfield JG. General pathology of nerve cell and neuroglia. In: Greenfield JG, Blackwood W, Meyer A, McMenemey WH, Norman RM, eds. *Neuropathology.* London: Ed Arnold, 1958;1–66.

17. Hirano A. The fine structure of brain in edema. In: Bourne GH, ed. *The structure and function of the nervous tissue.* New York: Academic Press, 1969;69–135.

18. Janeczko K. Spatiotemporal patterns of the astroglial proliferation in the rat brain injured at the postmitotic stage of postnatal development: a combined immunocytochemical and autoradiographic study. *Brain Res* 1989;485:236–243.

19. Kao CC, Chang LW. The mechanism of spinal cord cavitation following spinal cord transection. Part 1: A correlative histochemical study. *J Neurosurg* 1977;46:197–206.

20. Klatzo I. Neuropathological aspects of brain edema. *J Neuropathol Exp Neurol* 1967;26:1–14.

21. Krikorian JG, Guth L, Donati E. The origin of connective tissue scar in the transected rat spinal cord. *Expt Neurol* 1981;72:698–707.

22. Lemmon V, Farr KL, Lagenaur C. L1-mediated axon outgrowth occurs via a homophilic binding mechanism. *Neuron* 1989;2:1597–1603.

23. Liesi P. Laminin-immunoreactive glia distinguish regenerative adult CNS system from nonregenerative ones. *EMBO J* 1985;4:683–686.

24. Lindsay RM, Barber PC, Sherwood MRC, Zimmer J, Raisman G. Astrocyte cultures from adult rat brain. Derivation, characterization and neurotrophic properties of pure astroglial cells from corpus callosum. *Brain Res* 1982;243:329–343.

25. Mansour H, Asher R, Dahl D, Labkovsky B, Perides G, Bignami A. Permissive and non-permissive reactive astrocytes: immunofluorescence study with antibodies to the glial hyaluronate-binding protein. *J Neurosci Res* 1990;25:300–311.

26. Miller RH, David S, Patel R, Abney RE, Raff MC. A quantitative immunohistochemical study of macroglial cell development in the rat optic nerve; *in vivo* evidences for two distinct astrocyte lineages. *Dev Biol* 1985;111:35–41.

27. Nieto-Sampedro M, Bussineau CM, Cotman CW. Optimal concentration of iodonitrotetrazolium for the isolation of junctional fractions from rat brain. *Neurochem Res* 1981;6:307–320.

28. Nieto-Sampedro M. Astrocytes mitogenic activity in aged normal and Alzheimer's human brain. *Neurobiol Aging* 1987;8:249–252.

29. Nieto-Sampedro M. Growth factor induction and order of events in CNS repair. In: Stein DG, Sabel B, eds. *Pharmacological approaches to the treatment of brain and spinal cord injury*. New York: Plenum, 1981;301–337.
30. Nieto-Sampedro M, Gomez-Pinilla F, Knauer DJ, Broderick JT. Epidermal growth factor receptor immunoreactivity in rat brain astrocytes. Response to injury. *Neurosci Lett* 1988;91:276–282.
31. Nieto-Sampedro M. Astrocyte mitogen inhibitor related to epidermal growth factor receptor. *Science* 1988;240:1784–1786.
32. Noble MN, Fok-Seang J, Cohen J. Glia are a unique substrate for the *in vitro* growth of central nervous system neurons. *J Neurosci* 1984;4:1892–1903.
33. Norton WT, Farooq M. Astrocytes cultured from mature brain derive from glial precursor cells. *J Neurosci* 1989;9:769–775.
34. Pixley SKR, Nieto-Sampedro M, Cotman CW. Preferential adhesion of brain astrocytes to laminin and central neurite to astrocytes. *J Neurosci Res* 1987;18:402–406.
35. Raff MC. Glial cell diversification in the rat optic nerve. *Science* 1989;243:1450–1455.
36. Raper JA, Kapfhammer JP. The enrichment of a neuronal growth cone collapsing activity from embryonic chick brain. *Neuron* 1990;4:21–29.
37. Reier PJ, Stensaas LJ, Guth L. The astrocytic scar as an impediment to regeneration in the central nervous system. In: Kao CC, Bunge RP, Reier PJ, eds. *Spinal cord reconstruction*. N.Y: Raven Press, 1983;163–198.
38. Richardson PM, McGuinness UM, Aguayo AJ. Axons from CNS neurons regenerate into PNS grafts. *Nature* 1980;284:264–265.
39. Schnell L, Schwab ME. Axonal regeneration in the rat spinal cord produced by an antibody against myelin associated neurite growth inhibitors. *Nature* 1990;343:269–272.
40. Schwab M, Caroni P. Oligodendrocytes and fibroblast spreading *in vitro*. *J Neurosci* 1988;8:2381–2393.
41. Silver J. Factors that govern directionality of axonal growth in the embryonic optic nerve and at the chiasm of mice. *J Comp Neurol* 1984;223:238–251.
42. Siman R, Card JP, Nelson R, Davis LG. Expression of β-amyloid precursor protein in reactive astrocytes following neuronal damage. *Neuron* 1989;3:275–285.
43. Tello F. La influencia del neurotropismo en la regeneracion de los centros nerviosos. *Trab Lab Invest Biol* 1911;9:123–159.
44. Tommaselli KJ, Neugebauer KM, Bixby JL, Lilien J, Reichardt LF. N-Cadherin and integrins: two receptor system that mediate neuronal process outgrowth on astrocyte surface. *Neuron* 1988;1:33–43.
45. Vanselow J, Schwab ME, Thanos S. Responses of regenerating rat retinal ganglion cell axons to contacts with central nervous myelin *in vitro*. *Eur J Neurosci* 1990;2:121–125.
46. Wandosell F, Bovolenta P, Nieto-Sampedro M. Reactive astrocytes and dBcAMP-treated astrocytes have different surface markers (*Abstr*). *Soc Neurosci Abst* 1990;16:351
47. Windle WF. Regeneration of axons in the vertebrate central nervous system. *Physiol Rev* 1956;36:427–440.

The Nerve Growth Cone, edited by P. C. Letourneau, S. B. Kater, and E. R. Macagno, Raven Press, Ltd., New York © 1992.

36

Growth and Differentiation of Regenerating CNS Axons in Adult Mammals

Garth M. Bray, Manuel Vidal-Sanz, Maria Paz Villegas-Pérez, David A. Carter, Thomas Zwimpfer, and Albert J. Aguayo

Centre for Research in Neuroscience, The Montreal General Hospital and McGill University, Montreal, Quebec, Canada, H3G 1A4

The growth of axons in the embryo is influenced by interactions of their growth cones with cells, extracellular substrates, and diffusible molecules expressed along their pathways and in their targets (e.g., refs. 1–5; see chapter by Lumsden et al.). Growth cones are not merely passive partners in these interactions. Indeed, the observation that inhibition of proteases released by growth cones affect their extension *in vitro* (6; see chapter by Seeds et al.) provides one example of how axonal tips can modify the different environments to which they are exposed. For retinal ganglion cell (RGC) axons, which are the subject of this review of neuronal responses to CNS injury, *in vivo* and *in vitro* studies in several species illustrate some of the interactions that involve RGC growth cones during development.

Along their pathway in the developing optic nerve (ON) and tract, RGC growth cones follow stereotyped projection patterns that lead them to specific regions of the brain. Several molecules have been suggested to play a role in the extension and guidance of these axons. In *Xenopus*, evidence has been presented for local positional cues in the neuroepithelium (7,8). In chicks, growing RGC axons are responsive to laminin within finite time limits (9,10). *In vitro*, axons from the temporal retina of chicks show preferences for growth with axons from the same region and are repelled by axons from the nasal retina, suggesting that, as in invertebrates (e.g., ref. 11), selective fasciculation is an axonal guidance mechanism (12,13). At the optic chiasm, crossing and uncrossed RGC axons respond differently to undefined "cues" at the midline (14; see chapter by Mason et al.).

Retinal ganglion cell growth cones presumably encounter different sets of signals within their *targets* (e.g., the superior colliculus, the dorso-lateral geniculate nucleus, the pretectum, and the suprachiasmatic nucleus). By analogy with the developing cortico-spinal projections (3), such influences may induce the primary axons to form collateral branches that innervate specific groups of nerve cells. Short-range guidance of RGC growth cones to the major divisions of the tectum appear to be provided by molecules in this field of innervation that attract or repulse growth cones from specific regions of the retina (15–17; see chapter by Bonhoeffer et al). Certain growth factors can also influence the direction of axonal growth; for peripheral sympathetic neurons, nerve growth factor (NGF) plays such a role (for reviews, see refs. 18,19). Target-derived influences also lead to the elimination and remodeling of axons or their branches that are initially widely distributed in the superior colliculus (e.g., refs. 20–22). Finally, activity-dependent mechanisms refine and stabilize synaptic contacts; in amphibians, this interaction appears to involve NMDA receptors (23).

After interruption of the optic nerve or tract in anamniotes (e.g., goldfish), the retino-tectal pathway, including the topographic order of its reformed connections, can be restored (for reviews, see refs. 24,25). In such circumstances, the growth cones of the regrowing axons presumably encounter and respond to signals similar to those present during early development. In adult mammals, however, interruption of axons in the ON is not followed by axonal regrowth, and many axotomized RGCs die (e.g., refs. 26,27). Thus, in the mature mammalian CNS, interactions between growth cones and the nonneuronal milieu do not lead to the extension and reconnection of axons, a phenomenon that may involve inhibitory molecules expressed in white matter (for review, see ref. 28), a lack of appropriate levels of growth factors (29), or even the formation of premature synapses (30,31).

The lack of regenerative axonal growth by CNS axons in adult animals precludes both functional recovery after injury and the assessment of the capacity of such axons for appropriate synaptogenesis. However, with the documentation that neurons axotomized in the CNS of adult rodents could elongate for several centimeters in peripheral nerve (PN) grafts (32), it became possible to guide the axons of CNS neurons to selected targets and to investigate the capacity of the growth cones of CNS neurons and differing neuronal or nonneuronal components in adult mammals to recapitulate interactions that promote appropriate axonal guidance and target specificity during development. In this review, we discuss the regrowth of axotomized RGCs in terms of the responses of their growth cones in the novel pathway formed by a PN graft and, beyond the graft, in the targeted superior colliculus (SC) or cerebellum.

REGROWTH OF AXONS INJURED IN THE CNS OF ADULT MAMMALS: EXPERIMENTAL STRATEGY

Neuronal survival and synaptogenesis are critical to the study of growth cone function and differentiation as the basis of CNS axonal regeneration and restoration of connectivity. To explore the extent and selectivity of the connections that can be regenerated by axons in the injured mammalian CNS, we have used PN grafts to rejoin the eye and the SC or the cerebellum after ON transection in adult rats or hamsters. In addition, because axotomy close to the cell body is necessary to induce the growth cones of CNS neurons to grow into PN grafts (33), the effects of such lesions on RGC survival after axotomy were also studied (27,34,35).

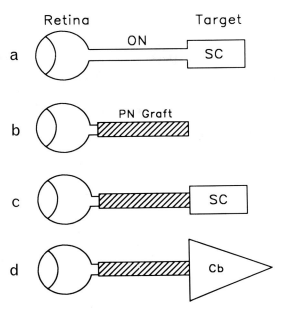

FIG. 1. a: Diagram of the retina, optic nerve (ON), and superior colliculus (SC). **b:** One end of a peripheral nerve (PN) graft (*hatched*) attached to the ocular stump of the ON transected near the eye and the other end of the PN graft left blind-ended over the skull. **c:** Distal end of the PN graft inserted into the SC. **d:** Distal end of the PN graft inserted into the cerebellum (Cb).

For these investigations of the responses of the growth cones of RGC axons to different neuronal and nonneuronal environments (Fig. 1), an autologous segment of PN was attached to the ocular stump of the ON transected near the eye and the remainder of the PN graft placed beneath the scalp (36). At various times after graft placement, some of these animals were used to study the growth (36,37) or survival (27,34,35) of axons within blind-ended grafts in the absence of terminal connectivity. In other animals, the distal end of the graft was inserted into the SC (36,38,39) or the cerebellum (31) to study the possibility of terminal connectivity.

Retrogradely and orthogradely transported neuronal tracers [horseradish peroxidase (HRP), the fluorescent tracers DiI and rhodamine (RITC), or ^{3}H-labeled leucine and proline] and immunocytochemical markers for intermediate filaments (RT-97, GFAP) were used to investigate (a) axonal growth from retinal ganglion cells; (b) the course of regenerated RGC axons along the PN graft and through the junctions of the graft with the ON on one end and with the target on the other; (c) the light and electron microscopic structure of regenerating RGC axons extending along these PN grafts; and (d) the penetration, arborization, and terminal connectivity of regenerated RGC axons in the SC or cerebellum. In some animals, the PN grafts or the portions of the SC near the termination of the grafts were studied electrophysiologically for responses to illumination of the retina (40). Molecular changes that accompany the injury and regrowth of RGC axons were also investigated (41–43).

GROWTH CONE INTERACTIONS ALONG THE REGENERATING RETINO-COLLICULAR PATHWAY

When the eye and a targeted region of the CNS are connected by a PN graft after interruption of the ON, axons proximal to the site of injury and their growth cones interact with different environments in the retina, the ocular stump of the transected ON, at the ON-PN graft junction, within the PN graft, at the PN graft–CNS junction, and in CNS targets (Fig. 1). Our findings are discussed in relation to these different portions of the experimentally created pathway and the selected targets.

Within the Retina

In normal retinas, RGC axons course in bundles toward the optic disc. When these axons are interrupted, either within the retina or in the ON close to the optic disc, many of the RGCs die (26,27,34,35), but some develop growth cones that extend in meandering patterns for a few hundred microns within the fiber layer of the retina (44–46; M. Vidal-Sanz, *unpublished observations*) or across the retinal layers (47). The extension of these axons, which is also observed in retinal explants (R.P. Bunge, *personal communication*), suggests that RGC growth cones can elongate better in the intraretinal environment than in the ON. In addition, axon-like processes with growth cones can develop from the dendrites or somata of axotomized RGCs. These "dendro-axons" also grow within the nerve fiber layer of the retina (M. Vidal-Sanz, *unpublished observations*) and can enter PN grafts inserted directly into the retina, where they extend for 1 to 2 cm (48).

At the Optic Nerve–PN Graft Junction

Seven days after PN graft attachment, orthogradely labeled RGC axons were observed to enter the PN graft from the proximal stump of the transected ON (37,49). As they invaded the PN graft, they tended to be grouped in bundles. In sections sequentially immunoreacted for RT-97 (to delineate axons) and GFAP (to visualize astrocytes and their processes), the ON-PN graft junction was clearly demarcated by the intense GFAP immunoreactivity in the retina and the ocular stump of the ON (Fig. 2).

Within the PN Graft

Groups of RGC axons, identified by the presence of tracer substances transported orthogradely from the eye, grew along the PN grafts without apparent branching at

The Nerve Growth Cone, edited by P. C. Letourneau,
S. B. Kater, and E. R. Macagno, Raven Press, Ltd.,
New York © 1992.

37

Fate of Axons of Embryonic Purkinje Cells Grafted in the Adult Cerebellum of the PCD Mutant Mouse

Constantino Sotelo, Rosa-Magda Alvarado-Mallart, and
Marcus Keep

Hôpital de la Salpétrière, 75651 Paris Cedex 13, France

In the mammalian adult CNS, neurons are highly differentiated cells that have lost their ability to proliferate. Moreover, they are particularly sensitive to pathologic influences. Perturbations beyond tolerable limits provoke losses of neurons, and when this loss reaches a critical level, irreversible functional deficits are set up. Because of its morphology, one of the most vulnerable parts of the neuron is the axon. Axotomy, whatever its cause, can produce the retrograde death of its parent neuron, or if it survives, its disconnection from its postsynaptic targets disrupts the neural network of which it was a part. Indeed, in the mammalian CNS, despite "ephemeral and frustrated regenerative attempts" (1), axotomized neurons are unable to reconstitute the selective patterns of previous connections.

Without considering the overwhelming amount of literature about this abortive behavior, let us argue that the process of axonal regeneration, which can lead to the reconstruction of the disrupted networks, results from three different processes: axonal elongation, growth cone navigation, and synaptogenesis with appropriate target neurons. At least the first two are dependent on external conditions, dictated by the local microenvironment in which the proximal stump must grow. The presence of a permissive microenvironment, as, for instance, the one provided by an aneural peripheral nerve graft (2), allows axonal elongation of axotomized neurons for several centimeters, distances greater than those required to reach their normal targets. Although very little is known about growth cone navigation in the adult CNS, by analogy with this process during development, the axonal growth could be oriented by axon–axon interactions and local and/or diffusible cues along the pathway (3). It is obvious that the cues are at least partially different during development and adulthood. Suffice it to mention the presence of myelinated fibers in the adult CNS and the presumptive inhibitory role of oligodendroglial cell surface molecules in growth cone attraction and adhesion (4). Finally, the necessary instructions for synaptogenesis between adult neurons seem to be preserved, as indicated by the great number of examples of reactive synaptogenesis reported since the original work of Raisman (5). Furthermore, Aguayo and collaborators (6) have shown that if the problems of axonal elongation and navigation are overcome by the use of bridges of peripheral nerve grafts, for instance, from the retina to the superior colliculus, the regenerating axons are able to establish functional synapses on collicular target cells. These observations suggest that synaptic target recognition cues that determine the specific pattern of connections during development can be expressed in the adult CNS during regeneration.

From the above-mentioned considerations, the limiting factors for self-repair of damaged central networks can be (a) in the case of massive neuronal cell death, the absence of precursors and/or dedifferentiated neuroblast-like cells capable of proliferative activity; and (b) In the case of surviving axotomized neurons, the nonpermissive microenvironment encountered by the growth cones formed at the tips of the axonal proximal segments, that can hinder their normal adhesion—preventing the axonal elongation—and their orientation. Several lines of research have been developed to provide regenerative axonal growth cones with permissive microenvironments that would allow regeneration. Some of these lines have been reviewed in this section of the book (see chapters by Bray et al. and by Nieto-Sampedro et al.). In any case, they are beyond the scope of our chapter.

Recent advances in the technology of neural grafting in the adult mammalian CNS have provided one experimental way to palliate the loss of precise neuronal populations in the adult CNS by replacing the missing neurons by homotopic, young postmitotic neurons, taken from isogeneic embryos. In systems organized in a "point-to-point" manner (7), neuronal replacement is only effective when the grafted neurons succeed in reestablishing the anatomical integrity of the damaged networks, by constituting equivalent synaptic circuits. Such a reconstitution is only possible when the grafted, immature neurons are able to pursue their developmental program in such a way that the cell-to-cell interactions between immature and adult neural cells recapitulate those that occurred during normal development. The prospective end result of the neuronal replacement is, therefore, the complete synaptic integration of the grafted neurons. That is to say, they need to be able to receive similar classes of synaptic inputs as the missing neurons and to make specific efferent connections on the postsynaptic targets. Hence, the restoration of the damaged circuit is not only based on the survival and normal development of the grafted neurons but also on two different types of oriented axonal growth and subsequent synaptogenesis: from the adult neurons of the host, and from the grafted neurons themselves. The possibilities and the underlying mechanisms involved in these two types of axonal growth and navigation are the matter of the present study.

NEURONAL GRAFTING IN THE CEREBELLUM AS A MODEL FOR NETWORK REPAIR IN "POINT-TO-POINT" SYSTEMS

The cerebellum of small rodents such as the rat and the mouse offers one of the most adequate models for the study of the nature of the reciprocal interactions be-the mutant cerebellum penetrated by the grafted Purkinje cells. Our morphometric analysis indicates that the volume of the mutant molecular layer containing the grafted neurons varies from 5 to 17% of the total volume of this layer (13).

To obtain functional recovery, it is imperative that the information processed by the repaired cortex reaches its target neurons. In other words, the reestablishment of a new corticonuclear projection is needed. The latter implies a process of oriented axonal growth that, owing to the nature of the neurons involved and to their cellular environment, will share some of the mechanisms underlying axonal pathfinding in developing brain, as well as axonal regeneration in the adult CNS. Indeed, the similarities and differences between these two processes emerge from the peculiarity of the situation created by the grafting, in which embryonic neurons need to interact with adult neural cells. Thus:

1. The distance to be covered by the growing axons of the grafted Purkinje cells and the cellular milieu faced by their growth cones are those offered by the adult host cerebellum. The obstacles that these axonal growth cones must overcome are those encountered by regenerating axons.

2. Purkinje cells in solid pieces of E12 cerebellar primordium are grafted either as precursor cells, conserving their proliferative ability and devoid of neuritic expansions, or as young postmitotic neurons, whose neurites are contained within the solid implants. Hence, because these neurons are not axotomized, the molecular signals involved in the fate of their axons would be different than those guiding regenerating axons. Moreover, the immaturity of those transplanted neurons would confer on them a greater plasticity than adult neurons.

3. The target domains, the denervated neurons in the deep cerebellar nuclei of the host cerebellum, have a mature stage of differentiation. If, as our results suggest, these neurons generate gradients of chemoattractant molecules involved in the orientation of the Purkinje cell axonal outgrowth (see below), it is most probable that such molecules differ from those generated by immature neurons.

All these peculiarities strongly suggest that the reestablishment of the corticonuclear projection is a difficult task. The results obtained in our experiments are in accord with this expectation. Indeed, the vast majority of the axons emerging from grafted Purkinje cells grow for long distances, up to 1 mm, in the host molecular layer parallel to the bundles of parallel fibers (Fig. 3A–D), but only a few of them succeed in innervating their specific target. Some of the axons, running in the molecular layer, are smooth and thick, and at the upper subpial region they can fasciculate into small bundles (Fig. 3A). Some others are beaded and thinner (Fig. 3A), suggesting that they can form synaptic contacts with other grafted Purkinje cells (Fig. 3B) or with interneurons of the host molecular layer. Frequently, the axons of these grafted Purkinje cells orient themselves toward the granule cell layer but do not penetrate it, ending instead in hypertrophic aberrant plexuses at the interface of the molecular and the granule cell layers (Fig. 3D), as if they are lost in their search for appropriate target neurons. Occasionally, some of these axons penetrate the

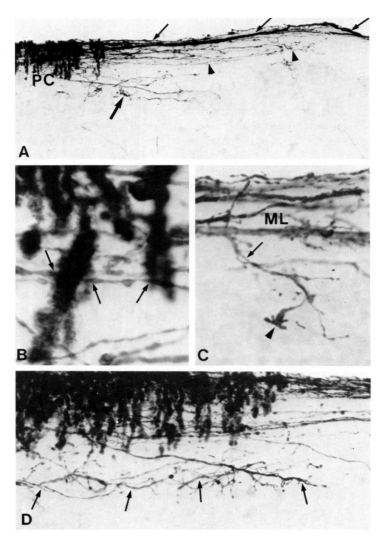

FIG. 3. Homotopic cerebellar transplantation in the cerebellum of the adult *pcd* mouse stained with anti-calbindin antiserum. Frontal sections; 1-month survival. **A:** Low magnification illustrating the extreme area where grafted Purkinje cells (PC) are found in the host molecular layer. Immunostained axons, fasciculated at the upper surface of the molecular layer (*small arrows*) and defasciculated at deeper regions (*arrowheads*), run for long distances, parallel to bundles of host parallel fibers. *Large arrow* points to an axonal plexus located at the interface between the molecular and granule cell layers. (X200.) **B:** Higher magnification of varicose Purkinje cell axons running parallel to the folium surface. Note that some of the axonal varicosities are in the vicinity of grafted Purkinje cell dendrites (*arrows*). (X1,500.) **C:** Grafted Purkinje cell axons run in the host molecular layer (ML). One of these axons follows an oblique direction (*arrow*) and penetrates into the granule cell layer, where it terminates in a large growth cone–like structure (*arrowhead*). (X600.) **D:** *Arrows* point to hypertrophic axonal plexus located at the interface between the molecular and granule cell layers. (X300.)

upper half of the granule cell layer, terminating in hypertrophic growth cone–like structures provided with filopodia, as the one illustrated in Fig. 3C.

In a few cases, a small minority of grafted Purkinje cell axons, for unknown reasons, succeeds in leaving the molecular layer and in perpendicularly crossing the granule cell layer (see Fig. 6C in ref. 15). Once in the white matter axis of the folium, these axons are able to grow for long distances, suggesting that one of the main problems for reestablishing a corticonuclear projection is the nonpermissive environment of the granule cell layer. The fate of these few axons of grafted Purkinje cells depends on their situation with respect to the donor deep cerebellar neurons (almost constantly present in the graft remnants), as well as to those of the host. If the implanted Purkinje cells within the host molecular layer remain in the neighborhood of the graft remnant, the donor deep nuclear neurons seem to exert a powerful chemoattraction, because most of their axons terminate by axonal arbors bearing presynaptic varicosities, covering the somata and part of the dendrites of these deep nuclear neurons (see Figs. 5 and 7 in ref. 7). If, conversely, the axons of grafted Purkinje cells are far from the graft remnants and within a maximum of 600 μm from the host deep nuclei, they grow in the host white matter, forming small bundles of fasciculated axons (Fig. 4A) directed toward the nearest host deep nucleus. When the bundles of immunoreactive Purkinje cell axons reach this territory, they differentiate into branched terminal arborizations of defasciculated fibers, bearing abundant varicosities (Fig. 4B). The terminal axonal plexuses can establish intricate nests, partially covering the somata and dendritic processes of immunonegative nuclear neurons (Fig. 4C). The electron microscopic analysis of one preparation immunostained with anti-calbindin antibodies has provided ultrastructural evidence that grafted Purkinje cell axons can establish appropriate synaptic contacts with the host deep nuclear neurons (see Fig. 31 in ref. 7), reconstituting a corticonuclear projection.

The results obtained in these grafting experiments suggest that the axonal navigation is regulated by two complementary mechanisms: first, interactions between axonal growth cones and local cellular elements, provided with specific cues, that stimulate (permissive) or inhibit (nonpermissive) the oriented axonal outgrowth; and second, chemoattractant molecules regulating the navigation of axons. Concerning the first mechanisms, our observations, showing that a great number of axons of the grafted Purkinje cells are unable to cross the host granule cell layer but that once they reach the white matter they can navigate for long distances and even reach their specific targets, raise an interesting question. In a recent study, Caroni and Schwab (4) identified inhibitory oligodendroglial surface molecules responsible for the nonpermissivity of CNS myelin *in vitro*. However, it is obvious that in our *in vivo* material the presumptive inhibitory role of oligodendroglial surface membranes is much less important than the almost total impossibility for the Purkinje cell axons to cross the host granule cell layer. Thus the essential problem for future investigations is to disclose which are the chemical cues that are missing or have changed in the granule cell layer (or in the gray matter in general) that prevent axons of grafted embryonic neurons from finding their ways toward the white matter and, later on, their specific target neurons.

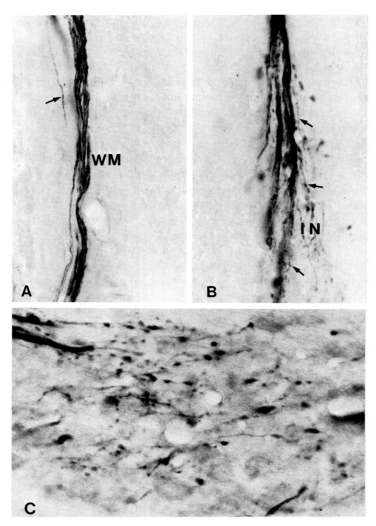

FIG. 4. Homotopic cerebellar transplant in the cerebellum of an adult *pcd* mouse stained with anti-cGK antiserum. Sagittal sections; 2-month survival. **A:** A bundle of immunostained axons, belonging to grafted Purkinje cells integrated in the host molecular layer, runs in the white matter (WM) axis of the folium. The *arrow* points to one thin defasciculated axon. (X400.) **B:** The axonal bundle illustrated in Fig. 4A reaching the dorsal pole of the nucleus interpositus anterior (IN). The bundle defasciculates within its terminal territory, and thin axons (*arrows*) emerge from it. Note that the axon bears some varicosities. (X400.) **C:** Higher magnification of the terminal arborizations of grafted Purkinje cell axons, where they reached their specific target neurons within the nucleus interpositus anterior. Note that the axons, thin and highly varicose, spread between the deep nuclear neurons. (X650.)

Subject Index

Subject Index